Dr Nick Read, MA, MD, FRCP, is a consultant physician and psychoanalytical psychotherapist who works to help people cope with illnesses that have no clear cause or pathology. He is also a Medical Adviser to the IBS Network, an independent charity set up to support, inform and advise people with irritable bowel syndrome. During his academic career, Nick held university chairs in Gastrointestinal Physiology, Human Nutrition and Integrated Medicine, published over five hundred original papers and review articles, and edited eleven medical books on gut function, eating behaviour, mind–body connections and unexplained gastrointestinal disease. He currently lives in the Yorkshire Dales and enjoys running on the moors and cooking vegetarian and fish dishes. Nick has a passion for the wilderness and wildlife and is a longstanding supporter of Sheffield Wednesday Football Club. His five children keep his feet on the ground. His website can be visited at www.nickread.co.uk.

sick and
tired

*Healing the illnesses doctors
cannot cure*

Dr Nick Read

PHOENIX

A PHOENIX PAPERBACK

First published in Great Britain in 2005
by Weidenfeld & Nicolson
This paperback edition published in 2006
by Phoenix,
an imprint of Orion Books Ltd,
Orion House, 5 Upper St Martin's Lane,
London WC2H 9EA

1 3 5 7 9 10 8 6 4 2

A CIP catalogue record for this book
is available from the British Library.

ISBN-13 978-0-7538-1714-8
ISBN-10 0-7538-1714-4

Printed and bound in Great Britain by
Mackays of Chatham plc, Chatham, Kent

The Orion Publishing Group's policy is to use papers that
are natural, renewable and recyclable products and
made from wood grown in sustainable forests. The logging
and manufacturing processes are expected to conform to
the environmental regulations of the country of origin.

www.orionbooks.co.uk

I owe a considerable debt of gratitude to my partner, Dr Joan Ransley. Not only has she been a constant source of support and encouragement, but she has carried out literature searches on my behalf, read several versions of the chapters and made numerous valuable suggestions.

I would like to dedicate this book to the many brave people who have entrusted me with their life story. They made me see how important it was to write it, and I hope I have done justice to their experience.

Although the cases presented in this book are informed by the narratives related in my clinic (I could not invent such a richness of personal experience), they do not represent any single patient. Moreover, I have directed my narrative spotlight on particular themes in order to illustrate my points and have changed the names and many of the details to protect confidentiality.

Contents

Preface

As a junior doctor, I was fortunate to work in Sheffield for a young gastroenterologist with an incisive mind and formidable research reputation. He ran a busy practice with great efficiency, devising problem lists to aid diagnosis and care plans to rationalise treatment. Wanting to prioritise and concentrate his expertise where it was most needed, he organised his clinics into illness categories and assigned his staff accordingly. I got the Friday afternoon clinic. Some said it was the short straw. It was full of people who suffered with abdominal discomfort and bowel disturbance, for which there was no clear explanation, as well as a whole raft of mysterious symptoms affecting other parts of the body. The experience was intriguing but frustrating. With little under twenty minutes per patient, there was barely enough time to check that they did not have any obvious disease and to prescribe treatment that was unlikely to relieve their suffering.

The frustration I felt during those clinics led me to devote much of the next twenty years to trying to find out what manner of illness they were suffering from. Assisted by a team of diligent and enthusiastic young scientists, I searched for the elusive disturbance in function that would lead to an effective treatment. Needless to say, we never found it, but all the time I felt that there must be another way.

This would come from an unexpected direction. My colleague Carmel Donnelly, who carried out the physiological tests on our patients, would often tell me of the tragic and difficult circumstances affecting the lives of so many of our patients. At first I dismissed this information with a feeling of irritation; there was just too much work to do. In time, however, I began listening to my patients more. And it was with a sense of shock that I realised how much their symptoms seemed to represent the changes that had taken place in their lives. They all had their story to tell and when they had told it, their illness became so much easier to understand and often seemed to improve.

This was nothing new – Dr Thomas Sydenham had said much the same thing over three hundred years ago and so, some time later, had Sigmund Freud – but for somebody indoctrinated in medical determinism, the idea was devastating. It changed the way I thought and altered the way I practised medicine. For the first time I felt I understood my patients and could help them get better. It was this experience that drove me to write this book.

The truth is I feel passionate about the way patients with medically unexplained illnesses tend to be exiled to a medical wilderness with a shrug of the shoulders and faint reassurance that there is nothing seriously wrong. *Sick and Tired* exposes the lack of balance in orthodox Western medicine. I feel that the focus on scientific evidence and physical cure has caused doctors to lose sight of the 'narrative' and meaning of illness.

My intention, however, is not to criticise the undeniable skill and dedication of most doctors and nurses, but to challenge the model of current medical practice, with its dependence on the pharmaceutical industry and manipulation by government and media. By emphasising medically unexplained or functional illnesses, *Sick and Tired* creates a vision of a future health care system where illness is viewed not only in terms of a physical 'malfunction' but also as the meaningful reaction of the *whole* person – mind, body and soul – to changes in their social and physical environment. The challenge of this book is to explore the meaning of illness while maintaining the necessary scientific underpinning.

The arguments I have constructed are supported by evidence, but this is not simply the statistical analysis of ill people; it also includes case histories, patient testimony, and both popular and philosophical literature. And in order to satisfy those readers who wish to explore in detail the themes and topics discussed in this book, there are endnotes and an extensive bibliography.

I sincerely hope that *Sick and Tired* will stimulate a lively debate that may in time help to achieve a more healthy society and more balanced system of health care that is responsive to the real needs of ill people.

Introduction

Little over a century ago, when most of our medical institutions were established, living conditions in the industrial cities of Europe were overcrowded and dirty. A large percentage of the population was poor and malnourished. Vitamin deficiencies, such as scurvy, rickets and anaemia, were commonplace. Scarlet fever, rheumatic fever, typhoid, typhus and diphtheria, which most doctors now only read about in the musty pages of medical tomes, were major causes of misery and death. Thousands of mothers died in childbirth every year. Dysentery frequently caused death in infants and among the old and infirm. People feared the inexorable wasting of tuberculosis as they fear cancer today. Syphilis led to madness and paralysis. Lunatic asylums were full of tormented souls, suffering not only with the psychiatric illnesses that we recognise today, but with epilepsy, neurosyphilis and Parkinson's disease. There were no reliable, specific and safe treatments for any of these conditions. Doctors could do little except offer support and try to suppress the worst symptoms.

Most of the diseases that affected Western communities in the early part of the twentieth century have either vanished or at least declined dramatically.[1] Gone are the infectious diseases that used to plague the lives of our grandparents and great-grandparents. Gone is the debility of widespread malnutrition. Even the so-called lifestyle diseases, such as heart attacks, strokes and peptic ulcers, have declined. Tens of thousands of British people died of bronchitis in the smog-ridden winters of the 1950s. This disease, like the smog that caused it, has evaporated. Cancer remains a significant cause of mortality, but now there are cures for some cancers and many more can be prevented. One hundred years ago, life expectancy was not much greater than about forty years among women and fifty in men, and 40 per cent of deaths occurred before the age of five. Now it has risen dramatically to eighty years in women and seventy-five years in men, and infant mortality is less than 1 per cent.

By every objective measure, people now have less disease and are living longer than at any time since records were kept. This is due in large measure to vast improvements in wealth, nutrition, housing and sanitation, although it is the advances in medical therapy that have captured the public imagination. But creating new treatments for previously incurable diseases also fosters the illusion that all human disease will soon be vanquished.[2] For example, immunisation has all but abolished many of the killer infections of the past and those that do get through the net can be quickly treated with powerful antibiotics. New imaging methods – for example, computer-assisted radiology, isotope scans and nuclear magnetic resonance – have allowed doctors to detect tiny tumours in organs and remove them before they cause serious illness. Hearts, livers and kidneys can be transplanted into people who would otherwise die. Organs can be repaired, blood vessels dilated and tumours removed while body functions are maintained by machines. Worn-out joints can be replaced with titanium ones, enabling the lame to walk again. Cataract surgery has restored sight to those who had become blind. And now operations can even be conducted through fibreoptic endoscopes without opening the body. These technological achievements in health care are little short of miraculous. It is, however, the advances in pharmacological treatments that have made the greatest impact. Drugs are now available to treat arthritis, angina, blood pressure, ulcers, colitis and many other diseases. People with diabetes can now expect to enjoy a near normal life-span on regular insulin treatment. The horrors of the asylums are no longer with us as many mental and neurological illnesses can be controlled with drugs. Tablets can even reduce the threat of disease by lowering high cholesterol, sugar and uric acid, and supplementing body stores of essential minerals and vitamins.

In the West, these miracles of medical science are now taken for granted. We view access to the latest treatments as a human right. So, in the last half century, governments have invested heavily in health care, increasing the numbers of doctors and nurses, opening new wards, building new hospitals and modernising diagnostic and therapeutic procedures – just to keep up with popular demand. The cost of the British National Health Service rocketed from £28 billion in 1982 to £65 billion a year in 2002 and is set to go up to an astronomical

£96 billion by 2008. This will bring it into line with other European countries, but it will still lag behind the enormous cost of health in the United States.[3]

With such vast investment in health care, such amazing advances in medical technology and the availability of effective treatments for many serious diseases, you would think that people living in Western countries would be healthier than ever before. Not a bit of it. Like anorexics starving in the midst of plenty, more and more people seem to be feeling ill. When people were interviewed for the 2002 UK General Household Survey, 35 per cent of them claimed to be suffering from a chronic or long-standing illness, an increase of 13 per cent since 1972. Comparable rates of chronic illness have been reported by consumer surveys across the European Union, from 45 per cent in Norway and Sweden to just 17 per cent in Switzerland. In Australia, a recent survey on self-reported health revealed that as many as 87 per cent of people over the age of fifteen had one or more long-standing health conditions, although these figures included short-sightedness and deafness as well as headaches and backache. The data from America, however, is conflicting. While government surveys indicate that three-quarters of Americans rate their health as excellent to good with very little change since the 1970s, figures derived from consumer research detailing how people feel about their health showed that only 55 per cent of Americans agreed with the statement 'I am in good physical condition' compared with 76 per cent twenty-five years ago.[4]

This apparent decline in self-reported health across the Western world cannot just be explained by the fact that older people are living longer in a state of ill health. One in four young British people aged between sixteen and forty-four report that they have a long-standing illness, nearly doubling the rate reported in 1972. And a study conducted in children from five Nordic countries showed that the prevalence of long-term illness had increased from 8 per cent to 15 per cent in the twelve years from 1984 to 1996. Across the European Union, over a third of teenage girls report they have a headache at least once a week, and nearly a quarter of them report weekly stomachaches and backaches.[5] A quarter of our children are now overweight or obese, a 100 per cent increase since 1995. The rate of childhood asthma in Western countries doubled between 1980 and 1995 but there are now some signs that this trend has plateaued. If health in children is a useful predictor of health through the life cycle, these figures would suggest that we are sitting on a public health time bomb.

Bearing in mind the apparent increase in self-reported illness, it is not surprising that more people throughout the developed world are visiting their doctors than ever before. Data from the UK Office of Health Economics has reported an increase of 38 million consultations with general practitioners, a rise of 15.9 per cent between 1985 and 2000, but records kept by some practices suggest the figure could be much higher.[6] During the same period of time, there has been a 50 per cent increase in the proportion of people attending outpatients or casualty departments. Nearly all of the adult population in the UK have visited their GP in the last five years and three out of five have been to hospital as an outpatient. And the annual number of prescriptions dispensed in the UK rose by 38 per cent between 1989 and 1999, while GP prescriptions have risen again by nearly 6 per cent a year from 2000 to 2004. Indeed, the demand for health care has increased so much that waiting times and bed availability have become major political issues in the last three general elections.

But what are the illnesses that people are suffering from day in and day out for years on end? Some are the heart problems, the strokes, the debilitating cancers and chronic inflammatory conditions such as rheumatoid arthritis or colitis, but many more are much less easy to characterise. Surveys from different countries throughout the Western world have shown that on average between 30 and 40 per cent of people who seek health care have illnesses that have no clear cause and no obvious basis in pathology.[7] And they are getting commoner. As the prevalence of diseases with a definitive pathological basis have been declining, so rates of medically unexplained illnesses have been going up. This is nowhere more striking than in Japan, arguably the most healthy westernised country, where rates of identifiable disease are among the lowest in the world yet levels of self-reported health are relatively poor.[8] And in his scholarly synthesis from the data from large social surveys, Robert Putnam wrote that the percentage of young Americans who suffer regular symptoms of 'ill-defined malaise' has increased from 30 to 45 per cent since 1975.[9] Similar rates exist among young Europeans. Literally millions of people are racked by back pains, tormented by abdominal gripes, alarmed by ringing in the ears, tortured by headaches, exhausted with sleep deprivation, frustrated with constipation, debilitated with nausea or faintness or anorexia, overwhelmed by the burden of obesity, terrified by shortness of breath or palpitations or just too sick and too tired to cope. And while, for many people, such everyday illnesses constitute an inconvenience that does not seriously disrupt their lives, they should not be dismissed as trivial. Medically unexplained illnesses can undermine people's comfort, mobility, happiness and sheer quality of life as much and sometimes more than life-threatening conditions, such as diabetes or renal failure.

These are the illnesses that the doctor cannot cure. The people who suffer from them not only go to their doctors more frequently than those with more well-defined medical conditions, they are also more likely to be referred to hospital. As many as a third to a half of all referrals to medical outpatient clinics are for common symptoms for which a pathological diagnosis cannot be established. According to recent reports, such frequent attenders suffer more from anxiety, loneliness, deprivation and unhappiness than other people, and are more likely to regard common bodily symptoms as indicative of serious disease.[10]

This is such a strange phenomenon. By all objective measures, people living in modern Western democracies are more prosperous and healthy than ever before. We have a state-of-the-art health service that claims to diagnose and offer treatment for any disease, yet we are afflicted by enormously high rates of illness that doctors seem unable to manage. As Susan, one of my patients, expressed it: 'How is it that modern scientific medicine can make a baby in a test tube and transplant a heart but cannot do anything for my abdominal pain?'

Our health services have no effective solutions for this modern epidemic, short of creating new diagnoses. In the last thirty years, a vast range of new and unexplained illnesses has appeared, from irritable bowel syndrome to attention deficit disorder to chronic fatigue syndrome. But despite the efforts of teams of medical experts from all over the world, we are no closer to finding a treatable cause for any of these conditions. The dramatic contrast between the declining rates of most pathological diseases and the increasing rates of unexplained illness leads to the inevitable conclusion that our medical system is expending more effort for fewer ill people. So, frustrated with the failure of orthodox medical services to cure their illness, more and more people are assuming control of their own health or turning to alternative medical practitioners. Within the last twenty-five years, self-help organisations, national charities and patient advocacy groups have been established for every illness from bladder pain to cyclical vomiting.[11] Health food shops and outlets for herbal remedies have become a prominent feature on the high streets and shopping malls of

Western towns and cities. At the last count, 41 per cent of people in the UK and more than 50 per cent in the United States were treating themselves on a regular basis with herbal remedies, tonics, vitamin supplements and designer foods.[12] And across the Western world, enormous numbers of people are seeking help for their illnesses from healers and therapists.[13] The number of complementary practitioners in Britain now exceeds the number of GPs and more visits are paid to complementary therapists than to casualty units. And in America, more visits are made to providers of complementary and alternative medicine than to primary care physicians, and more is spent on the services of complementary healers than on hospital admissions. Overall, recent figures suggest that between a quarter and three-quarters of people living in Western countries undertake some form of complementary therapy. American figures are around 40 per cent, but when prayer is specifically used for health reasons, the figure rises to 62 per cent. In Australia, nearly half the population uses some kind of complementary therapy, while in Germany the figure is nearer 65 per cent, an increase of 13 per cent since 1970.

The sheer magnitude of unexplained illness in our society must cause us to reappraise our assumptions regarding the nature of illness. Throughout the last three hundred years, Western societies have been conditioned by scientific discoveries to perceive illness as a distinct entity that attacks us from outside our 'selves' and produces definite pathological changes that need to be treated with specific medicines or surgery. Science has raised medicine out of the realm of faith and superstition to become a rational procedure supported by evidence. Yet here we are at the very acme of scientific discovery in medicine and most of the population is suffering from illnesses that have no obvious basis or external cause and are, more often than not, quite resistant to treatment.

So what does this mean? What kind of illnesses are these? Why do they seem to be getting more common? And what does this have to say about the way we lead our lives and about the society in which we live? These are some of the questions that I shall attempt to address in this book.

1

What kind of illness are we suffering from?

Denise looks a picture of misery. Her skin has an unhealthy yellowish tinge, her hair is greasy and lank, there are deep rings under her eyes and her body is so braced with tension it looks as if she could snap in half. She leans forward in her seat and fixes me with wild eyes. Her words seem to tumble over each other as she tells me, in a voice hoarse and dry with emotion, 'I feel dreadful every single day of my life. I get this gnawing feeling like an emptiness in the pit of my stomach, just here.' She bunches the hem of her blouse into her fist. 'But as soon as I try to eat something to relieve it, I immediately feel so sick and bloated I have to stop. And the skin of my stomach gets so itchy I want to scratch it to pieces. And sometimes I get this horrible pain around my eye and the right side of my head. It makes me feel so sick and awful I have to lie down. And I'm just tired all the time. I get so cross and frustrated that I snap at Charlie [her four-year-old] and he's done nothing wrong.' Her face crumples up and she starts to cry. 'He looks so upset and confused. I just can't bear it.'

As the sobbing subsides and the tension slowly ebbs away, Denise continues: 'I have had to take so much time off work that I am surprised I still have a job. The only relief I get is when the children are in bed and I can settle down with a glass or two of sherry, but it doesn't last. By four o'clock in the morning I'm awake again. My heart is thumping, I am sweating and I start to panic about whether I am going to get through the day. Why can nobody seem to help me? I've tried so hard, but nothing ever works.'

It's true. Denise has been back and forth to the doctor countless times over the years. She has been referred to gastroenterologists for her stomach complaints, neurologists for her head pains, she has seen a dermatologist about her skin and her hair, and she has even been sent to a psychiatrist, who said that there was nothing wrong with her mind. She has spent days in hospital undergoing all kinds of humiliating and uncomfortable tests. She has had scans of her abdomen, her pelvis and her brain. She has had a barium meal and several barium enemas. She has had a camera down her throat, which made her sick for days, and another inserted into her colon, which was, she told me, 'the most embarrassing and traumatic experience of my life.' She has had tests on her pancreas, her liver and her kidneys, but all were negative. So despite all the time and discomfort, she was no further forward.

With no definitive diagnosis, the doctors had tried to control her symptoms with drugs, but none worked; in fact, they just seemed to make her worse. The headache tablets made her stomach feel sore, the ones for sickness made her dizzy, the grey and green capsules she took for diarrhoea brought on such awful pain and bloating that it was better to do without, and the antidepressants just made her feel like a zombie.

In desperation, her GP had referred her to a dietician, who said she probably had a food allergy. So she went on a wheat-free diet, then a milk-free diet, then she cut out meat, fish and tomatoes. Every time she removed another item from the diet, she was better for a few days, but the symptoms always came back and she lost so much weight that her doctor was very concerned. Disillusioned with the medical profession, Denise sought help from complementary practitioners. Acupuncture, reflexology and homeopathy each helped for a time, but the benefit didn't last and eventually she lost faith.

Denise is literally at her wits' end. She pleads with me to help her. 'I will try anything, be a guinea pig, even go to a surgeon, if you think it would help!'

Denise's story is more severe than most, but it is not unusual. Medical clinics and surgeries throughout the Western world contain many people with similar illnesses. She and others like her are part of an enormous public health problem that doctors seem incapable of resolving.

So what is responsible for this insidious epidemic that has come to afflict us just when we thought 'we had it so good'? Have we fallen victim to some elusive micro-organism that may linger in our body, slowly undermining our health? Certainly the increasing mobility of human populations has brought us into more contact with animal reservoirs of infection, releasing new diseases such as AIDS, the Ebola virus and legionnaires disease on populations that have no natural resistance.[1] But despite enormous media coverage and public concern, such infections, at least in Western countries, are rare and, once suspected, readily diagnosed. AIDS, for example, has as yet never achieved the endemic proportions in the West that were feared. There are, however, worrying reports of antibiotic resistance, notably in the staphylococcal infections that seem to lurk in hospital wards and the new strains of tuberculosis. Even the common 'flu' virus can undergo alarming mutations, which challenge the adaptability of the immune system and can cause serious illnesses. But such outbreaks are usually rapidly identified and contained.

Discoveries of human immunodeficiency virus (HIV) that causes AIDS, and the prion responsible for new variant Creutzfeld-Jacob disease (the human variant of mad cow disease) has reminded us that such organisms can lurk dormant for years, like time bombs, before some change in our immune tolerance triggers them to instruct our own genetic machinery to manufacture trillions of new infective particles. We harbour more bacteria and fungi in our bodies than the cells that make up our organs and tissues. The vast majority of these coexist with us in a mutually beneficial manner. But has something happened to disrupt that peaceful coexistence? Has the rich diet that we consume encouraged an overgrowth of yeasts like *candida albicans*, making the gut more leaky and poisoning the blood with toxic products?[2] Has the large quantity of meat that we consume or the sulphur compounds that we use to preserve our foods encouraged an overgrowth of sulphur-reducing bacteria in our colons that poison us with toxic hydrogen sulphide?[3] As Gail Vines reported in *New Scientist*: 'If you thought junk food would merely make you fat, think again. You could also be fattening a hungry mass of alien gut bacteria that may repay you with bowel disease and even cancer.'

Or perhaps we are slowly being poisoned by contaminants in our water or food or pollution of the atmosphere?[4] We are undoubtedly living in a very artificial environment and exposed on a daily basis to a whole range of potentially toxic contaminants and additives. In the last fifty years, medical scientists have discovered how smoking causes lung cancer, how exposure to asbestos causes serious lung disease and how certain dyestuffs can cause bladder cancer. They have also suggested plausible hypotheses to implicate dietary fat in coronary heart disease, and red meat and lack of leafy green vegetables in colonic cancer. The pages of health magazines are full of many other putative health risks – food contamination, daily exposure to high lead and sulphur emissions, mercury poisoning from dental amalgam, fluoride intoxication from tea, toothpaste and domestic water supplies,[5] and electromagnetic radiation from power lines or mobile phones – but the contention that any of these might be responsible for an erosion of our health on such an enormous scale is just not supported by sufficient scientific evidence.

Or have we become allergic to modern life?[6] A recent report from the UK Royal College of Physicians reported that the prevalence of allergies has increased threefold in the last twenty years. The latest estimates suggest that one-third of the total UK population will develop an allergy at some stage in their lives. In the UK, allergic disease currently accounts for 6 per cent of general practice consultations, 0.6 per cent of hospital admissions and 10 per cent of the GP prescribing budget. Much of this increased load comprises asthma and hay fever, although food allergies have also increased. There is, however, a poor correlation between self-reported food allergy and the results of allergy testing. In recent years, there has been a rapidly accumulating body of evidence showing that emotional stress can trigger hay fever, asthma, eczema and food allergy.[7] People are more likely to report allergies if they are suffering from psychological distress or medically unexplained illness, both of which are often characterised by enhanced organ or tissue sensitivity and enhanced reactions to foods and other environmental triggers.

Each of these possibilities is plausible and may well be responsible for some cases of otherwise unexplained illness, but there is no data to substantiate the contention that they account for the sheer scale and variety of our current malaise. However, there *is* a very strong body of evidence to indicate that the mysterious illnesses that have come to afflict so many people in Western countries are associated with what has been happening in their lives. The problem is that modern medicine is not equipped to deal with such illness.

Western orthodox medicine was designed to detect and treat diseases that have a well-defined pathology and, in most cases, an obvious cause. Its development was conditioned by the infectious and nutritional diseases that afflicted such large numbers of people in the nineteenth century and was further modified by the lifestyle diseases of the twentieth – the ulcers, heart attacks, strokes, bronchitis, cancer and high blood pressure. The meticulous disease history, the careful physical examination and the detailed investigations were refined throughout the last century to facilitate the detection of any one of several thousand known diseases, which could then be extirpated by the appropriate drug or operation. Doctors are very good at this. Years of training and more years of practice have honed their diagnostic skills to an exquisite acuity. There is very little pathology that escapes the diagnostic net of the modern doctor, and very few organic diseases that cannot be treated, but as more and more organic diseases have submitted to the might of surgery and pharmacotherapy, their places, like the broomsticks in *The Sorcerer's Apprentice*, have been taken by a multiplicity of unexplained ailments for which orthodox medicine has no magic solutions.

These conditions are often known as '*functional illnesses*'. The term was coined by Dr James Braid in the middle of the nineteenth century to describe maladies caused by disturbances in the function of specific organs or systems that were not accompanied by any structural or pathological change.[8]

By contrast, illnesses with a definitive pathology and cause are known as '*organic diseases*'.

Illness defines how a person feels, how his body reacts and how he then behaves. It is the subjective state of being unwell. Disease, on the other hand, is usually taken to indicate an objective pathological change. So, illness is what the patient has, but disease is what the doctor diagnoses. Sometimes the two match, but increasingly, the patient's illness cannot be translated into a disease. Doctors are trained to diagnose and treat organic disease, not to understand the 'meaning' of illness. This may explain why many of the millions of people who suffer from functional illnesses end up feeling blamed and rejected for not having a 'proper' disease.

In an attempt to contain the epidemic of functional illness, the opinion leaders of orthodox Western medicine have created artificial diagnoses out of groups of unexplained symptoms as if awaiting the discovery of a definitive cause. So over the last fifty years there has been a proliferation of syndromes and various other non-specific, atypical and unexplained disorders. We not only have chronic fatigue syndrome, irritable bowel syndrome, bulimic syndrome, globus syndrome, premenstrual syndrome, temporo-mandibular syndrome, fibromyalgia syndrome, burning semen syndrome and even Stendhal's syndrome (a sense of dizziness and disorientation caused by visiting art galleries),[9] we also have 'atypical' or non-cardiac chest pain, atypical facial pain, non-specific abdominal pain, non-ulcer dyspepsia, unexplained back pain and tension headaches. The list is endless.

But what is regarded as a functional or an unexplained illness is a subject of lively controversy and territorial infighting, as different experts make claims on different illnesses as distinct diseases. While most doctors would agree that irritable bowel syndrome and fibromyalgia are functional illnesses, chronic fatigue syndrome is still controversial and regarded, at least by those who suffer severely from it, as being caused by the ingestion of toxic substances or an undiagnosed infection. Other conditions such as asthma, epilepsy, migraine and high blood pressure would tend to be regarded as organic diseases because there is either a clear pathological or physiological basis. But what about anorexia nervosa, bulimia nervosa and binge eating disorder? They are included here as unexplained disturbances of the function of eating, just as insomnia is a disturbance of the function of sleep. But the boundary between functional illness and organic disease is not always distinct. For example, both high blood pressure and asthma start as a physiological change and only later develop distinct pathological changes. Obesity is also rather like that. What may start as a disorder of eating behaviour or energy balance results in clear pathological accumulation of body fat. And even the classic 'functional illnesses', such as fibromyalgia, chronic fatigue, and irritable bowel, have evidence of mild inflammation in the affected organs.[10]

But can there really be so many separate specific diseases without a cause? Many would think not and so collections of otherwise unexplained symptoms have been grouped by some alternative practitioners under a single attribution, such as *candidiasis* hypersensitivity syndrome, hypoglycaemia syndrome, multiple chemical sensitivity and total allergy syndrome. The problem is that when the symptoms of these conditions are listed, they are so protean and non-specific that they could apply to *any* illness. For example, the symptoms of *candidiasis* hypersensitivity syndrome are listed as tiredness, headaches, mood swings, breathlessness, earache, nausea, vomiting, weight loss (or unexpected weight gain), diarrhoea, abdominal bloating, stomachache, impotence, infertility, muscular pains, arthritis and many more. The same list can be found in descriptions of multiple chemical sensitivity, food allergies, fluoride toxicity and hypoglycaemia syndrome. Although these attributions rarely stand up to scientific scrutiny, they can seem quite plausible and may become established in a person's mind, providing both meaning and reason for their illness.

One example that continues to excite fierce controversy is the Gulf War syndrome.[11] More than one in twenty UK servicemen, and as many as 25 to 30 per cent of US veterans who served in the First Gulf War, continue to suffer from a variety of unexplained medical symptoms, which include mood swings, memory loss, lack of concentration, night sweats, muscular pains, general fatigue, skin allergies and sexual problems. A variety of reasons have been suggested. These include exposure to depleted uranium, pesticides, smoke from burning oil wells, and the drugs and vaccines the troops were given to protect them against bacterial or chemical weapons. Nevertheless, the symptoms are very non-specific and essentially similar to symptoms experienced by veterans who did not serve in the Gulf War. They are just reported at higher frequencies. Sixty-one per cent of Gulf War veterans reported at least one new symptom since 1990, compared with 37 per cent who did not serve in the Gulf. Despite the assertions of the veterans, a recent report from the Medical Research Council concluded that there is no evidence for a single syndrome related specifically to service in the Gulf. Instead they accepted that Gulf War veterans were at increased risk of suffering from post-traumatic stress disorder and suggested that depression and alcohol were also very important risk factors. The debate continues.

Examine the records from any medical speciality and you will find alarming increases in consultations for every type of functional illness.[12] For example, in the UK, five times as many people seek specialist medical help for headaches now compared with the 1970s, yet the vast majority of headaches are not caused by any demonstrable pathology. Consultation for indigestion has increased by more than 25 per cent since 1982, but only a small proportion of these patients have cancer, ulcers or gallstones. By far and away the greatest number have functional dyspepsia – in other words, indigestion of uncertain cause. The number of surgical admissions for unexplained abdominal pain has more than doubled since 1968, but rates of appendicitis have shown a dramatic decline over the same period. Unexplained chronic back pain has increased six- to sevenfold over the last fifty years. Fibromyalgia, persistent niggling pains and tender areas in the large muscles of the back, neck and shoulders, has become the second most common cause of referral to rheumatologists after arthritis, comprising about 20 per cent of cases. Chest pain is the most common reason for referral to a cardiologist, but in over half the cases, no cause can be found. Rates of anorexia nervosa continue to cause concern, but bulimia nervosa, unknown before 1979, is now the commonest cause for referral to eating disorder clinics, with nine times the rate of anorexia. On the other side of the coin, the prevalence of obesity has tripled in Britain and America since 1980 and binge eating disorder was coined as a separate condition in the 1990s.

It is hard to grasp the sheer enormity of the problem that this poses for our Western health services. While organic diseases are declining across the Western world, functional illnesses are on the march. And since functional illnesses express themselves through the same repertoire of feelings and bodily reactions as organic disease, a system of medical practice that is based on the identification of pathology is bound to be incredibly wasteful of resource. For example, health care costs for irritable bowel syndrome in England and Wales have now risen to £50 million a year.[13] Although IBS is not regarded by doctors as a dangerous condition, it can still take vast numbers of negative X-rays, endoscopies and blood tests to exclude beyond all reasonable doubt the possibility of bowel inflammation or colonic cancer, especially if we factor in the concerns of a health-conscious population and doctors' fears of litigation if they miss a serious disease. And it can take several speculative trials of treatment before the doctor finally admits he cannot cure it.

Other illnesses are more expensive. For example, by 2000, back pain was costing the British taxpayer over £1.5 billion a year to treat with an additional £10 billion indirect costs due to absenteeism and loss of productivity, while the total annual cost of migraines was estimated at nearly £2 billion in the UK and $14 billion in the USA. Finally, it costs the UK National Health Service over a billion pounds to treat obesity and related illnesses. But with an estimated 80 million working days being lost per year in the UK because of sickness related to being overweight and the high risk of premature mortality, the total cost of obesity by 2003 was nearer £4 billion, about 7 per cent of the total health budget. In the United States, the economic costs of obesity in 2001 was $117 billion.

If we were to add together the figures for all the 'medically unexplained' illnesses, the cost to the state becomes truly vast. As some indication of this, by the last years of the twentieth century in Britain, the illness category 'symptoms and signs of ill-defined conditions' had the highest outpatient expenditure of any other single category, while in the United States, patients with multiple unexplained physical complaints had 50 per cent more office visits than patients with organic disease, 80 per cent more specialist referrals, four times the number of hospital admissions and consumed nine times the cost of health care.[14]

But what are functional illnesses? Are they really a whole variety of different unexplained illnesses awaiting the discovery of definitive causes and cures or are they, as Simon Wessley, Professor of Psychological Medicine at King's College, London, put it, 'like the elephant to the blind man – simply different parts of a larger animal'?[15] The evidence suggests that they are. Although the symptoms of functional illnesses can show enormous variability, there are also common features that are quite distinct from the bulk of organic diseases.

Firstly, functional illnesses are much more common than most organic diseases. For example, between 20 and 40 per cent of the British population say that they feel tired all the time while chronic fatigue is the commonest cause of chronic ill health in our secondary schoolchildren.[16] Fibromyalgia, which frequently coexists with chronic fatigue syndrome, affects between 6 to 8 million people in the USA. About 15 per cent of the UK population are disabled by chronic backache, yet in less than a tenth of these cases is there an obvious basis in pathology. No fewer than 5 million people in Britain consult their GP with digestive and bowel complaints every year and in less than a quarter of them can any organic diagnosis be established. Irritable bowel syndrome affects between 15 and 20 per cent of Western populations, and 'functional' dyspepsia up to 40 per cent. Migraine is said to afflict 25 to 30 million people in the United States alone and tension headaches are three times as common. Thirteen per cent of British people suffer from breathlessness, but in most, the cause cannot be confirmed. Over 20 per cent of Americans and Britons suffer from unexplained chest pain. By contrast, angina, one of the commonest organic diseases, affects just 1.4 million people in the UK, less than 3 per cent of the population.

Second, unlike organic disease, the same functional illness can have a variety of different symptoms. This fact was brought home to me when I ran my first therapeutic group for patients with irritable bowel syndrome. Although they all fulfilled the diagnostic criteria for IBS, their illnesses appeared to be very different from each other. For example, one patient developed constipation at the time of an operation on his back. After a few weeks this changed to diarrhoea and he experienced abdominal pain. His symptoms got worse if he ate pork. Another had severe pain low down on the left side of the abdomen associated with diarrhoea. This started at the time of the miners' strike in 1984 and had stopped him from seeking further employment. He spoke with a stammer and also complained of heavy legs and depression. A third suffered severe abdominal pain and constipation. Her abdominal pain was associated with severe backache and both symptoms were identical to the symptoms she experienced when her son was born. This son had recently been convicted of aggravated burglary and sent to prison. She was very depressed. The fourth patient experienced bloating and an alternating bowel habit. She often found it difficult to pass her stools, but after a few days, this would give way to frequent loose bowel actions. Her symptoms were associated with an aversion to food and came on for the first time after she left home to live with her boyfriend. The next patient had smelly wind, rumbling noises in her stomach, abdominal cramps and occasional diarrhoea. Her symptoms started when she was cramming for her exams at school in Tokyo and seem to be associated with feelings of loneliness. The sixth patient, a teacher, suffered episodic abdominal pain and bowel looseness that was made worse by carrying heavy bags, and started when she had her hysterectomy. The final patient in this group, a social worker, complained of a feeling of bloating and emptiness, but developed severe abdominal pain when she ate. She was also troubled with constipation, had suffered from anorexia and remained angrily attached to her elderly parents. The symptoms of each patient's illness were so distinct that each of them seriously questioned whether they really had the same diagnosis. They were right to question it. The variation in the way their illness occurred suggested that they were less like a specific disease and more the expression of the individual, as unique as a fingerprint or a DNA profile.

Doctors rely on a stereotypical pattern of symptoms in order to make a clinical diagnosis of organic disease. For example, if a man has a sharp boring pain at one spot under the breast bone and this pain is relieved for about two hours by eating and can wake him up at night, then the doctor can be pretty sure he has a duodenal ulcer. And if a woman reports a soreness in the right upper quadrant of her abdomen which seems to go through to the back just below the right shoulder blade and this soreness is associated with vomiting and fever and made worse by eating a fatty meal, then she almost certainly has an inflamed gall bladder. Functional illness, on the other hand, never has such a stereotypical presentation, which explains why it can tend to be a diagnosis made after other conditions have been ruled out.

The symptoms of functional illness do not just vary between individuals, they also vary within the same individual over time. Patients can change their symptoms as often as they change their wardrobe. It is not so much that symptoms disappear completely to be replaced by other symptoms – they are probably always there – but like an Escher engraving, sometimes certain features appear to be in the forefront of the patient's problems, at other times they are in the background. So a patient who presents with bowel complaints one year may complain of indigestion and headaches the next and extreme tiredness the year after. No wonder those with severe functional illness can end up being seen by a score of different specialists, each of whom conducts their own specific 'battery' of investigations before suggesting they might need to see another type of specialist. As the referrals and the investigations accumulate, such patients may be unkindly labelled as suffering from 'thick file syndrome'.

In view of this variability, it is not surprising that there is considerable overlap.[17] When Professor Simon Wessley reviewed the published definitions of twelve different functional syndromes, he found that bloating, headache and fatigue featured in over half of them. Most patients with specific functional syndromes, like chronic fatigue syndrome or irritable bowel syndrome would fulfil diagnostic criteria for several other syndromes. In my experience, a history of anorexia nervosa is so common in patients with severe constipation that they might usefully be considered together in what I have termed 'the nothing in, nothing out syndrome'.

The variability and overlap between diagnoses might create the impression of a vague kind of malaise where anything goes, but this would be misleading. The various functional syndromes and unexplained illnesses share a range of specific features that distinguish them from most organic diseases. For example, throughout the developed world, functional illnesses such as migraine, atypical facial pain, irritable bowel syndrome, functional dyspepsia, temporomandibular joint dysfunction, lump in the throat (globus syndrome) and unexplained urinary frequency tend to occur more frequently and more severely in women than men.[18] Three times as many women than men suffer from chronic fatigue syndrome, four times as many suffer from bulimia nervosa and ten times as many have fibromyalgia. The female predominance of anorexia nervosa or severe constipation is so great that until recently they were considered 'diseases of women'. There are, however, a few exceptions to this rule. Cluster headaches, atypical chest pain and frozen shoulder syndrome are more common in men. By and large, organic disease does not show nearly the same predisposition for women, with the notable exception of allergies and other disorders of the immune system, such as rheumatoid arthritis, lupus and thyrotoxicosis.[19]

In addition, although functional illnesses can occur at any stage in life, most people tend to seek medical help for the first time in their late teens and early twenties. This contrasts strikingly with the great majority of chronic organic diseases, which tend to come on much later in life. Erratic eating and sleeping and feeling tired all the time are so common among teenagers and college students that they are almost defining features. Anorexia nervosa is a disease of adolescence and severe idiopathic constipation often develops at around the same time. Chronic fatigue syndrome also tends to present for the first time in teenage, often in association with the pressures of college examinations. And finally, my experience is that the symptoms of 'irritable bowels' often start shortly after young men and women leave home to go to college or university.

Finally, many surveys have clearly shown that patients with functional syndromes score more highly for anxiety and depression than healthy people or patients with organic illness.[20] They also tend to have experienced more threatening life events. For example, psychological distress is more prevalent in fibromyalgia than rheumatoid arthritis, and in irritable bowel syndrome compared with Crohn's disease or ulcerative colitis. Patients who have unexplained food intolerances have higher rates of psychiatric disorder than those with established allergy, while depression is a common feature of patients with chronic fatigue syndrome. Not only do patients with functional illness have abnormally high rates of psychological distress and psychiatric disorder, but patients attending psychiatric clinics for emotional distress have more than twice the prevalence of unexplained bodily symptoms than healthy people. The association between psychological distress and functional illness is so strong that the number of functional symptoms that a person suffers from correlates with the number of episodes of anxiety and depression they have experienced.

So does that mean that functional illness is all in the mind? Not at all. But neither is it all in the body. When things upset, annoy or frighten us, we 'feel' it as both a physical upset and an emotional disturbance. Indeed Ian Deary, Professor of Differential Psychiatry at Edinburgh University, has proposed that functional illness stems from a state of dysphoria that affects both mind and body, a reaction of the whole person to life situations.[21] So it is not surprising to find that psychological disorders, such as anxiety and depression, are also extremely common, tend to affect women more than men, young people more than middle-aged, can wax and wane according to what is happening in a person's life and have increased quite dramatically within the last fifty years.[22] What might surprise you, however, is that, like psychological disorders, functional illness is not a modern phenomenon.

Physicians and healers have for centuries described illness that expresses itself in various bodily and emotional symptoms, and changes in relation to the vicissitudes of life. What is modern is the way it is configured. So the afflictions that might now be grouped under headings of chronic fatigue syndrome, irritable bowel syndrome, food allergy, fibromyalgia syndrome and candidiasis bear a remarkable resemblance to what in the past were variously known as hysteria, melancholy, the spleen, the vapours, hypochondriasis, spinal irritation, reflex neurosis and neurasthenia.[23] Like their modern counterparts, these ancient illnesses also tended to be more prevalent in women rather than men, in the young rather than the old and in city-dwellers rather than those who lived a traditional rural life.

For example, Hippocrates wrote how people suffering from melancholy 'were lean, withered, hollow-eyed and wrinkled with dry bellies and hard dejected looks'. They were 'much troubled with wind and griping in their bellies, and they belched frequently'. They also had 'flaggy beards, singing in the ears, vertigo, and were light headed. The little sleep that they had was interrupted by terrible and fearful dreams.' I am not at all sure about the flaggy beards, but the other symptoms might nowadays be diagnosed as chronic fatigue syndrome, irritable bowel syndrome or any number of functional illnesses.

But it is in the writings of the physician Thomas Sydenham (1624–89), 'the English Hippocrates', that we find the most striking connection between illness concepts of the past and the functional illnesses of the present day.

> Of all chronic diseases, hysteria – unless I err – is the commonest . . . As to females, if we except those who lead a hard and hardy life, there is rarely one who is wholly free of them [hysterical complaints], and male subjects, such as those that lead sedentary and studious lives and grow pale over their books and papers, are similarly afflicted . . . The frequency of hysteria is no less remarkable for the multiformity of shapes that it puts on; violent headaches, occasionally followed by vomiting, violent coughing and spasms of the colon, continuous vomiting and diarrhoea, pain in the jaws, shoulders, hands, legs and particularly the back and polyuria [the frequent passage of urine]. Few of the maladies of miserable mortality are not imitated by it. Whatever part of the body it attacks, it would create the proper symptom of that part. Hence without skill and sagacity, the physician will be deceived so as to refer the symptoms to some essential disease of the part in question and not to the effects of hysteria.
>   . . . The remote or external causes of hysteria are overordinate actions of the body; and still oftener over-ordinate commotions of the mind, arising from sudden bursts of anger, pain, fear and other emotions. Hence, as often as females consult me concerning such, or such bodily ailments as are difficult to be determined by the usual rules for diagnosis, I never fail to carefully inquire whether they are not worse sufferers when trouble, low spirits or any mental perturbation takes hold of them.[24]

In his description of hysteria, Sydenham encapsulated most of the features of modern functional syndromes: the variability of the symptoms; the ability to mimic organic diseases; the gender predisposition for women; and the links with emotional disturbance and life events. Unencumbered by systems of classification and diagnostic algorithms, physicians probably had greater insight into the phenomenon of functional illness over three hundred years ago than they do today. Then such illness was understood less in terms of pathological changes and more in relation to the trials of living in contemporary society.

By the beginning of the eighteenth century, several terms, all derived from adaptations of classical Greco-Roman medicine, were used as a diagnostic rag-bag for all kinds of unexplained symptoms, such as colic, bowel upsets, tremors, fits, spasms, headaches, palpitations, heartburn, swooning, anxiety, sighing, short breath, coughing, even laughing. The spleen – otherwise known as the hype or hypochondria because it was situated in the hypochondrium, the region of the abdomen that lies underneath the diaphragm – was widely considered to be the source of the black humours or 'vapours' that produced melancholia. In women, the same black vapours were thought to emanate from the retention of semen or menstrual blood in an obstructed uterus and were considered responsible for 'hysterick fits' or 'fits of the mother'. These conditions were so prevalent in England at the time that they came to be called 'the English malady'.[25]

By the nineteenth century, otherwise unexplained illnesses were attributed to irritable weakness and 'nervous exhaustion' brought about by the pace, noise and busy and overcrowded nature of contemporary urban life. A patient of Dr Alfred Bottiger, a nerve doctor working in Hamburg, described his symptoms as follows:

I feel as though my head is in a vice or I feel as if someone is trying to bore with a key through my skull or I feel as if a saddle is tied about my nose or I feel as if my arms are being tied down with sandbags or I feel as if my back is about to wrench loose or I feel as if the skin is falling off my thighs or I feel as if a rope is being tied around my throat or I feel as if a ball is climbing up from my stomach or I feel as if a stone was lying in my stomach or I feel as though someone had jumbled my intestines all up or as though there were a blockage somewhere.

People afflicted by such a complicated jumble of symptoms would often say that they suffered from their nerves, but it was the electrophysiologist, George Beard, who coined the term 'neurasthenia' to describe the profound physical and mental exhaustion, difficulties in concentration and memory loss, muscular aches and pains, gastrointestinal problems and sleep disturbance that busy people seemed to suffer from.[26] Beard proposed that the brain 'undergoes slight, undetectable, morbid changes in its chemical structure as a result of the stresses of contemporary life and as a consequence becomes more or less impoverished in the quantity and quality of nervous force'. This concept was amazingly prescient. Recent discoveries in neuroscience have shown how sleep deprivation and chronic stress can affect both the function and the structure of the brain through modulation of neurotransmitters and growth factors. In a recent article written in the prestigious *Annals of Internal Medicine*, Dr Michael Sharpe, Senior Lecturer in Psychological Medicine at the University of Edinburgh, suggested that neurasthenia or functional disease of the nervous system might offer a more coherent explanation for the riot of medically unexplained symptoms that occupy our outpatient clinics today than the overlapping confusion of functional syndromes. So why did it drop out of favour? The answer is that concepts of illness like hysteria, melancholy and neurasthenia were considered too vague and undefined at a time when medical science was discovering specific concrete causes and treatments for so many diseases.[27] In other words, it did not fit with the culture. By the 1960s, it was widely believed that if the cause of a specific illness was not known, the rapid advances in neuroscience and molecular biology would soon reveal it.

But now the pendulum has swung too much the other way. Illness tends to be seen almost exclusively as a matter of chance, a combination of unfortunate genes, poor diet and exposure to noxious agents, with patients as its passive victims. But that perspective is limited by its objectivity. There is little understanding of the role of the individual, of the way our lives have moulded us and the impact of the various challenges of modern life on the illnesses that we suffer from. Yet our subjective experience and intuition informs us how life events, difficult life situations, loneliness and the sheer pressure and pace of life can affect how our bodies feel and function.[28] We have all experienced exhaustion when we are struggling to do something we would rather not do. We can all suffer from headaches if we feel under pressure. We can all get a lump in the throat or feel breathless and wheezy if we are upset. We can all get indigestion if we make ourselves too busy to allow ourselves sufficient time to relax and enjoy our meals. We can all remember times when we felt so anxious and needy that we pigged out or when we were angry and didn't feel like anything to eat at all. And what about our bowel habits? Are these always as regular as clockwork? Not at all; they are exquisitely responsive to how things make us feel. It is no coincidence that threatening situations can 'give us the shits' or that constipation is associated with feeling uptight.

The difference between the everyday symptoms that we all experience and severe functional illness is simply an order of magnitude. Such symptoms become a problem when they are so persistent, severe and worrying that the sufferer becomes preoccupied with fears of being ill, has a considerable impairment in quality of life and has to seek medical care.

The proportion of people said to be worried about their health has more than tripled since the 1960s to comprise about 50 per cent of the population. But this does not mean half of us are suffering from psychiatric illness. Neither does it mean that we are weak and not up to the demands of normal life. It just means that we are human, and when human beings are exposed to severe dilemmas that they cannot resolve, the more likely it is that their 'stress' symptoms will persist and become consolidated as illness. So it is wrong to dismiss patients with unexplained illness as the 'worried well', over-sensitive souls whose anxieties about their health have been elevated by media scares. It is wrong to suggest that they are hypochondriacs. Such insults diminish the severity of the illness and call into question the integrity of the patient. Neither is it appropriate to indict patients with functional illness for exhibiting abnormal illness behaviour.[29] They feel ill, damn it! How else are they expected to behave? Illness focuses our attention and organises our behaviour. When I have a toothache, my whole being is concentrated around the pain in my tooth. So for people with persistent painful and disabling illness, irrespective of whether or not it has a pathological basis, their symptoms are an ever-present handicap, making even the most simple tasks difficult. And for some they can be so debilitating that they control their lives, confining them to their homes, restricting their diets, and even limiting the normal intimate relations with their partners. This was how Jane, a young, intelligent solicitor with a three-year-old daughter, described her symptoms:

I seem to toss and turn all night and start the day exhausted. I feel the tension like a tight band around my head and am often too nauseous to eat any breakfast. I try to be cheerful for Alexandra, but more often than not I end up shouting at her and leave her at nursery sad and upset. And then the pain starts, a gnawing ache just below my breast bone, which seems to grow until it becomes like a big, empty hole. I just have to eat something so I grab a sandwich or a pasty at the service station on the way to work, but after two mouthfuls I feel stuffed and a bit sick all over again. At work it is as much as I can do to concentrate. The telephone is ringing all the time and everybody seems to be complaining. I know I am not coping, but what can I do? I just feel so ill. I sometimes have to go out for lunch with clients, but that is purgatory; the pain is dreadful and I just have to smile through it. By the end of the afternoon I have had it. I can barely keep awake and I have this awful ache in my back and round my shoulders. I don't know how I cope with Alexandra but as soon as Jim comes home I just feel like throwing her at him and going to bed. And then it starts all over again the next morning. We haven't gone out in weeks and I never want sex. I feel too awful. And I don't dare to go on holiday. I can't bear the heat and the food always seems to upset me. I have no life at all – and nobody can find out what's wrong.

Many of the people that come to my clinic claim that their illness has cost them their job, wrecked their marriage, made them irritable with their children and even caused them to have car accidents.

Just because there is no pathological evidence of disease does not mean that the patient is not ill. People suffering from chronic fatigue can feel weaker and more disabled than many patients with cancer or heart failure, and those with unexplained bowel cramps can experience more pain and a greater impairment of quality of life than those with colitis, Crohn's disease or even cancer.[30] People don't have to be riddled with cancer or severe inflammation to justify illness behaviour. Some people can be so severely afflicted with unexplained abdominal pains and bowel disturbances that they do not dare to leave the house without knowing where all the toilets are. I have visited patients suffering with chronic fatigue syndrome who spend their time sitting in a chair or lying in bed, too tired to get up and cook themselves a meal. I have counselled patients with food intolerances who are unable to sit down and enjoy a meal without doubling up with pain. I have seen people so tormented with nagging pains in their back and shoulders that they can never seem to get comfortable or have a good night's sleep.

These people are not making it up to gain attention. They are ill. And if they have to justify this fact every time they go and see the doctor it is hardly going to make them feel better. Patients with severe functional illness are often desperate for some relief or at least some understanding. It is said that no patient ever died from a functional illness. Not true. What about patients with anorexia nervosa, or those with food intolerance so severe that they can eat nothing? What about patients so tortured with pain that they take their own lives? And finally, what about those people who are so stressed and upset that they develop heart failure? A recent study published in the *New England Journal of Medicine* showed that a severely stressful life event can damage the cardiac muscle in people with normal coronary arteries, probably due to the toxic effect of adrenaline and noradrenaline released from the sympathetic nervous system.[31] It seems that people can literally be scared to death.

If any infection was so prevalent and caused such serious disruption to everyday life, there would be widespread panic and gloomy predictions of the end of mankind. But because the conditions we are describing are so familiar to us, so much part and parcel of life, and because they manifest themselves in such a variable and protean manner, we fail to identify them as a specific threat. Instead they remain as insidious camp followers of the march of progress, the hidden epidemic that saps the will and takes away the everyday pleasures that other people take for granted.

The healing professions urgently need to view functional illnesses from a different perspective. Although it is undoubtedly important to rule out serious organic disease, an exclusively biomedical approach to medically unexplained symptoms and functional illness obscures the impact of personal disharmony and can leave people feeling that they have not been understood.[32] The greater amount of human illness may well be caused by the stress and the loneliness of modern living, but such factors cannot be measured, catalogued and assessed by the systematic approach of biomedicine. Seen from this perspective, we may well wonder whether molecular biology with its worrying potential for gene therapy is a brave new world of disease conquest or the last desperate gasp of medical determinism and pharmaceutical dominance?

In Idries Shah's *The Exploits of the Incomparable Mullah Nasrudin* the Mullah was observed looking on the ground outside his house for a key he had lost indoors. When asked to explain his strange behaviour, he replied that there was more light there than inside his house. Although Nasrudin's behaviour may seem absurd, it is exactly how our orthodox biomedical system approaches the enigma of functional illness. The more successful and efficient modern medicine has become in diagnosing and treating biological diseases, the less able it is to understand and help people suffering with functional illness. It has quite literally 'lost the key' and it will never find it 'outside the house'.

2

What makes people ill?

Kath was only twenty-nine when Gerald killed himself, but it altered the course of her life. She had been divorced from her first husband, Alan, for three years and was struggling to bring up her two boys. She met Gerald in the pub where she worked. He was a married salesman and worked in Leeds during the week, returning to London at the weekend. They found they had much in common. Gerald was urbane and knowledgeable. Kath had always been artistic. They were both lonely. Kath suggested that Gerald could stay in her house during the week; she had a spare room and she would enjoy the company and so would the boys. Their relationship intensified, but the weekends, when Gerald went home to his family, were dreadful for Kath. On Friday evening, she always felt physically ill.

Gerald wanted to leave his family and live with Kath but he couldn't bring himself to do it. Kath pleaded with him to make up his mind. So Gerald screwed up his courage and told his wife, who angrily told him to leave and changed the locks on the doors. Stricken with guilt, Gerald went to his garden shed and swallowed a large amount of weedkiller straight from the bottle. The doctors struggled to save him but he died in hospital three days later. When Kath first heard about it, she felt nothing except a strange sense of relief. She was not invited to his funeral; their relationship had always been a secret and she did not know Gerald's family. So she tried to blot out her feelings by keeping busy. She redecorated the house, landscaped the garden, took on extra typing work at home and looked after the boys. She literally worked herself to a standstill. After a few weeks, her body just seemed to pack up. She couldn't swallow, her bowels stopped working, even her kidneys failed to function. She felt so awful she just wanted to die. So she was taken into hospital and put on sedation. She slept for a whole week and when she woke up, she decided that she owed it to her boys to keep herself together.

But Kath could never come to terms with the loss of Gerald. And because this was a secret relationship, she could not work through her feelings of pain, anger and rejection by talking to anybody else. On the surface, her life continued as if nothing had happened. But she had a pain behind her breastbone that was so intense it took her breath away and made it difficult to swallow. Indigestion medicines helped a bit, but more often than not she just had to try to relax and wait for the discomfort to lift so she could swallow small amounts of food. Slowly, and with the help of medication from her doctor, her pain became less severe, but she still had to be careful what she ate.

Two years later she married a man who was kind and looked after her, and her life settled into a quiet routine. Kath might have put her experience with Gerald behind her, but every so often, her symptoms returned – and were always much worse at the weekend. Invariably, her husband would upset her by forgetting to do something he promised to or by being late. She would feel cross and upset and try to keep her anger and her symptoms at bay by throwing herself into a frenzy of housework until gradually all her physiological systems would shut down all over again. At first she couldn't swallow, then she had difficulty breathing, became constipated, stopped passing urine, and her fingers and face became puffy with retained fluid. Medications just didn't seem to help her. All she could do was put herself to bed and sleep. By the next day, she would feel better. Her kidneys and her bowels would start working again, she was able to swallow fluids and her breathing became easier.

This was the pattern for over twenty years. Then, last year, everything changed. Kath met Sally, a widow who lived by herself in a cottage in the next village. They formed a close friendship and soon became inseparable. For a time, Kath was perfectly well, but then Sally became alarmed at the intensity of their relationship and tried to cool it off. Kath became seriously ill. She could not eat and lost 2 stone in weight. She became severely constipated, her blood pressure rocketed and she couldn't sleep. She was convinced that she would have died were it not for her son and his family telling her how much they needed her. She could well have been right.

Kath was my patient for a long time and I got to know her very well. When she first came to see me in 1985, she had been seen by a score of consultants and had a string of diagnoses: labile hypertension; idiopathic constipation; acute urinary retention; oesophageal spasm; gastro-oesophageal reflux with oesophagitis. But none of these conditions had responded very well to medical treatment. It was only

when Kath began to understand the meaning of her illness in the light
of what had happened all those years ago that she began to regain
some control.

Kath's story demonstrates in the most powerful and poignant way
how illness can be both instigated and shaped by a particularly tragic
episode in life. Because the death of her secret lover could never be
properly acknowledged, it remained locked away as a symptom
memory and was only replayed in situations that reminded her of her
devastating loss. Indeed, her experience had so sensitised her to
rejection that even the slightest lack of thought by her husband could
trigger a bodily shutdown, and to this day, she still tends to feel unwell
on Friday evenings. Nevertheless, something compels her to seek out
situations – like her friendship with Sally – in which she is likely to be
rejected.[1]

Western medicine tends to view patients as victims of fate and doctors
as the only people who can make them well. That notion may suffice
for people with serious organic disease, but it does not help many
people with functional illness. On the contrary, the failure to see illness
in the context of what has happened can cast patients into a
therapeutic wilderness.

Studies of people with chronic functional illness have shown that
they have experienced more severe loss, more deprivation and more
disruption in childhood than healthy people and patients with organic
disease.[2] They are also more likely to report a history of physical and
sexual abuse. This is not new. In the mid-nineteenth century, the
French psychiatrist Pierre Briquet reported that out of a series of 501
patients with physical symptoms that had no clear cause and were
thought to be 'hysterical' in origin, 381 were instigated by a specific
traumatic event.[3]

The link between life events and illness is particularly compelling when
we study people who have been affected by the same traumatic event.
At the beginning of their book on the subject,[4] George Brown and
Tirril Harris described how, on a spring morning in 1957, an oil
tanker collided with a freighter in the Delaware River. Eight men were
killed instantly, but the rest of the crew survived in spite of being
surrounded by fire on the ship and in the water. All of them suffered
short-term psychological symptoms, but when the men were seen a
few years later, three-quarters of them had received some form of

medical help for severe non-specific physical illnesses. Most complained of continuous disabling headaches and sleep disturbance, and a third of them suffered with gastrointestinal illnesses.

A similar phenomenon has been reported by victims of natural disasters.[5] In October 1985, Puerto Rico was hit by severe flash floods and mudslides, leaving 180 people dead and thousands injured. In the years following the disaster, those who were injured or lost relatives and property had a higher prevalence of unexplained symptoms affecting the gut (abdominal pain, nausea, vomiting and excessive gas) and the nervous system (amnesia, paralysis, fainting and double vision) than those who had not suffered such losses. As I mentioned in Chapter One, abnormally high rates of physical illness have also been reported by combat veterans.[6] In the 1970s, Dr Finn Askevold interviewed Norwegian sailors who had served with the Allies during the Second World War. Over 90 per cent of them suffered from extreme exhaustion, 50 per cent had chronic dyspepsia, 75 per cent experienced pains, 62 per cent dizziness and 80 per cent were impotent. He called this the war sailor syndrome. Such long-term medical illness among military veterans is more likely if they had experienced terror on the battlefield and suffered nightmares, flashbacks and panic attacks afterwards.[7]

The most dramatic evidence of illness caused by collective experience of trauma has been reported by survivors of the Nazi Holocaust, many of whom suffered from chronic ill health for up to forty years or more after their liberation.[8] Long-term illness in Holocaust survivors is so specific it has been termed concentration camp syndrome or holocaust survivor syndrome. Other such illnesses might include shell shock for the shakings and fits of invalids of the First World War, soldier's heart for the chest pains and palpitations of veterans of the American Civil War, railway spine for the effects of Victorian railway accidents, and even the South Sea vomits for the distempers caused by the collapse of the South Sea Bubble in 1720.[9]

These days psychologists call the illness following a single episode of trauma 'post traumatic stress disorder' (PTSD). The initial symptoms are predominantly psychological. In the weeks after the event, the scenario is played over and over again in the mind like a loop of videotape, preoccupying thought processes, blocking concentration and causing a state of extreme arousal commensurate with the original trauma.[10] Sleep is difficult and often interrupted by horrific re-enactments in the form of nightmares. People with PTSD are said to suffer from 'the tyranny of past events'. Tense, exhausted and demoralised, otherwise minor setbacks can become major frustrations, amplifying feelings of tension to levels that are manifested, for example, as heart palpitations, pressure in the chest, aches in the muscles, diarrhoea, sickness, headaches and difficulty in sleeping.

Trauma is like a shock to the system, a state of panic that suppresses the ability to resolve what has happened. Victims of PTSD deal with it in different ways. Some find relief in food, alcohol or drugs. Others withdraw and avoid contact with other people, develop phobias and intolerances to foods. If the feelings evoked by the memory of what happened cannot be resolved, many gain respite by blocking the memory from conscious thought and going into a state of amnesia or denial. In such cases, the traumatic memory does not completely disappear. It hides, primed to effect a terrorist campaign of sabotage on the body when rekindled by association. Thus, as the psychoanalyst Henry Krystal noted from his observations on Holocaust survivors in 1999, 'traumatised people come to experience emotional reactions as somatic states without being able to interpret the meaning of what they are feeling and so suffer from bodily feelings and reactions that have no illness and must be interpreted as medical disease'.[11] For them it is no longer the memory that persecutes their every living moment, but their own body! They are afraid of going to bed, because they wake up tense and sweating with palpitations. They avoid going out because of the threat of incontinence. They cannot go to work because they are feeling so ill, or sit down to a family meal because everything upsets them. Time does not necessarily resolve the illness. The memory of what happened lives on in the symptoms and ruthlessly dictates how its victims organise their lives.

The varied symptoms of post-traumatic stress disorder are not just observed in the context of disasters and war. They can occur after any dramatic, life-changing emotional experience, even falling in love, and especially after being rejected. In the romantic novels of the nineteenth and twentieth centuries, young people who were 'crossed in love', showed an unerring tendency to contract tuberculosis.[12] In modern-day reality they are more likely to get asthma or bowel upset. Large numbers of people attended their GPs with the physical and emotional symptoms of PTSD after the shockingly tragic death of Princess Diana in 1997. And in a study from the Royal United Hospital in Bath, a third of all children involved in road traffic accidents suffered from PTSD.[13] But during peacetime, PTSD has been most frequently investigated in the context of physical and sexual abuse.

There can be nothing more damaging to a person than the experience of being abused.[14] The feelings of being overpowered and invaded can leave the victim feeling humiliated, depersonalised and extremely vulnerable. Victims of abuse talk of being reduced to the status of a used and discarded object. The loss of innocence and identity can shatter self-confidence and self-esteem. It is like a murder of the soul. It is hardly surprising, therefore, that physical and sexual abuse can lead to all the features of PTSD – the intrusive memories, hyperarousal, sleep disturbances, and phobias. These initial features of PTSD may be followed by a period of denial, but later – sometimes years later – many abuse victims seek medical treatment with symptoms of abdominal pain, headaches, dizzy spells, and bowel and bladder disturbance, but they rarely acknowledge any association, symbolic or otherwise, with the abusive experience.

Research has shown that people who have had a history of physical or sexual abuse suffer more pain, spend more days in bed through illness and experience greater impairment of daily activities than those who have not been abused.[15] They also have a greater prevalence of depression, eating disorders, sleep disturbance, headaches, obesity and alcohol and drug abuse. Reports of severe abdominal and pelvic pain, bowel disturbance and urinary symptoms are particularly common in women who have been sexually abused. They also undergo four times as much pelvic surgery, especially hysterectomy, as healthy non-abused controls. Many of these operations are quite unnecessary.

Jessica's mother never seemed to care for her. She was always telling her off and never seemed to acknowledge her feelings. Jessica formed a much closer relationship with her father, who seemed to understand her unhappiness. Puberty came early for Jessica and by the age of twelve her father's regard for her seemed to change into something more than just paternal affection. At first she didn't mind him touching her. He had told her how unhappy he was with her mother so Jessica felt that she and her father could console each other. Jessica had an intimate relationship with her father for four years. Many times, she tried to stop it, but she couldn't.

Then her mother found out and sent her away. Jessica was devastated and suffered a serious mental breakdown. She told me that she was saved by her religious faith, but from her mid-twenties onwards, she suffered with severe constipation and pelvic pain, which prevented any sexual relationship and could not be helped by any medications. She repeatedly requested referral to surgeons to have 'what was bad cut out of her'. By the age of thirty she had had five abdominal operations and her uterus, ovaries and half of her colon had been removed. Despite this, no pathology had been found and she had been referred to a colorectal surgeon for consideration of a total colectomy. I suggested that she delay this operation while we arranged some therapy sessions. She reluctantly agreed, but by the end of our fifth session, she announced that although He knew I was doing my best, Jesus had told her that she had to have another operation. What could I say?

Jessica's pain seemed to represent all the wickedness that she felt was inside her. She had to have it cut out, even if this meant another symbolic abuse, this time at the hands of the (male) surgeon.

What is it about such trauma that causes such profound mental and physical illness? The answer, I believe, is that trauma creates a severe crisis of identity. It confronts people with extreme dilemmas that challenge the image they have created of themselves.[16] The threat of physical or psychological annihilation prompts desperate and extreme measures to survive. Wars are said to brutalise people. They strip from us the veneer of civilisation that separates us from animals. Wrongs are committed, often more out of cowardice than malice. Victims bear the tension of grievance and the need for retribution for years afterwards. And the perpetrators may be stricken with guilt and shame because of the atrocities they felt forced to commit or the colleagues whom they abandoned to die. In the Korean War, a platoon of American soldiers were reputedly ordered by their commanding officers to shoot civilians, including women and children, at a place called No Gun-Ri.[17] According to anecdotal reports, many of them went on to suffer with the emotional and physical symptoms of PTSD for many, many years afterwards. And survivors of the Nazi Holocaust have written of the guilt they feel in having lived when so many died, when living often meant collaborating with their persecutors or at least repressing the rage they felt.[18] In a similar way, victims of sexual abuse often report the guilt they feel for colluding in their own humiliation.

Angela had married Tom to get away from her family. She had been both sexually and physically abused by her stepfather since she was twelve and her mother had turned a blind eye to it. So when Tom promised to look after her, she jumped at the chance, even though she was unsure that she loved him. Tom needed her but was very possessive. He refused to let her go out to work, insisted on the house being kept clean and tidy, kicked up a big fuss if his meal was not on the table when he came home and forced her to have sex whenever he wanted. Angela bore all of this with fortitude, though she was frequently ill with stomach pains and sickness. She worked hard to look after their daughters but things just got worse. Tom began to consort openly with other women but still insisted on sex with her. When she refused, he beat her up. But when Claire, her eldest daughter, came home covered in bruises and told her that her boyfriend had beaten her up and raped her, Angela collapsed and was admitted to hospital.

Angela had convinced herself that she had to keep the family together, but when Claire was also abused she could not bear the pain and the guilt and collapsed.

In the ten years between 1993 and 2003, I conducted detailed assessment interviews on over a thousand people who suffered from chronic unexplained medical symptoms. Over 90 per cent revealed that their illness had been preceded by changes in their life, which they could not come to terms with. A few had been involved in accidents, a small proportion had been victims of physical, sexual or emotional abuse, but, for many, the events that seemed to instigate their illness were more prosaic and could perhaps be characterised as the loss, or the threat of loss, of the people, objects or beliefs around which they had constructed their sense of identity.[19]

The renowned physician and psychiatrist George Engel documented how real, threatened or even symbolic losses could induce feelings of hopelessness that led to a deterioration of a person's physical health. A paper written by one of his associates reported as many as forty-one out of forty-two admissions to the medical ward of a general hospital had experienced loss and hopelessness just prior to the onset of the illness.[20] Many of these patients had also suffered painful losses and separations during their formative years and it was as if their recent loss had rekindled all their painful feelings. In another study of seventy-two widows under the age of fifty-six, nearly half of them reported their health had been worse since the death of their partner. Their illnesses included loss of weight, rheumatism, fibrositis, asthma, bronchitis, chest pains, peptic ulcers, skin rashes, abscesses of the gums, headaches and dizziness. It's even worse for widowers, many of whom become ill with cardiovascular disease – one might say they suffer from a broken heart.[21] This risk is mitigated in men who re-marry, but strange to relate, there is little statistical evidence to suggest that the health of widows is improved by getting married again, though forming a close relationship with another woman seems to help. You might conclude from this that relationships with women make people feel better than relationships with men!

When you lose somebody with whom you have not only shared your most intense and intimate bodily pleasures but also your innermost fears and thoughts, it is as though a whole segment of your identity has been removed. But while it is easy to understand how the loss of a beloved partner can leave a person feeling bereft and susceptible to illness, people also get ill when they lose a partner with whom they had a difficult relationship.

Rose had suffered Frank for years. She hated the way he just dropped his dirty clothes on the bedroom floor for her to pick up, never changed the loo roll, left beer cans and papers around the sitting room, and never seemed to talk about anything else but football and cars. She had threatened to leave him on many occasions, but Frank had just laughed and asked her what was for supper. She always seemed to be nagging him and never stopped complaining to her friends about him. Even when he became ill, she said he was 'making a real song and dance about it'. So when he dropped dead on the way back from the pub, everybody thought that after a short but appropriate period of time, she would live the life of a merry widow. How wrong they were. Rose was inconsolable. She couldn't eat or sleep, her house became a tip and she wallowed in the mess, persecuting herself for the way she had treated Frank.

In the early stages of a relationship, partners project all their hopes, aspirations and yearnings onto their partners in a kind of mutual idealisation; this might be why falling in love is so seductive and so exhilarating. But unfortunately reality soon dawns; their prince was a frog after all and couples who have perhaps built up their expectations too high may come to feel badly disappointed. All too many marriages seem to assume a kind of stability in mutual projection as couples trade accusations of laziness, fecklessness, untidiness, unreliability, mental instability and being taken for granted. The real problems can arise when one partner leaves or dies. Lonely and embittered, unable to trust another person enough to go through it again and bereft of a suitable vehicle for negative projections, the remaining partner can turn all their frustration on themselves and become ill.

While death of a partner is almost always traumatic, at least there is finality. The deceased can be grieved and, in time, the pain of the loss will fade.[22] Divorce is different. Your best friend may be transformed overnight into your worst enemy and a relationship that was once creative is now destructive, considerably undermining your sense of self-worth. Moreover, the loss of a once beloved partner can be accompanied by a whole raft of other losses or potential losses: home, family, children, friends, income – to say nothing of the losses of intimacy, companionship, friendship, pride, honour, status and self-confidence. The desolation can all but destroy a person. And the threat and pain of rejection and disintegration are constantly rekindled in protracted legalised grievances over joint assets, custody and access to children. Such devastating attacks on the self can so drain both physical and mental resources that it is not surprising many people experience a profound deterioration of health after separation or divorce.[23]

Even without divorce, the loss of a person's home can be a major cause of illness. For example, during the Bristol floods of 1968, people whose homes had been flooded suffered more illness and a 50 per cent increase in mortality compared with those whose homes had been spared.[24] A more recent comprehensive survey involving face-to-face interviews with 1,510 people in thirty locations that had been subjected to flooding throughout England and Wales found that over 70 per cent of those whose properties had been flooded suffered a deterioration of health at the time of the flood, and a third were still suffering from illness three months later. Other studies had shown that the disaster continued adversely to affect health four years later. Some illnesses, such as the 'flu', colds and bowel upsets, were probably related to the direct effect of chilling and contamination; others, such as headaches, 'shock', aches and pains in muscles and joints, muscle weakness, insomnia and depression, were probably more related to the stress of the event. Health effects were more likely when there were problems with the insurers and in those who had needed to be evacuated from their homes. Women suffered more health problems than men. There is the same appalling sense of devastation, disorientation and loss, most recently evident in the horrifying images of the 2004 Boxing Day tsunami in the Indian Ocean.

Home is more than bricks and mortar or even comfortable furniture, a well equipped kitchen and a nice garden. It is family, community, friends and culture. So it is not just the destruction of one's house, it is also the displacement from one's community. Even moving house can make some people ill.

Heather was always quiet even as a child. Her mother was rather anxious and over-protective, but her father was more relaxed and 'loved her to bits'. Her brother, James, was boisterous and excitable and Heather was a bit frightened of him. They all lived comfortably in a big house. Heather would spend hours playing with her pets and her toys in their walled garden. You could say she lived a charmed life.

Peter was the first boy whom she had gone out with. He lived in the next street and they met at a dance in the church hall. Within a year they were married and went to live just a few miles from her family home in Bury St Edmunds. For a time they were very happy. Heather's bowel problems started when her husband got a new job in Durham and they had to move. You might say that although she moved her bowels didn't. She became constipated. She was seven months pregnant at the time. The birth was traumatic; she hated staying in hospital and didn't go to the toilet for the whole of the three weeks that she was on the ward.

Although Heather and Peter live in a lovely house in a picturesque village in the Cleveland Hills, Heather does not feel at home and her neighbours seem intrusive. Any interruptions of her routine cause her bowels to seize up; holidays are a nightmare. The only time she has a normal bowel action is when she goes to stay with her parents. She is sure that if she could move south permanently she would be well.

Home is where the heart is – and, it seems, the large intestine! Heather's sheltered upbringing did not really equip her to deal with the realities of the outside world. Consequently the move to Durham felt threatening and caused her to retreat into herself.

It has been known for a long time that the prevalence of illness in refugees and first-generation immigrants is much higher than in the indigenous population.[25] This has often been ascribed to a change in diet, overcrowding and relative poverty, but a crucial factor that is so often ignored in epidemiological studies is the stress of being detached from a familiar community to live in an isolated and alien environment, a condition that was originally captured by the term 'nostalgia'.[26]

Another cause of illness for many people is the loss of their job. For many men and women, their hopes, ambitions, status, self-esteem and purpose in life are centred on their occupation. They are what they do. So losing their job, failing to get the expected promotion, being assigned a smaller office or a less expensive company car may constitute such a severe blow to their self-esteem that it can lead to prolonged sense of grievance and physical illness.

Vincent is a barrister. He has done very well, considering his upbringing in the poorest area of Liverpool. His brother is a lawyer, too, a solicitor in London. As a child, Vincent felt his big brother was the favoured one, and that he had to work hard to be noticed by his parents. He sailed through law school, always coming near the top, but had great difficulty in getting a partnership in chambers. Vincent had done his training in Manchester and felt he was always the token provincial candidate, likely to be overlooked in favour of less able candidates who had trained in Oxbridge and London. It was during his struggles to get into chambers that Vincent first began to suffer from the stomach pain that gnawed at his gut incessantly and kept him awake at night. That was around the time he married Rachel, also a lawyer. He describes her as more capable and efficient than him, but at times a little distant.

Vincent is still a junior partner; Rachel has done better and is a senior. They have three children and have just bought a house that cost £1 million. On the face of things they are doing very well, but he still has severe abdominal pain. Vincent has been investigated by several gastroenterologists and all that has been found is some patchy inflammation towards the outlet of his stomach. He has been treated with numerous courses of acid-blockers; each has worked for a week or so, but the pain has always returned. It was during his third visit that Vincent told me that he thought his stomachache was caused by his head of chambers, who seemed to favour the juniors ahead of him, and the solicitors, who did not refer enough cases to him, and even his rather distant wife. He could feel the churning and discomfort as soon as he thought about them. Vincent felt that he had always been ignored, but despite those feelings or perhaps because of them, he continued to work extremely hard, doubling the case load of the previous incumbent, and writing articles for specialist publications. He rarely had any time to relax at home. He and his wife hardly ever spent a night out together and he couldn't remember the last time they had made love.

So what was causing Vincent's pain? Yes, it was partly the pressure of work and the unreasonable demands that others made on him, but it was deeper than that. Vincent's experience of being ignored in favour of his older brother had inculcated a need for love and a deep fear of rejection. So to deserve love and offset rejection, he had to work harder than anybody else. He could never be satisfied with himself. Unfortunately, his surrogate parents – the senior partners in chambers

– seemed insatiable as well, demanding more and more from him but giving nothing back except criticism. So Vincent's feelings of being overlooked at work and his relative lack of affection at home rekindled the painful memories of childhood, churning his stomach, stimulating acid secretion and eroding both his self-esteem and the lining of his stomach.[27]

It is not just the obvious setbacks and major losses of life that bring about illness. Even events that most would perceive as positive can make some people ill. It is the change itself that upsets them, probably because change always incurs the risk of separation or loss, which sensitive and vulnerable people may find frightening. The arrival of a new baby is generally seen as a joyous event, but in our modern nuclear families, it can constitute a difficult adjustment, incurring the loss of personal freedom and often employment, not to mention time for oneself, sleep and marital intimacy. These massive changes can threaten the stability of many a young parent, and their effects are magnified for many mothers if they are socially isolated. No wonder so many women suffer from depression and functional illness after childbirth.

For similar reasons, getting married can be equally stressful to some people.

Jemima's illness commenced on her honeymoon. Her parents had doted on her from the day she was born and had given her anything that she wanted. She had bags of confidence and by her mid-twenties had become quite a successful businesswoman. She met Reg at a nightclub in town. As she later related to her friends, he had the sort of smouldering good looks that made her legs turn to jelly. She had to have him. Reg may have been Wath-on-Dearne's answer to Harrison Ford, but he worked as a miner and Jemima could run rings round him intellectually. Her parents thought the marriage was a bad idea but they stumped up the cash and gave Jemima a fairy-tale send-off. Jemima looked beautiful and Reg and his friends looked like film stars in their sky-blue morning suits. The happy couple spent their honeymoon on the island of Barbados, but this was not the romantic idyll that Jemima had dreamed about. Instead of being transported by passion into paroxysms of pleasure, she spent their wedding night on the toilet, tortured by spasms of vomiting and diarrhoea. Her illness continued throughout the honeymoon, and on and off for the next three years. It only seemed to improve when she spent a few days with her parents.

When Jemima went away on her honeymoon, she not only lost the protection of her family, but the prospect of sexual intimacy threatened to disrupt her fragile personal integrity. Although Reg loved her and tried to be understanding and caring, he was frustrated by her illness and unable to calm her fears. Fearful of his rejection, Jemima would try her best, but she couldn't control her guts.

And family holidays are not always a pleasurable opportunity to relax in the sun away from the everyday stresses of work and domestic responsibilities. For some people, the annual family holiday can be a cauldron of emotion, bubbling with tension as the participants struggle to come to terms with the loss of privacy and independence. Issues that are normally defused by talking about them with the wider family and friends, become concentrated on holiday when there are no friends to confide in. Things often boil over and, not infrequently, somebody gets ill.

Julie was dreading the holiday. She hated Benidorm, she didn't know how she was going to cope with James for two weeks and she knew the children would drive her mad. To make the prospect even more horrendous, it was only a month ago that James had found out about her affair with Bob. After bitter scenes of recrimination, they agreed they owed it to the children to stay together and try to make a go of it. Julie promised she would not see Bob again – a promise she broke within three days. So she embarked on the holiday in a turmoil of emotion. She missed Bob desperately, hated James for dragging her away, felt ashamed of herself and horribly guilty about the children. So when James told her that it was clear she didn't want to be there and that she was spoiling the holiday, she felt so dreadful she developed a pounding headache that went on for days and forced her to rest quietly by the hotel pool while James and the children went out.

For Julie the tension of being somewhere she just didn't want to be was unbearable, but at least her illness allowed her space to think and rest.

Even Christmas can make people feel ill. In contemporary Western culture, the enforced and often guilt-ridden reunion of a divided family at Christmas has a potent capability to rekindle old grievances, while for people who are isolated Christmas can just intensify their loneliness. Reports of illness always seem to go up around Christmas time, notwithstanding the weather.

The capacity for certain situations to cause illness in some people but not in others depends on their associations – in other words, what they mean to an individual. It is for this reason that people tend to suffer a recurrence of their illness on the anniversary of a traumatic event. In the same way, a minor car accident would be of little significance to most people but it could cause major distress and physical upset to somebody whose husband was killed in a car accident. The minor accident 'rekindles' all the shock and emotion of their sudden and tragic loss. And I have observed that many of my patients who suffer from severe unexplained abdominal symptoms have lost a close relative through bowel cancer. And finally, some people are more likely to become ill after success than failure, probably because they have learnt that success leads to change and social isolation, and attracts the envy of others.

But for many of us, it is not what has happened that inhibits our sleep, ties knots in our muscles and wrenches our guts out of kilter, it is the prospect of what *could* happen. We may well be able to deal with what *has* happened, but the only thing we do about what *might* happen is to worry about it. Anxious people suffer that inner sense of loss which can never be grieved and mourned because it has not yet happened. When Drs Lawrence Hinkle and Harold Wolff from Cornell University examined the long-term relationship between life events and physical illness in a large number of telephone company employees in the 1950s, they found that episodes of illness were concentrated in the same 25 per cent of subjects and tended to occur when individuals were experiencing life situations as threatening. More recent research has shown that fluctuations in the severity of functional gastrointestinal symptoms is almost entirely accounted for by the presence and intensity of worrying life situations.[28]

To find a term that captured the impact of life events on a person's health, the physiologist Hans Selye (1907–82) coined the term 'stress' in the 1930s, using an analogy derived from mechanical engineering. So in medicine as well as engineering, stress is something that causes strain to a physical body.[29] In metal bars, it is measured by the degree to which it is deformed; in the human body by disturbances in physiological function. Since Selye invented the term, stress tends to be used to indicate the effect of threatening situations. We talk about being under a lot of stress when we are short of money, working for examinations, not getting on with our spouse, or have more responsibilities than we can cope with. In all of those situations, we are suffering from fear of loss – of home and possessions, of a future, of our marriage, job and self-esteem.

But stress is a misleading term. So many of my patients almost seem to invite stress. They perversely take on extra responsibilities just to keep themselves busy. This occupies the mind, gives them a role and stops them from fretting. It's only when they stop that their worry and regret return to pain and exhaust them.[30]

Joyce was sent to see me because of muscular aching and abdominal pains that tended to come on late in the evening and always on Sundays. 'I know I work too hard,' she told me, 'but this can't be stress because I am fine when I am working. It's when I stop that it hurts.' Joyce works as a company secretary for a small manufacturing business in Stoke-on-Trent. She arranges appointments, purchases the raw materials and components, arranges the advertising and marketing, sends out the invoices and organises the budget. She literally does everything. Her manager depends on her absolutely. Years ago, however, they had an affair and she had a child. He couldn't leave his wife and so she brought up the boy alone. At the time she came to see me, her son was serving a three-year prison sentence for drug dealing and robbery with violence. Joyce was mortified. The burden of guilt and gut-wrenching futility of all those years serving the man who could never be the father her son needed was more than she could bear. She could bury it all while she was working, but as soon as she stopped, she was racked with despair and anger.

Fear of change can also stress people and undermine their health. Some may remain for years in a job where they feel they are not valued, but cannot take the risk of trying to find something different. Others may feel trapped in a relationship, too afraid to strike out alone.

Rob and Jen had been going out for ten years. For the first two years of their relationship, he was married, then his wife, Denise, found out and so he left home. They were in love, and thought the love they had for each other could overcome the bitter recriminations of his wife, the enormous maintenance payments Rob was forced to make and his guilt about abandoning his children. The divorce went through and Denise remarried, moving to another part of the country. In the meantime, Rob and Jen have come to realise that they are never going to get married or have children. Rob is too scared to risk it again and Jen values her independence too much. So they stay together on the margins of separation, neither working together for a future nor cutting their losses and

moving apart. Every day of their lives, each of them in secret goes through the awful scenario of separation, the risk of loneliness, how they can't bear to hurt the other, how upset their parents would be, how they would ever find anybody else and 'what is wrong with me?'. Rob has been getting headaches and is sleeping badly. Jen has premenstrual pains that now seem to last all month. They both feel too ill to sort things out. Both know that they either need to make the commitment and stay together or split up and move on, but the risk of loneliness is too great.

Rob and Jen are in a double bind. They are unable to make a commitment to each other and unable to break free. Both fear dependency, because that would make the risk of separation much more painful, yet they fear the loneliness more. And the more they torment themselves with the threat of loneliness on the one hand and intrusion to their fragile identity on the other, the more they feel ill and stuck. But their illnesses have allowed them to avoid the issue: 'I can't possibly think of leaving now; I feel so ill. I'll think about it when I'm better.'

For Rob and Jen, their personal history has caused both of them to feel ambivalent about commitment. Jen was scarred early in life by her own parents' acrimonious separation while Rob has gone through a painful divorce. Both are so sensitised to the shame and the risk of separation that they experience it in everything they do (or don't do) together.

If failure to adapt to change, or even the prospect of it, can cause us to become ill, it follows therefore that those members of society that have to confront the most change are more likely to get ill and their illness will often occur at times of greatest change.

In many respects, life for a woman is more complicated than for a man. For large parts of their lives, many women change roles several times every day from wife to mother to housekeeper to employee to lover. The modern woman can be required to 'do it all' – hold down a competitive career and run a home and care for children all at the same time – but that cannot always be sustained without stress and illness. Fulfilling these roles effectively requires a sophisticated application of diplomacy and social skill, but every adjustment can mean the erosion of one identity in favour of another. And since the attachments a woman makes with her mother, lover, husband, children and friends are often said to be closer, more dependent and intimate than those which men form, those losses may also be more deeply felt. Many women who are referred to me suffer illness in their late teens when they leave home and go to college or university, perhaps in their twenties, when they might get married and have children, and in their thirties when they are struggling to cope with the conflicting demands of growing family and a more responsible job. For some the late forties and early fifties are another time of illness. Not only is there 'the change' itself – implying a loss of reproductive capacity – but there is also the loss of children as they leave home, the loss of one or both parents, perhaps the loss of husband through separation and divorce, and, possibly, the symbolic losses represented by mastectomy or hysterectomy. All of these changes are potentially threatening and could lead to illness. For example, about 10 per cent of women develop chronic abdominal pains and bowel disturbance for the first time after hysterectomy. Research carried out in my laboratory in Sheffield showed that this was more likely to occur in those women who were depressed just before the operation.[31] Hysterectomy can carry enormous emotional significance for a woman. The surgical removal of her womb may represent the loss of her femininity, the loss of her ability to bear children and even from a psychoanalytical perspective, the loss of the inner child. If she can no longer be a mother, who is she?

Every loss is a loss of identity. This is why it can hurt so much. We construct our identity from our experience. Who we are, the attitudes we have, the food we like, the house we live in, the type of job we do, the things we like doing and the way we treat our children are not just a matter of chance – they are related to our previous experience of those things. The same applies to the situations that make us ill. Illness is more likely to be caused by situations that undermine those aspects of life that we have come to trust. So public disgrace may be quite life-threatening to a proud man who had constructed his life around concepts of honour and reliability. A spouse's infidelity is a disaster to a woman who was brought up to believe in the sanctity of marriage. The realisation that working hard and acting honourably does not automatically bring the rewards we were brought up to expect can cause a considerable and prolonged sense of grievance. But it is often not just one event or situation that makes people ill, but a whole cascade of setbacks.

Peter was referred to me with a series of symptoms. He was unsteady on his feet, suffered from shaking of his limbs, had abdominal pain and frequent belching, was constipated and ate very little food. He had lost 3 stone in weight in the previous year and seemed intolerant to most of the foods he used to like. Hospital investigations had failed to reveal any obvious disease and allergy-testing had proved unhelpful. But as I got to know Peter better through therapy, he gradually came to recognise the events that triggered his symptoms. Social encounters made him fearful of rejection and tended to induce shaking. Feeling controlled by others would cause belching and rejection of food. Hypocrisy, especially in authority figures, could bring on attacks of diarrhoea because this reminded him of his strict father. Recently, while watching the prime minister on television, he felt so furious that only the urgency of his bowels prevented him from throwing an ashtray through the screen. Peter did not feel in control of his emotional and physiological responses and that terrified him.

Peter had been brought up in a Roman Catholic household. He was devoted to his mother but feared his father, an elder in the Church. He was a rather sickly boy and was bullied at school, but he enjoyed his time at university, and within a few years of leaving had married and settled down to life as a teacher and a father. After a devastating sequence of losses and life crises, however, he lost the ability to cope and became ill. First there was the collapse of his marriage after years of bitterness and character assassination. This led to a rather distant relationship with his teenage children and months of wrangling through solicitors. Then, the same year, his mother, to whom he had always been very close, collapsed and died. A few months later he took early retirement from his teaching job on the grounds of ill health.

So, within a short period of just over a year, the key components of Peter's identity had been systematically dismantled. But he survived the desolation of it all, helped by his strong religious faith and his interests in rambling and bird-watching. Five years later, Peter got married again. Although their relationship was close and happy, marriage to a non-Catholic brought rejection from the Church and the disapproval of his father. An intensely proud and private man, Peter tortured himself with the shame of his rejection, his guilt about not helping his children through his divorce, and spasms of irritation with Mary. Was he just not good at relationships? He keenly felt the injustice of his father's behaviour and the hypocrisy of the Roman Catholic Church in not recognising his second marriage. He could not enjoy the pleasure and companionship that Mary offered him. He felt he didn't deserve it. The feelings of shame, guilt and grievance went round and round in his head, wearing him down and leaving him unable to relax and see things in perspective. He felt under attack the whole time – not so much from his father, the Church or his children, but from his own feelings of

unworthiness. There seemed to be no escape. Like a man under siege, he was constantly on edge and vigilant, reacting swiftly and dramatically to new events as if his life depended upon it.

People, it seems, can cope with almost anything so long as they feel robust enough to retain a sense of self-worth. The devastating sequence of life changes that Peter had experienced seriously challenged his sense of identity, but he still had his religion and the support of his father to sustain him. But when even they failed to endorse his last chance of happiness, Peter 'lost faith'. He would interpret every change as a possible disaster and react with extreme anxiety and anger, while at other times he condemned himself to such an onslaught of self-recrimination that he was overwhelmed with feelings of hopelessness and helplessness.

Peter's illness was, I would argue, brought about by a crisis of identity. He was unable to accept and grieve the loss of the things that he had relied on to hold him together because without them there would be nothing left. Neither was he able to trust the safety of his new relationship and home. And so his feelings of anger and disappointment were kept alive as the destructive effects of grievance and shame that engendered a sense of hopelessness which made him dread that it would all go wrong again.

When people's confidence in themselves and their world has been undermined, then even minor setbacks can upset them and make them ill. They become so sensitised to the threat of loss they see it everywhere. Events that might seem quite minor to other people – such as arguing with a work colleague, or receiving a parking ticket – can cause them to feel so unwell that they have to take time off work.[32] They fret about what will happen when their daughter leaves home, or their husband or wife retires. They can worry themselves sick about the faulty switch in the bathroom, the damp patch on the ceiling, and the brakes on the car. They can die a thousand painful deaths in their minds as they worry about getting an incurable illness, or live through the most painful scenario of rejection when their son forgets to ring. They might suffer the extreme humiliation of abject failure waiting for their examination results to arrive. Such everyday worry 'domesticates' a much more terrifying existential insecurity. People with chronic functional illness are more likely to perceive life changes as negative and worry about what may seem to others to be relatively trivial problems. The risk of everyday life can seem so great that even pleasurable events that disrupt the routine of life – a holiday, for example – are seen as threatening.

Peter had converted his fear and anger into a martyrdom that not only made everything seem negative and hopeless, but also infected everybody close to him.[33] We all know people who can wallow in such misery, like the character Victor Meldrew in the sitcom *One Foot in the Grave*. Perhaps we can all be like it. At bad times it seems better to wallow in the mess of one's life; at least things cannot get any worse and there is a perversely heroic quality in such a martyred existence. It is much riskier to accept change and the option of life, because it could all go so badly wrong and how on earth would one survive such a devastating blow?

The body cannot withstand such sustained levels of threat without becoming ill. Not only can the prolonged tension cause sensitivity and inflammation in many parts of the body but, as George Engel pointed out, the sheer mental and physical exhaustion that accompanies feelings of hopelessness and helplessness can deplete our physical resources.[34]

But paradoxically, the very same people who fret about what might happen often deal with real crises very well. They will arrange the funeral, get the car repaired, get the builders in to sort out the leaking roof and forward cash to their son who has run out of money. It is like having a treatable organic disease, something tangible that can be dealt with and justify one's distress. If I had £10 for every person with irritable bowel syndrome who has told me how they wished they had a serious disease that could be resolved by surgery, I would be rich.

In this chapter, I have attempted to illustrate how it is the episodes in life that challenge a person's sense of their own identity which are most likely to result in illness. These require a dismantling of previous assumptions and a reconstruction of the self, which cannot be conducted without feelings of disharmony and illness. Sometimes the damage cannot be properly repaired and the ego remains disrupted. So the guilt that cannot be absolved, the shame that cannot be forgotten and the grievance that we cannot let go of can all cause an unremitting and debilitating state of depression that chronically exhausts a person.

Peter is recovering from his illness. Slowly, through many sessions of therapy, he has begun to see his illness not as a threat in itself but the representation of the way his identity had been threatened by the accumulation of personal challenges. He has realised that he doesn't have to be a victim of his own persecution and that he could put his life together without relying on the approval of the Church and his parents. He has regained confidence in himself, taken more responsibility for his relationship with Mary and learnt to manage his father rather than feel threatened by him. He left the Roman Catholic Church and worships with Mary at the local Anglican church. His illness still has a tendency to return whenever he feels rejected, but he is able to recognise this and discuss it with Mary, so allowing the feelings to recede into the background.

When we are exposed to 'stress', we react as a whole person. And when we recover, we need to reconfigure both our emotional and bodily responses. But exactly how life situations cause illness and how recovery can take place has until recently been the subject of mystery and conjecture. The next chapter summarises recent developments in our understanding of emotional responses to certain situations and shows how this issue can leave people suffering from chronic illness.

3

Emotional regulation and
the development of illness

It was the summer of 1895, on a hot, humid day in New York. Tom, just nine years old, was playing in the backyard when his father returned from a political rally carrying a full beer 'growler'. Hot and thirsty, Tom followed his father into the house. Seeing the pitcher on the stove, and thinking it was full of cold beer, he grasped it by the top, which was still cool, and without looking inside, took a very large mouthful. But it wasn't beer that was in the pitcher; it was scalding clam chowder. Fearing the wrath of his mother who was in the next room, he didn't spit it out but swallowed it and immediately collapsed to the floor. Tom was rushed to hospital. He was very ill. He couldn't eat a thing and drinking was agony. Over the next few weeks the whole of his oesophagus scarred and narrowed to the size of a straw. There was nothing the surgeons could do except make a permanent hole in his stomach so that he could feed himself.

Tom learned to cope with his disability remarkably well. He blocked the hole with a pad held in place with a binder. And when he ate, he chewed his food thoroughly and then spat the masticated contents into a funnel connected to a rubber tube, which he inserted through the hole in his abdominal wall, and swilled them through with water. Despite his unusual way of eating, Tom grew up quite normally. He was able to work, he courted and married a woman somewhat older than him with a family of her own and they had a daughter together.

It was not until he was well into his thirties that Tom's predicament came to the notice of Dr Stewart Wolf, then working as a resident at the New York Hospital. The two became friends. Wolf helped Tom cope with his gastrostomy and in return was able to make direct observations of what was going on in Tom's stomach over a period of twenty years.

Tom had a somewhat volatile temperament. When he was agitated about something, Wolf observed his stomach turned red, produced copious amounts of acid and was churned by strong contractions. But when he was more quiet and withdrawn, it became pallid and dry and the contractions were weak and infrequent. Things came to crisis for Tom and his stomach at the time of his daughter's wedding. Not only did he have the usual worries of arranging a wedding to contend with, but he had fallen over and fractured his wrist. In addition his landlord had informed them he was going to sell their house. Throughout this time, Tom's stomach was consistently red and swollen, acid secretion was sustained at a high level and in places the lining had broken down into erosions, which bled copiously. Tom took large amounts of milk of magnesia to suppress the soreness, but it was not for a couple of weeks after the wedding ceremonies, when he had been able to negotiate an extension of his tenancy with his landlord and his arm had healed, that Tom's gastric functions subsided to their usual level.

The circumstances of Tom's tragic accident gave Stewart Wolf a rare opportunity to observe how the events in Tom's life were played out in his stomach.[1] Not only were changes in emotional tension associated with quite dramatic alternations in gastric physiology, but the physiological fluctuations differed according to the nature of the emotional response. And when Tom was upset by a sequence of difficult situations, the stomach lining actually broke down with much bleeding.

Our 'emotional' body is exquisitely responsive to changes in the external environment. Anything that breaks the routine induces a state of arousal, a rise in physiological tension that can be measured as an increase in muscle tone, a rise in heart rate, an elevation in blood pressure, increases in the rate and depth of respiration, changes in visceral sensitivity and alterations in the activity of organs such as the stomach, colon, bladder or bronchi. Indeed, as I start to write this chapter, the thought of not making the date set for delivery of the manuscript is causing my heart to speed up, quickening my breathing and causing my muscles to tense. I sense a mild anxiety. Then as I begin to get into the writing, the way the ideas are coming together relaxes me, slows the pulse, generates one or two satisfying gurgles in the stomach and relieves the tension in my back and shoulders. These are the minute-by-minute changes that occur in everybody. They make us aware of how things affect us. More serious events induce more dramatic visceral reactions and more severe physical and emotional symptoms.

Jill was eating her supper when the telephone rang. It was the police. Her husband, Ron, had been injured in a car accident. Jill's reaction was immediate. She was so overcome with dizziness and faintness that she almost blacked out. This was followed by an irrepressible urge to be sick. These symptoms continued for the next few days and only subsided when Ron's injuries had healed and he was back home again. Nevertheless, she still feels sick whenever Ron has to go on a journey.

Different emotions are often associated with different bodily responses. Anything that induces fear causes the heart to beat faster, increases the tension in our back and neck muscles, enhances the sensitivity of the bladder, which makes us want to wee, and causes our hands to tremble. When something makes us sad, our eyes water and the upper oesophageal sphincter goes into spasm, producing the sensation of a lump in the throat. And when we are angry, not only do we experience the sensation of our heart thumping, but studies have shown that the colon contracts vigorously and the lining of the stomach becomes suffused with blood.[2] The idea that emotion is associated with particular bodily feelings is supported by recent experiments with functional brain mapping. The neurologist Antonio Damasio has demonstrated that when subjects recalled and re-experienced different emotions, such as sadness, happiness, anger and fear, they engaged particular regions of the brain involved in the control of certain bodily functions. This suggests that certain feelings are grounded in neural maps that are not only specific to certain emotions but also show subtle differences from one person to another.[3]

On a more humanistic level, the association of physiological changes with certain emotions is also supported by the worldwide use of visceral metaphors to express emotional states. For example, in English, if we don't feel like doing something, we might say that we don't have the heart for it, or that we can't swallow or stomach it. If somebody annoys us, they may make us sick, or we may feel 'pissed off'. If something frightens us, it might be described as spine-tingling, or causing butterflies in the stomach or even giving us 'the shits'. We can be breathless with anticipation, faint with desire and, if something really upsets us, 'gutted'. Even the less descriptive medical terms for emotional states, like anxiety and depression, are derived from bodily sensations of squeezing tight or pressing down. And the ancient humoural doctrine of medicine made important connections between feeling and bodily states, which survive in emotional adjectives such as choleric, phlegmatic, melancholic and sanguine.[4] Such metaphors have achieved common usage because the feelings associated with certain fundamental emotional states are experienced by most if not all of us.

Our faces, of course, are particularly expressive. The whole gamut of human emotions is eloquently expressed by combinations of involuntary changes in blood flow to the skin, secretion from the sweat and lacrimal glands and subtle alterations in the contractions of the tiny muscles of the face.[5] These changes can not only signal joy, sadness, fear and anger, but more complex emotions such as shame, guilt and jealousy, and they can even betray our clumsy attempts to conceal our true feelings with false smiles and masks of concern. Facial expressions (and changes in bodily posture) signal our emotional responses to others, whereas bodily sensations and reactions tell us how *we* feel about the everyday events in our lives, what they mean to us. But how are such responses generated?

Whenever something happens to us, its meaning is evaluated in the executive offices of our emotional brain which occupy the mezzanine of the skull behind the forehead and above the eyes. This region of brain is known as the orbitofrontal cortex and is the apex of a highly sophisticated emotional intelligence network.[6] Not only does it contain a gigabyte memory of every significant experience that has ever affected us but it also possesses a comprehensive and integrated map of the body state. With the aid of these databases, the orbitofrontal cortex processes sensory information to determine the meaning of what is happening with reference to prior experience, and executes the most appropriate bodily responses. So without even thinking about it, a particular event may cause a rapid and specific unconscious change in physiological function that informs us how we 'feel' about it.[7]

Changes in bodily function are brought about largely through a combination of two parallel emotional brain circuits that are linked to the sympathetic and parasympathetic branches of the autonomic or visceral nervous system. These neural networks coordinate quite different strategies for coping with what happens to us.

The *sympathetic* response is a high-energy strategy geared towards helping us escape or defend ourselves from danger (flight or fight), and to maintaining vital functions in the face of severe injury. It speeds up the heart, increases the blood pressure, increases respiration, redistributes blood to the heart, lungs and muscle (where it is needed most), and shuts down areas such as the gut, liver and kidneys. It also releases readily available chemical energy in the form of glucose and fat from body stores, stimulates the immune system, and increases the acuity of sense organs.

The *parasympathetic* system, by contrast, is geared towards conservation, restoration and recovery. This induces a state of rest and calm, promotes sleep, stimulates the digestion, and supports tissue growth and repair. Unlike the sympathetic system, it slows the heart, steadies the respiration and promotes the function of the gut, liver and kidneys.

Sympathetic and parasympathetic responses to change are often supported by the release of the 'stress hormone' cortisol from the adrenal glands situated just above each kidney.[8] Cortisol's release is prompted by injury, infection, starvation and exhaustion – anything that threatens to overwhelm us. Its role is to maintain energy resources and defend the stability of the body's internal environment in response to threat. So, among its many actions, cortisol releases glucose from bodily stores of glycogen and breaks down fat and protein in order to replenish those same stores. It also redistributes body fat to abdominal sites, making it more accessible as an energy source, helps to retain salt and water in the body, and suppresses the immune response.

The same strategies that maintain vital functions in the face of tissue damage and injury can be deployed to deal with threats from the external environment. So anger and fear cause the same physiological manifestations of sympathetic arousal as an acute injury. And disappointment may activate the parasympathetic nervous system in the same way as a chronic infection, encouraging withdrawal and recuperation. But if such threats cannot be resolved either by 'sympathetic' action or 'parasympathetic' withdrawal, then prolonged activation of these strategies will inevitably result in exhaustion, demoralisation and illness.[9]

To illustrate this, let us return to Kath who introduced Chapter Two. Her illness was instigated by the tragic suicide of her lover, which left her feeling abandoned and desolate. And even twenty years later, anything that caused her to feel rejected rekindled the traumatic memory and triggered the same extreme protective response from the sympathetic nervous system. The pattern was always the same. She would try to close her mind and pretend it didn't matter, throwing herself into a frenzy of work, but her body closed up, too. The surge in sympathetic nervous activity made it difficult for her to eat by drying up the saliva, causing spasms of the gullet and arresting the emptying of her stomach. And at the other end of the gut, it reduced peristalsis in the colon and constricted the anal sphincter, leading to constipation. It also tightened up the muscles around her larynx, and contracted the urethral sphincter, making it difficult for her to pass urine. Most alarmingly, it narrowed the arteries that supplied blood to the kidney, which reduced urine production, increased her blood pressure and caused her skin to become puffy with retained fluid. Even her frequent attacks of arthritis, skin rashes, laryngitis and oesophagitis can be explained by the sympathetic nervous system's sensitisation of the immune system. But activation of the sympathetic nervous system not only affected Kath's bodily functions, it also induced a state of extreme arousal, causing anxiety and insomnia and pain. In these various ways, Kath's over-active sympathetic nervous system enacted a last-ditch defence of her self on the territory of the body. If this continued, the sustained tension would undoubtedly cause serious increases in blood pressure, strain on the heart and inflammatory illness. But Kath has an in-built survival strategy. After a few days, she would collapse with exhaustion and submit to the persuasive recuperative functions of the parasympathetic nervous system. She experienced an overwhelming desire to rest and sleep for thirty-six hours. When she woke up, she would often feel very upset and weep 'buckets of tears'. Then she passed a large volume of urine, the swelling of her hands and feet went down, her bowels started working, her breathing eased and she found she could swallow fluids and feel like something to eat.

While the parasympathetic system and the release of cortisol helped Kath recover from her extreme levels of tension, such adaptive responses are not always so recuperative. For people weighed down with seemingly hopeless and irreconcilable situations, the persistent exhaustion and demoralisation are accompanied by abnormally high levels of plasma cortisol, and when these are sustained for weeks or months, they can lead to physical illness. High cortisols are found in people who work too hard, in those struggling to survive in impoverished circumstances, or suffering with sleep deprivation; they are associated with the loneliness of old age and the depression of the young, and they are found in those who attempt to compensate for their feelings by drinking or smoking heavily.[10] George Engel and his colleagues, working in Rochester, Minnesota, recognised that high cortisol levels often accompanied a state of hopelessness or 'giving up and giving in' and could predispose to many different types of illness, not only functional ailments but also physical illness like heart attacks, duodenal ulcers and strokes.

It started the day Sam learnt that the herd had foot and mouth disease. They received some compensation from the Ministry of Agriculture, but it was never enough. They were already struggling. The fields down by the river were flooded three times the previous winter and the fences had needed repairing, then there was Jess's college fees and Susie's marriage to Dave. It had all come at once, but the loss of the herd was the final straw. Even if they were able to re-stock now, it would take another three years before they could hope to make any profit. There was no other alternative; they just could not hope to keep up the tenancy on the farm and they would have to go. It was heartbreaking; Sam had been born in the house, he had taken over the tenancy from his father and had reared his own family there. How could they leave?

They took out a mortgage on a little terraced house in town and looked for work. Marjorie got a job cleaning at the local hospital, but there was nothing for Sam. Nobody seemed to want to take on a man in his fifties and he was only trained for farming. In any case, every time he tried to do anything he got such severe tiredness and pains in his chest, there was no point. Sam felt so ashamed; he didn't know what to do. He was washed up, finished, and he spent his days drinking at the local pub while Marjorie worked longer and longer hours just to make ends meet, but the pains and stiffness in her joints was making this more and more difficult.

Three years after they left the farm, Sam was weaving an unsteady course home when he was gripped with a chest pain stronger than he had ever experienced and he collapsed in the road. By the time they got him to the hospital it was too late. He had died of a massive heart attack. Marjorie reckoned he didn't want to live anyway. The heart had gone out of him the day they lost the farm.

Sam's decline may have been a coincidence. It might have happened anyway; heart trouble was in the family. But Marjorie was convinced that Sam had just lost the will to carry on. His feelings of hopelessness would have undoubtedly induced an exaggerated increase in cortisol. While this may have helped him cope at first, the longer it continued, the more it would have raised his blood pressure, encouraged weight gain, increased plasma levels of fat and cholesterol, and increased the stickiness of his blood. All of these factors could well have led to the clot that eventually blocked his left coronary artery, leading to the irregularity in heartbeat that killed him. Exaggerated cortisol secretion does not only raise blood pressure and predispose to heart attacks, it also leads to obesity, diabetes, encourages infections, ulcers and is associated with the whole range of functional ailments.[11]

Impaired regulation of the sympathetic and parasympathetic nervous systems and the release of cortisol are implicated in all kinds of illness, playing fundamental roles in the function of the immune system, protection against cancer, inflammation, the metabolism of fats and sugars and the day-to-day function of all the organs of the body. So while the circumscribed tensions and upsets in our lives can cause transient alterations in the function of different parts of the body – elevating the blood pressure, inducing intestinal spasm, increasing acid secretion and causing a variety of otherwise unexplained symptoms – if these situations cannot be resolved and the tension and depression goes on for months or years, then this can even instigate the structural changes of organic disease. The art of medicine is to know when illness is reversible and may respond to support, counselling, rest and relaxation, and when the illness has caused changes in structure and more physical treatment is required.

But stressful life events do not always make us ill. Most people can usually cope with the majority of difficult situations without getting sick. All of us possess an emotional immune response that functions in a manner similar to the way our biological immune system deals with infections.

When bacteria invade the body, some of them are enveloped by large white blood cells called *macrophages*. These digest the invader and display its proteins like a talisman on their cell surface. This then attracts other immune cells called *lymphocytes*, some of which recognise the marker by virtue of a complementary protein on their cell surface. These stimulate a clone of identical lymphocytes that home in and attack everything they find with the same chemical configuration. In this way the infection is suppressed, but sufficient members of the clone return to their home base in the regional lymph glands, where they form the nucleus of a specific rapid reaction force –

an immune memory – should this particular organism have the temerity to invade again.

In the emotional immune response, it is the meaning of a particular life change, in relation to the database of prior experience stored in the brain, that is expressed in physiological responses. These 'feelings' are recognised by the brain and brought together with the context that caused them. The emotion created by this brings the meaning of what has happened to our attention and encourages an appropriate cognitive response to deal with what is happening. It also generates the 'charge' that allows this situation to be stored in long-term memory so that the person may recognise and react promptly to similar situations in the future. So just as the recovery from infections, such as measles and chickenpox early in life, leads to life-long immunity, so a wide experience of dealing successfully with the trials of life allows us to deal with most situations without getting ill. We might therefore conclude that some people have a particular predisposition to illness because their emotional immune system has not been sufficiently 'primed' by the successful resolution of past events.

This notion of a 'psychological immune system' tends to assume that emotions emanate from bodily feelings and reactions. We feel sad because we cry, happy because we laugh, or feel desire because we have an erection.[12] But is this true?

Feelings akin to emotion can certainly be generated by artificial stimulation of certain regions of the body. When fat emulsions are covertly infused through tubes into the small intestine, volunteers feel calm, relaxed and sleepy. Sugar solutions, in contrast, make them feel tense and excited.[13] Similarly, when the chemicals released from damaged tissue are isolated and injected into healthy volunteers, they induce 'feelings' of lethargy.[14] And stimulation of the skin can convey a whole range of quasi-emotional experience from relaxation to alarm to excitement and desire.[15] But are such bodily feelings emotions? I would say not, but they are a component of emotion. Emotions are feelings put into context. They are about situations and relationships. We feel angry with someone. We are sad because of something that happened. We feel ashamed of something we did, guilty about hurting somebody, disgusted at something, in love with somebody. It is impossible to experience emotion without relating it to a context that encompasses what the situation means to an individual, according to his own personal attitudes, beliefs, ideas and previous life experience.[16]

When I am lecturing, I sometimes illustrate this with the following scenario:

> Suppose a young woman marched into the lecture theatre and stood here where I am standing and scrutinised all of you in the audience. Most of you would think it a little curious, funny even; a few might even start to laugh. It would certainly liven up the lecture. But if you were the person who was having an affair with her husband, you would probably be stricken with a thumping heart, acute nausea and an intense desire to go to the toilet, which you would recognise as the fear caused by the encounter.

Emotion does not *just* inform us of how we feel about the things that happen to us, it also creates the motivation for adaptation and change.[17] When we fall in love, it is that frisson of joy and desire that can make the most fundamental life changes not only possible but imperative. When somebody ignores us or attacks us, anger provokes us to defend ourselves. When danger threatens, fear makes us take avoiding action. And when somebody dies, it is our grief that not only encourages others to give us support, but also preoccupies our thoughts, giving us the opportunity to think things through and modify our life to manage without that person.

Thus, to paraphrase, the creation of an emotion stages what has happened to us in the 'theatre of the body'. The director, situated in the frontal lobes of our brain, sets the scene, arranges the players, organises the lighting and stages it all in a visceral setting. The drama captures the attention and conveys the meaning of what has happened, leading to a successful denouement that we remember and learn from.

Just stop reading a moment and think about what has happened to you last week: what you ate, whom you met, where you went, how you felt. You can probably remember three or four events really clearly and there are big gaps of time where you cannot remember what you were doing at all. What you remember are the things that are important to you – maybe some of the people you met, a meeting you went to, an altercation with a neighbour – in other words, the events that are layered with emotional significance.[18] Warring couples often accuse each other of having selective memories, but in reality, memory is always selective, we only remember those events or aspects of situations that *affect* us, and the more profoundly they affect us, the more clearly we remember them. I can remember so vividly the time I nearly put out the eye of my son with a boomerang. It is like a video-clip played in slow motion in my head. The boomerang whirling horizontal, head height, out of the bright sun. Alex looking around, excited, 'Where is it, Dad?' A dull thud, silence, people running, his eyes screwed tight with a single tear of blood emerging from one corner and an awful, sick, sinking feeling in the pit of my stomach. The boomerang cut his tear duct and detached his retina. Thankfully his sight in that eye is only slightly impaired, but you can bet your bottom dollar, I will never try to throw a boomerang again. Such emotionally loaded experience controls our future behaviour.

The impact of an emotional event on future behaviour is likely to be greatest if it is associated with an intense physical experience. When Virgil wrote of how the Queen of Carthage on seeing her ex-lover, 'felt traces of the old flame creep beneath her limbs', it helps to explain how the intensity of 'feeling' can encourage lovers to overcome the most extreme of obstacles and human couples to stay together for the birth of their children and for many years beyond. Moreover, the bond between a mother and her child is thought to be consolidated by that unique blend of physical pain and joy that accompanies natural childbirth.

Our memories are constructed from the joys, tragedies, disappointments, fears and irritations of life. What we take in from emotionally laden experience are the lens through which we view life, what psychoanalysts call our 'internal object relations'. This emotional chart of our social world defines how we feel about the people, institutions and the things that have happened to us, and it is by reference to this internal map that a new situation is given a visceral shade or hue of feeling that forms a major part of what we call intuition, guiding our attitudes, judgement and behaviour.[19] That's why psychotherapists tend to ask, 'And how did that make you feel?'

So we are not the rational, detached and objective individuals we like to think we are. We are emotional creatures, ruled by feelings and prejudices that we may not completely understand. As the French philosopher Blaise Pascal (1623–62) wrote, 'The heart has its reasons that reason doesn't know.' We all tend to see the world through the 'spectacles of our experience': some are rose-tinted, others shaded; some give us a broad vision, others make us short-sighted.[20] For people who have been brought up to feel safe and comfortable in the company of others, social contacts make them feel alive and reinforce their self-confidence, while constantly fine-tuning the view they have of themselves. It's quite a different matter for the many, many people whose life experience has been much less consistent and secure. Ill equipped to deal confidently with social encounters, they find it difficult to trust people. This colours their internal world with suspicion, reinforcing the threat of social encounters and the chance of disappointment and illness.

Janice had suffered from severe bouts of abdominal pain for the last four years. She had seen several doctors and undergone a whole dossier of investigations and treatments. All to no avail. She was fed up. She hated her job and was struggling to run the home and look after her two energetic boys. We were not making any headway in therapy and, as the weeks went by, she became increasingly frustrated. Then I had to leave for two weeks to deal with a family crisis. When I came back she complained that while I was absent her stomach had been so bad she had had to go to casualty. I wondered whether the latest bout of illness might have been related to her anger with me for abandoning her therapy without sufficient notice. At that, she burst into tears and angrily exclaimed, 'It's always the same. People never take any notice of me.'

She went on to tell me that her father had left the family when she was very young and her mother never seemed to have any time for her after that, except when she was ill. So Janice would work so hard to be useful, cooking an evening meal for her mother when she came home, cleaning the house, doing the shopping, anything to make her mother notice her a little. But her mother rarely did, and Janice's frustrated needs gave her abdominal pain which elicited some sympathy. Twenty years on, she is married to Tim, who is heavily involved in running the local football team and has no real time to listen to Janice, and her line manager at work does not acknowledge how hard she works.

Exploring these issues allowed Janice to understand how she tended to perceive her world (including her relationship with me) through the filter of her childhood grudge and how she needed to break free from that and take responsibility for her own feelings. The knowledge empowered her to negotiate a part-time arrangement at work and a greater sharing of responsibilities at home. When I last saw her, she seemed more confident and assertive, and said that her pain had improved a lot. 'It must be that diet you put me on!' she added with a twinkle in her eye.

Emotion is potentially dangerous. Like electricity, it can be used to provide illumination and drive the motors of change. But when discharged without restraint, it can create an awful 'shock' and may cause damage.[21] So if we cannot put our feelings into context or if we are unable to resolve the emotions that are generated, then the tension can overload the system and make us ill.

Our ability to resolve our emotions and learn from experience requires the space to reflect on what has happened and create a 'social or cognitive buffer' that protects us and society from the consequences of acting on impulse. If somebody annoys us, we don't usually turn round and hit them. If we fancy somebody, we don't just jump on them. Our cognitive buffer enables us to live in the society of others by 'digesting and absorbing' what has happened and directing our emotional responses along more creative channels. As Plato wrote, 'Emotions are wild horses that have to be reined in by reason.'

Effective emotional regulation requires the integration of both right and left frontal cortices. The more *intuitive right side* puts the feelings we have about what happens into a personal context, generating emotion, while the more *analytical left side*, with its lexical database of ideas and knowledge, enables a person to think rationally about what has happened and discuss it with others.[22]

Language transforms emotional experience into a meaningful symbolic form that can be transmitted and received by others. Our facility for language therefore allows us to change our mind and adapt to changing situations by communicating with other people. Every encounter we have has the capacity to change us. For example, during the process of getting to know one another, couples compare personal attitudes and beliefs and relate their life experiences. The emotion that is generated by the interaction may encourage trust and confidence, or it may lead to an assertion of independence. Either way, their personal 'map' is changed by the encounter. That's what's so exciting and so scary about personal relationships.

People vary considerably according to how they deal with their emotions. Many are so skilled at controlling their emotional responses that they can manipulate others. These are the streetwise, the city slickers and the political operators, who can be seductive and persuasive but may at the same time engender distrust because we never see enough of their raw humanity. But there are others, in whom the veneer of civilisation is painted very thin, and who struggle to keep their emotions under control. It has been reported that patients with functional illnesses tend to use more ineffectual strategies, such as confrontation, avoidance and self-controlling, to cope with stressful situations. From clinical observations it would seem that the emotional strategies they use can influence the type of illnesses they suffer from.

Geraldine was nearly forty, and suffered with such severe constipation that she could go several weeks without a bowel movement. Even powerful laxatives failed to relieve her. Her specialist had subjected her to the full humiliating gamut of colonic investigation and tried many different combinations of dietary and medical treatments, all to no avail. He had just about reached the stage of referring her to a surgeon for an operation to remove her colon, when he decided to send her to me as 'a last resort'.

Geraldine told me that she had first become constipated when she was eighteen, after the death of her mother, but this improved after she got married. Unfortunately her marriage broke down after just four years and since then she had been severely constipated.

During our first meeting, Geraldine was painfully shy. She kept her overcoat tightly buttoned up even though it was early summer. She answered all my questions with brief comments while staring fixedly at a spot on the floor. It was a difficult interview. We never really engaged with each other. Nevertheless I learnt that not only was she constipated, but her eating behaviour was also quite restrained. She was a strict vegetarian, ate only organic produce and fretted about food contamination. Geraldine lived alone with her two cats and worked in the local library. The only people she seemed to mix with were her father and an older brother. She relied on them to help her deal with the outside world, but she was deeply embarrassed by the way they noisily assumed they could just take over her life.

She was the same during the second session. She looked so frightened I felt concerned and tried to rescue her by asking questions and lightening the conversation, but it was hard going. The third session started in much the same way, but I soon ran out of things to say. So I decided to give her the space to talk. We sat in silence for forty-five minutes. I lapsed into a peaceful reverie, occasionally looking up to smile at her. And when the bell rang for the end of the session, I quietly announced that it was time for her to go, whereupon she got up abruptly and almost ran out of the room. I admit that I felt some remorse about leaving her in silence for most of the session and wondered whether she would return the following week. To my surprise she did turn up but this was a different Geraldine. Without waiting for formalities, she sat down and berated me for my rudeness.

'Do you know how long it takes me to get from Mold to Sheffield?' she said. 'You have to get a bus into Chester, then catch the train to Manchester and then change onto another train that trundles across the Pennines, stopping at every flipping station on the way. Then even when you get to Sheffield, the hospital is miles away!'

I smiled and shook my head.

'Well, it took me three hours to get here last week and you just sat there and said nothing. I've got better things to do than come all the way to Sheffield just to sit in silence. I felt so angry! And I've had diarrhoea all week!'

Now this was the person who had been so seriously constipated for so many years that the only way her doctors could think of relieving her was to remove her colon. Yet, she had cured herself by daring to acknowledge how cross she felt with me! It may seem hard to believe, but expressing her anger had relaxed her bowels more than any of the laxatives and herbal remedies she had consumed.

There is often a moment in therapy when things change. For Geraldine that moment was truly cathartic. She became more open and talkative, she started to go out more, and she began to take more responsibility for herself. She appeared more confident and her bowels settled down into a much more regular pattern. She only came for twelve weeks, but I asked her if she would come back for a follow-up appointment after a year. What a change! She had given her overcoat to a charity shop, left her job in the library, bought herself some new clothes and had even had her hair styled. And, she announced with a big grin, 'I've met a man! We're getting married next year.' She seemed surprised when I asked about her bowels. 'Most of the time,' she replied, 'they are fine, once or maybe even twice a day, but whenever something upsets me, they can seize up. They are my barometer that tells me when there is trouble about!'

So Geraldine's reserve and defensiveness were associated with a corresponding restraint in her bowel function and eating behaviour. Her intense fear of social interaction and her anger at the intrusion of others created a build-up of emotional tension, which was associated with exaggerated activity in the sympathetic nervous system. And since this tension could not be worked through, it remained locked in and was acted out in the 'theatre of her body' with symptoms that seemed to represent control and restriction. But as soon as she felt sufficiently provoked to express her feelings, her bowels were also released from inhibition.

But not all people who have difficulty in regulating their emotions are so controlled. Some are quite the opposite. Like John Cleese's character, Basil Fawlty, they fly into a rage at the slightest provocation, fall in love at the bat of an eyelid, and experience the slightest setback as a major disaster that can make them feel dreadful. Their lives are taken over by chaotic surges of emotion, which cannot be properly resolved and therefore result in a riot of physical symptoms.

Sharon looked a wreck. There were bags under her eyes, her hair flopped over her face, she wore a dress that buttoned down the front, gaped at the midriff as she sat down and kept falling open at the thigh. She literally seemed to be coming apart at the seams. She spoke rapidly without pausing, assailing me with a confusing litany of symptoms – tiredness, bloating, itching, nausea, backache, bleeding gums, headaches and diarrhoea. She was sure these symptoms had to be due to food allergy, or some toxic substance in her home, but nobody could determine what it was. She told me her story with a breathless air of desperation, illustrating her points with dramatic gestures and frequently weeping with frustration and distress. The atmosphere in the room felt like the stifling humidity before a storm. I felt pressurised, and struggled to find a quiet place in my mind where I could think, but I guessed Sharon must feel like this most of the time.

'I can't bear this a moment longer. You have to do something to help,' she said. 'I feel awful as from when I wake up in the morning to when I go to bed at night. I can't sleep. I daren't go out anywhere because of this awful gut rot. It's just destroying my life. My husband won't look at me, my friends are fed up with me, even my little girl seems to avoid me. None of the tablets work. The diets are useless, and how is talking ever going to help? I've done all the talking. I've talked until I am blue in the face. Can't you understand? I'm not ill because I'm unhappy. I'm unhappy because I'm so ill.'

I let her continue until she literally ran out of steam. And then, relieved of the pressure to talk, she seemed to let go and her body, unsupported by the tension in her limbs, slumped back in the chair. After a few minutes, I asked her to tell me not so much about the illness, but about her.

Sharon told me she had always been nervous. She was a nervous child. She had been brought up by her mother. Her father had left home when she was very young and she has no recollection of him. Her mother struggled to support the two of them and, when she became exhausted with work and worry, would blame Sharon for the way her life had turned out. Sharon had left home at twenty and lived by herself for a few years until she met Andrew. Within three months she was pregnant. At the time I saw Sharon, her daughter, Isabella, was a demanding three-year-old and Sharon was still working full-time. She was exhausted. Andrew was supportive but could not cope with Sharon's volatile temperament and just switched off or went out. Sharon felt lonely and desperate. She wanted to be a good mother and wife, but she needed space for herself as well. She felt overwhelmed with the responsibility and so guilty that she could not manage it better.

I suggested that her illness expressed the enormous pressure she was under. I told her she was like an engine racing along in neutral, generating much heat and stress but doing little work. She was literally wearing herself out. She needed time to think and get things into perspective. If she could do that, then not only would she be able to feel better herself, but she would also be able to have the time to help Isabella and Andrew. At that she collapsed in floods of tears.

Sharon came to see me every week for about three months. Sometimes she was upset, but most of the time she was calm and sad. I didn't apply any specific intervention; I just created the space for her to think and the opportunity to talk things through. Within a few weeks she had negotiated with her employers the opportunity to work part-time, stopped losing her temper with Andrew, abandoned the gaping frock and wore a more close-fitting top and trousers. In every way, she seemed more contained and although her symptoms still emerged when things threatened to get on top of her, they no longer ruled her life.

Sharon had found it impossible to control her feelings. She was overwhelmed with panic, frustration and fear and a riot of physical symptoms. There was no respite and no hope. In the past, her expression of catastrophe and chaos would have been described as 'hysterical', but nowadays such labels all too often provide the excuse for institutionalised rejection. Her illness was not so much a medical condition with a clear cause and stereotyped clinical features, more a state of body and mind caused by an accumulation of life events and an overwhelming escalation of tension. Instead of helping her to sort out what was happening, her emotions just swamped her ability to think. And so the distress, which was out of all proportion to the nature of the symptoms, was attributed to her illness, while the social pressures that caused them were hidden from view.

Sharon's despair was like a child's cry. She was very frightened. She was so desperate and chaotic that she had tried to relieve the tension with food or alcohol or medications – anything that would provide a brief respite from intolerable reality. But all too often, these behaviours made things worse, undermining both the integrity of her body and the stability of her mind. Sharon desperately needed somebody to rescue her, but more often than not her desperation tended to induce a sense of panic in the people around her, including, of course, me. She could make me feel directly responsible for not making her better.[23] So, with my expertise and authority challenged and my mind numbed by the intensity of her distress, I needed to resist the easy option, which would be to prescribe more tablets and order more investigations just to make *me* feel better. I needed to keep thinking and talking. Over the course of the next few weeks, Sharon visibly relaxed and was able to find the mental space to sort her life out.

Although both Geraldine and Sharon experienced emotion, they differed in the way they dealt with it. Whereas Geraldine closed down and suppressed hers behind a mask of control, Sharon's distress broke out in a riot of physical symptoms and a desperate plea for help. Control and chaos were represented in their respective physical symptoms. In my experience, people who keep their emotions locked in tend to have symptoms that represent the pressure and control, such as constipation, headache, backache and muscular tension (mediated by the sympathetic nerves), while people who find it difficult to contain their emotions are more likely to experience expressive symptoms, such as diarrhoea, urgency, faecal or urinary incontinence, coughing and vomiting, which represent a lack of control (mediated predominantly by the parasympathetic nerves).[24]

Franz Alexander, founder of the Chicago Institute of Psychoanalysis and one of the foremost psychosomatic theorists in the 1930s and 1940s, suggested that patients with psychosomatic illness struggled with conflicts around dependency. When neglect or deprivation blocks dependency, he said, then energy is expended to the parasympathetic nervous system, but when autonomy is blocked by excessive control, symptoms are largely mediated by the sympathetic nervous system.[25] This pattern is probably most clearly seen in people with eating disorders. Those who binge or comfort eat often do so when they feel depressed and lonely and out of control, using food to help them feel better. In direct contrast, anorexia nervosa is associated with the physiological signature of sympathetic over-activity and represents the sheer power of the will to keep control of the self, even if it means the starvation of the body. *Hunger Strike* by Susie Orbach is a brilliant description of this situation.

The analogy between emotional expression and physiological function was documented scientifically in a study of bowel function that was carried out on the male inmates of an American prison at the height of popular enthusiasm for 'dietary fibre'.[26] Volunteers were put on diets containing different amounts of fibre, and underwent a series of investigations, including personality inventories. As expected, the bowels were certainly more active when people consumed more fibre, but this association was not as strong as that between personality and bowel function. People who scored highly on the extroversion scale passed large, soft and frequent stools, whereas those who were introverted and defended struggled to squeeze out a few small pellets. So it would seem that people suffering with diarrhoea that cannot be explained medically find it as difficult to contain their emotions as they do to contain their motions, while at least some of those with unexplained constipation may be, quite literally, uptight.

But bowel habit or eating behaviour are not fixed aspects of personality, of course; they can change according to the circumstances of a person's life. For example, people with irritable bowel syndrome tend to oscillate between diarrhoea and constipation as they swing from control to chaos and back again. The same dialectic may be represented in patients with bulimia nervosa by the cycles of bingeing, vomiting and restraint.

Jean, a schoolteacher who lives by herself in south-east London, either feels panicky and out of control or lonely and isolated. There is no middle ground. She doesn't have that sense of containment, which would allow her to regulate her emotions in the face of an ever-changing social environment. 'Whenever I feel lonely, I start to panic and then I feel like something to eat,' she told me. 'It calms me down, but the more I eat the more I want to eat. This continues for several days until I am so fed up with myself, I am sick. Then I tidy up, have a shower, put on some clean clothes, exercise in the gym, stop drinking and just eat salads – but the loneliness starts creeping back again.'

Like a house with a faulty thermostat, Jean suffers from a disturbance in emotional and physiological regulation, either blowing too hot or too cold.[27]

The people I have described in the last few pages all suffer from a surfeit of emotion caused by life situations which they cannot resolve. The difference in emotional expression – chaos or control – may be neatly explained by differences in the balance of sympathetic or parasympathetic activity while the high degree of emotional tension might imply elevated levels of cortisol.[28] But there is another way in which people react to traumatic situations that just cannot be resolved.

That is to switch off and behave as if nothing significant has happened. People who exhibit this strategy are not upset. They have blocked the creation of emotion and are just left with the disconnected feeling or bodily reaction.

Emotional detachment is a feature of post-traumatic stress disorder. It occurs in people who have been severely physically or sexually abused, those who have suffered extreme trauma, and those facing impossible situations, such as starvation, imprisonment, severe injury or death.[29] So in the same way that 'shutting off' helps people cope with severe injury, it also protects the self from the devastating effects of intolerable life situations.[30] Longer-term emotional detachment is a feature of autism, Asperger's syndrome and schizophrenia, and some people with particularly resistant and florid unexplained illnesses.

Psychologically, people with severe emotional detachment appear flat and devoid of personality. They express themselves in a very concrete, almost robotic way with no real sense of understanding or feeling. This state of being has been characterised by two American psychoanalysts, John Nemiah and Peter Sifneos, by the term 'alexithymia', which literally means 'absence of word emotion'.[31] Unable to work through the bodily reactions to life situations by connecting them to the context, people with such extreme emotional detachment exhibit the most obvious changes in physiology in response to what happens to them, and have the least insight.

Thomas was thirty-one. He lived with his parents, worked as a packer in his father's business and played drums for a local band. For years, he had been suffering with attacks of headaches and a severe difficulty in swallowing. A family friend who was a specialist had suggested he might have a brain tumour but investigations had failed to substantiate this or any other condition.

Thomas was difficult to talk to. When I asked him how he felt about his illness, his job, relationships with members of his family, he just wrinkled his mouth in a kind of scowl, shrugged and said it was all right. He did not appear to have any feelings about anything. I asked him about girlfriends. He shrugged again and replied that he had one once, about five years ago, but she left after a few months. He supposed another one would come along some time. 'Like a bus,' I added with a smile on my face. He furrowed his brow and seemed confused. He did not understand humour. After an hour of trying to establish an emotional link with Thomas, I invited his parents in and slowly explained that I suspected his illness was related to conflicts over leaving home, which he could not talk about.

Thomas said nothing, but watching him carefully, I noticed that although it was a warm day, his hands and forearms and also his ankles turned blue as if with cold. I commented on this and suggested that he might be feeling quite cross about what I was saying. He nodded and blushed, and his hands and arms turned pink again.

Thomas's physiology was remarkably responsive to activity in the sympathetic nervous system, causing the dramatic fluctuations in blood flow that made his skin turn from blue to pink. Dr Ian Wickramasekere, one-time President of the Association of Applied Psychophysiology and Biofeedback, has used a range of physiological recordings – including skin conductance, muscle tension, heart rate, blood pressure and hand temperature – to confirm that people who show little emotional response exhibit the most florid changes in physiology.[32] One explanation of this is that they lack the modulating role of cortisol, which is suppressed in people with such extreme emotional detachment. Activation of the sympathetic nervous system does not just alter blood flow, it also excites the immune system and causes inflammation. Thus people who exhibit a pattern of emotional detachment for long periods of time are susceptible to attacks of allergic or inflammatory diseases, such as ulcerative colitis, Crohn's disease, arthritis, asthma, eczema and those functional diseases that show some evidence of mild inflammation, such as fibromyalgia and chronic fatigue syndrome.[33]

The advent of functional brain imaging has confirmed that this remarkable combination of heightened physiological reactivity and emotional detachment is associated with diminished activity in the right frontal cortex.[34] So in people like Thomas, it seems that if the right brain cannot integrate the bodily reaction with the context through the creation of emotion, then it may be analysed with devastating logic by the left brain as an allergy, a novel infection or even a brain tumour that requires detailed investigation and treatment.

We need good integration between emotional and analytical brain functions in order to deal adequately with what happens to us. Although the differences between the function of the right and left frontal cortices are not as distinct as was once thought, it would seem valid to suggest that the more focused, analytical capabilities of the left frontal cortex exerts a restraining function on the emotionality of the right brain while the right frontal cortex injects some feeling and humanity into left brain efficiency. In support of that notion, clinical observations have shown that the same disturbances of emotional regulation that occur in people with severe functional and psychosomatic illness can be observed in patients who have sustained injury or strokes affecting the regions in the front of the brain that regulate emotion. One of the most vivid examples of this was the story of Phineas Gage, described by his doctor, John Harlow, and related in Antonio Damasio's book, *Descartes Error*.[35]

Phineas Gage was a construction foreman on the Rutland and Burlington Railroad in Vermont. One day, in the summer of 1848, he was preparing the charges for blasting when a premature explosion blew the tamping iron through the base of his skull and out through the top of his head. Gage survived the wound and the infection that followed, but he was not the same person. Before the accident, he was a responsible and reliable man with a shrewd eye for business and an energy and determination to succeed. Afterwards, he became difficult and obstinate, prone to attacks of rage at the slightest provocation, and totally unreliable. He indulged in long bouts of heavy drinking and the grossest profanity, distancing him from his one-time colleagues and friends. Gage had lost the cognitive buffer that allowed him to function in society; he was at the mercy of his emotions.

The orbitofrontal regions of the brain not only generate emotion but also modulate its expression. They are critically important for such functions as social adjustment, the control of mood, drive, responsibility and decision-making, the exercise of judgement, responsibility, empathy and intuition, and, of course, the regulation of bodily functions. If they are damaged, then feelings and emotions may be liberated from cognitive restraint or locked in (as in people like Thomas). Both extremes are associated with illness and difficulties in socialisation. Emotional incontinence, similar to that exhibited by Phineas Gage, is more likely to be seen in people with strokes involving the more analytical left frontal cortex, who often behave as if what has happened to them is a catastrophe, even if the disabilities they have suffered are relatively mild. In contrast, patients with right-sided frontal strokes or tumours tend to exhibit a pattern of emotional detachment similar to that described in patients with alexithymia. Unmoved by what has happened to them, they maintain a rather bland, detached attitude, even in the face of quite dreadful suffering.

In the same book, Damasio also described a young man called Elliott, who had a rapidly growing tumour removed from the front of his brain. With his tumour went his capacity to feel emotion. As Damasio expresses it, 'He was always controlled, always describing scenes as a dispassionate, uninvolved spectator. Nowhere was there a sense of his own suffering . . . he was not inhibiting the expression of internal emotional resonance or hushing inner turmoil. He simply did not have any turmoil to hush.'[36] The same kind of detachment is observed in patients who have had the connections between the right and left sides of the brain divided in operations to cure severe, drug-resistant epilepsy.

For hundreds of years, people (mainly men) have commented on ways in which men and women express and deal with emotion. The consensus is that women are more intuitive, emphatic, in touch with their feelings and emotionally expressive than men, who, it is suggested, are more focused, rational and decisive. Recent studies to map the activity of the brain have given some support for this observation by demonstrating that women tend to engage both left and right sides of the brain while dealing with emotional situations whereas men tend to use one side more than the other.[37] This might suggest that when confronted with traumatic events, women are more likely to be overwhelmed with feeling, whereas men can more readily detach themselves emotionally from the situation. There are also indications that women have a greater connectivity with the autonomic nervous system while processing emotional tasks. If this is indeed the case, it would offer a neurological explanation for why women suffer more from emotional and functional illnesses than men, and why, when men develop functional illness, they have a greater tendency to explain it in terms of physical disease.

This chapter has described how, when we are overwhelmed by situations in our lives, the feelings and physiological reactions that these situations induce remain in the body and are reconfigured as illness. People get sick when they cannot regulate, through the creation and resolution of emotion, these bodily reactions. Furthermore, clinical observations suggest that emotional resolution can be inhibited in three recognisable ways: detachment, where creation of the emotion is blocked and the burden of physical illnesses is borne with stoicism; resistance, where the expression of emotion is imprisoned behind a high tension barrier; and despair, where the emotion is present and ascribed to the unbearable physical symptoms. These different emotional strategies influence the kind of illnesses a person suffers through alterations in the balance of the autonomic nervous system and in the release of cortisol.

But it would be mistaken to regard these emotional strategies as distinctive aspects of personality; we each have the capability of employing all three and using them interchangeably. An initial attitude of resistance is frequently followed by collapse into despair, and despair may find respite in detachment.

But this should not lead people with functional illness to feel stigmatised as mentally fragile. None of us cope perfectly all of the time, and when we fail to cope, we can get ill. This is part of our human condition. People with functional illness are not mad or unstable. On the contrary, their illness is an adaptive process that protects them from feeling swamped by what has happened. So when any of us are forced by desire or circumstance into doing something that feels wrong, when we are persecuted by the threat of failure or stricken with inconsolable grief, that's when we may become ill. At those times we need support and a proper understanding of the nature of our illness, not rejection and criticism.

But not all people respond to the trials of life by getting ill. Some seem to be able to cope with the most catastrophic events without any problems at all, but others 'catch cold' at the slightest provocation. So why do some people seem to get ill so frequently while others rarely have a day's illness? Have they just been unlucky? Do they just have more to cope with? Or is there something about their constitution and the way they were brought up that makes them less capable of regulating their emotional responses than other people? This is the question that is explored in the next chapter.

4

Why some people get ill and others don't

Why do some people find it more difficult to regulate their emotional responses than others? Is it simply the way they are or does it have something to do with the way they were brought up? Is it nature or nurture?

I would argue it is predominantly nurture. Our genetic inheritance can only provide us with the biochemical and physiological potential to respond to what happens to us in certain ways, but it is the environment in which we live that develops that potential and steers it in a particular direction. So just as an alteration in the climate of East Africa may have conditioned the evolution of early man into an upright, tool-using hunter, so our social environment conditions the way our personality develops. And just as the shape of a tree is largely determined by the influences on it when it was a sapling, so the kind of person we become, what we believe in, how confident we are and how we respond to what happens to us, is mainly shaped by the relationship we had with our parents or primary carers during the first few years of life when our emotional brain was still developing.[1]

I have never met Elizabeth. She has never been well enough to come and see me in Sheffield, but we have corresponded for five years. For all of that time, she has hardly been able to eat without getting severe abdominal pains that are like a tight band right around her middle and into her back. She also feels sick, and is so exhausted she can barely cope. Medical investigations have failed to yield a diagnosis and she is currently living in a respite home with people much older than her. Once gregarious and out-going, her life has constricted to one of loneliness and pain. When we last corresponded, I asked her to write down the major events in her life history so I could more easily place her illness in context. This is a précis of what she wrote:

Age two: Father died. I have no recollection of him, but Mother's references were always derogatory. Apparently they didn't get on.

Age two to eleven: Mother worked full-time from 8 a.m. until 6 p.m., leaving me in the care of a succession of childminders. Suffered with tummy troubles a lot. The best time was age six during the London blitz when I was evacuated to Wolverhampton with a train full of children. I spent ten months there. It was my only experience of family.

Age eleven: Mother married my stepfather and we moved into his house in east London. I had a terrible life with him – no protection from Mother. This went on for six years. Stopped eating for a while.

Age seventeen: Left home and moved into a furnished bedsit, initially on my own.

Age twenty-three: Had a two-year relationship with a young man, but he went back to his ex-fiancée. Devastated and physically sick.

Age twenty-six: Moved again. Shared flat with divorced woman I met in Territorial Army. Many emotional problems, which were associated with abdominal pains and sickness. Had normal appendix removed.

Age twenty-eight: Moved again.

Age thirty: Became redundant and moved job to one with more responsibility. Started getting panic attacks. Gave up work for a while. Woke up at 3 a.m. every night. Treated with antidepressants and then with valium.

Age fifty-six: Retired early from work with abdominal pain, bowel upsets and anxiety, caused by bullying partner in legal firm. Began to find that certain foods caused pain and sickness.

Age sixty-five: Increasingly isolated and ill. Moved into residential home.

Clearly Elizabeth has been ill for much of her life, starting at the age of two. There has never been any evidence of obvious organic disease, but her bouts of illness have always been associated with situations inducing feelings of rejection and social exclusion. It is tempting therefore to think Elizabeth's unhappy and insecure childhood had compromised her ability to regulate her own physiological responses to separation, predisposing her to illness whenever she felt isolated, disappointed and bullied.

In support of Elizabeth's experience, a large comprehensive survey of 13,494 American adults, conducted in 1998, found strong, irrefutable correlations between adverse experience and family dysfunction during childhood and high-risk health behaviour and chronic disease during adulthood.[2] But how might this association have come about? To answer that question, we first need to understand how children acquire, through the sponsorship of their parents, the capacity to regulate their feelings and bodily responses and develop into healthy independent people.

A baby is born helpless. From the relative peace of the womb, it is squeezed through a narrow elastic channel, like a pig through a python, into an environment that is suddenly bright, noisy, rough, painful and totally inhospitable. Without the care of our mothers, we would get ill and die very quickly.[3] Mothers are complete intensive care providers. Not only do they feed their infants, control their fluid balance, regulate their body temperature, shelter them, protect them from danger, and keep them clean, they also function as external psychic regulators to calm the tensions, caused by countless discomforts and separations, instilling in their infants a sense of their own confidence.

Of course, our little darlings are never placid for very long! They are endearing and frustrating bundles of feelings, charming one minute, hot and screaming with anger the next, and withdrawn and apathetic after that. These changes in mood are mediated by the autonomic nervous system: angry protest by the sympathetic loop; despair and apathy by the parasympathetic loop. And since the autonomic nervous system regulates bodily function, infants respond to change through their bodies. Parents become quite adept at interpreting how changes in the colour of their baby's skin, alterations in their bowel habit and rate of respiration, and whether a feed is kept down or regurgitated can so eloquently reflect how they are feeling. They recognise anger in their attacks of colic, resistance in the refusal of food and constipation, rejection in their vomiting and despair in their wheeziness. And by sensitive response to the prevailing mood, parents learn how to rectify disturbances in their infants' bodily functions. So if their babies are upset, they hold, rock or feed them, or change their nappy, whatever is necessary to restore a state of peace and harmony. And when their infants are withdrawn, they engage them with smiles and vocal sounds while gently stimulating their interest with objects and toys. And as parents adjust their infants' emotional climate, so they regulate their bodily functions and facilitate the development of those parts of the brain that will allow their children eventually to do the same job for themselves.

Failure of the relationship between infants and their parents can compromise emotional regulation and make children vulnerable to change and susceptible to illness. In the aftermath of the Second World War, doctors observed that infants separated from their mothers at a very early stage of development, and brought up in institutions with high standards of nourishment and cleanliness, not only appeared withdrawn and depressed but were markedly under-weight and suffered a variety of illnesses.[4] These observations were recently confirmed in the tragic environment of Rumanian orpha-nages. As an illustration of this, the eminent physician and psychiatrist George Engel described the touching story of the infant Monica, who was born with a gastric fistula, a hole in her stomach connecting to the abdominal wall. Her mother refused to accept her and she was brought up in hospital, where she became apathetic and unresponsive. Unable to feed properly or produce gastric acid, she lost weight. It was only when one of Engel's staff took on the job of 'specialing' Monica that she began to improve. Whenever her surrogate mother appeared, Monica, who had previously been lying on her bed staring at the ceiling, became animated and responsive, would accept food and even started producing gastric acid. The recovery of Monica's impaired physiological and psychological disturbances emphasised that there is something more in the mother–baby interaction than catering for the infant's bodily requirements.

Failure of parenting at such a vulnerable stage of life can not only lead to illness in infants, it can also set the pattern for illness throughout life. Follow-up studies of orphaned, abandoned and neglected children show an abnormally high prevalence of long-term medical illness.[5] Studies of the post-natal records of middle-aged people with chronic illness showed that many were underweight during early infancy, suggesting inadequate nurturing.[6] And of course, disturbances in the mother–infant relationship are frequently revealed during the course of therapies conducted on people with both mental and physical illness. Finally, an impressive body of research conducted in experimental animals has shown that stress or separation early in life provokes a pattern of exaggerated behavioural and biochemical responses to stress, increased sensitivity to psychoactive drugs, and various kinds of illness throughout their life cycle.[7]

Parents instil the capacity for their infants to regulate their own bodily responses by a process of 'attunement' and 'imprinting'.[8] Shortly after birth, basic biological rhythms of sleep and feeding are entrained using touch and smell. Later, as visual capabilities develop, they are able to encourage ever more complex repertoires of behaviour in their infants through facial expression and tone of voice.

Like lovers, a mother and her infant can hold their gaze for quite long periods of time, establishing an intensity of communication through which they come to know each other. This intense visual interaction induces mutual activation of the sympathetic nervous system, causing the pupils to dilate and establishing an intense emotional connection, 'a communion of souls'.[9] Soon, fixed by eye contact, the communication broadens to include facial expression. An infant's first smile, albeit lopsided and apt to be confused with 'wind', is celebrated as the first instance of meaningful communication – a real 'E.T.' moment. So when a mother's smile causes their infant's face to light up, their pupils dilate and their eyes look bright, a signal has been transmitted, recognised and responded to, inducing a mutual sense of joy that reinforces desired behaviour.[10]

The smile is the first 'psychic organiser', as Spitz has termed it. It acts via the sympathetic and parasympathetic nerves to regulate an infant's responses and feelings, and becomes a reward for getting it right. The smile is followed by other facial communications – eyebrows raised in surprise, the boo response, the grumpy face – as messages are conveyed and copied. Humans have the most expressive faces of any animal. There are over thirty different facial muscle groups, each innervated by one or other branch of the autonomic nervous system. Thus, by subtle alterations in the balance of the sympathetic and parasympathetic nerves, bringing about small modulations in muscular activity and blood flow, infants mimic their parents' expressions and, as they do so, they 'feel' the expression in physiological changes induced by the same subtle modulation of the autonomic nerves elsewhere in the body.[11] By means of this eloquent facial dialogue, parents can instruct their infants how to 'feel' about certain situations.[12] But facial expression is not the only psychic organiser – otherwise how would children born blind ever develop feelings? Touch and tone of voice can also establish a feeling connection between infants and their parents.

By about six months, the sounds infants make are interpreted as meaningful utterances by their parents and returned, so 'aa' quickly becomes 'da' or 'ma' and is celebrated as the first word. Infants copy the sound and each time they get it right they are rewarded with a smile and an enthusiastic vocal response from either mother or father. Tagged with feeling, these situations are committed to the infant's memory. To put it simply, a child begins to learn through empathy and feeling. To illustrate the capacity for all of us to learn in this way, functional brain scans have demonstrated that when someone is watching another person transmit a certain facial expression or carry out a certain task, the same areas of brain 'light up' in both individuals.[13] But parents and infants cannot be on a 'high' all of the time. They would soon get exhausted. There have to be quiet times. So if an infant is getting too excited, a parent will look away and attempt to calm things down; ever the mimic, the infant will copy.

The infant psychiatrist Daniel Stern has described the attunement that exists between a mother and her infant as like that of dancing partners, who come to know and trust each other's responses so well that they can respond rapidly and consistently to minimal signals.[14] Thus by this process of attunement during a time of rapid brain growth, parents are able to programme their child's brain, facilitating the development of those parts that will be responsible for regulating emotional responses. As the psychoanalyst Margaret Mahler put it: 'The early mother–infant relationship functions as regulatory system that facilitates the emergence of a mind from the bodily experiences of the infant.'

The failure of a child to bond with his mother and father can have a big impact on their development.

Jason had always been a sickly child. Between the ages of six and ten, he suffered terribly with asthma and missed a lot of school. Then as the asthma got better, he began to get very fussy about food and became very thin. His attacks of arthritis and severe abdominal pain started at the age of sixteen. At first, his doctors thought he was suffering from irritable bowel syndrome, but when he began passing blood, it was clear that there was something else going on. The investigations revealed that Jason had Crohn's disease, but it failed to respond to medical treatment.

When I first saw Jason, he seemed a strange, somewhat detached young man. Thin and wearing a rather old-fashioned check sports jacket, he looked at his hands, avoiding eye contact with me. He described his symptoms and the type of stools he passed in meticulous detail, but when I asked him how his illness made him feel, he looked puzzled. Jason's emotional responses were characteristic of alexithymia (see page 67). I was not sure how to reach him, but I thought it might help if I talked to his mother. Although I might have guessed the essence of her story, I was surprised at its intensity.

Natalie had never really wanted to have Jason. She loved her job as an R&D director in a pharmaceutical firm and enjoyed the exciting lifestyle that went with it. But she had an affair with one of the managers and had become pregnant. She was sure that Ian, Jason's father, would stay with her, but when it came to the crunch, he could not leave his wife and Natalie was literally left holding the baby. From the beginning, Natalie could not bond with her infant. She felt his presence as a guilty reminder of her foolishness and would leave him for hours on end just playing by himself or sitting in front of the television. Even Sue, her childminder, seemed to spend more time cleaning and ironing than playing with Jason. But Jason never complained. For most of the time he was in a world of his own playing quietly with his toy soldiers. His symptoms, she added, seem to have got a lot worse since he had left home and gone to university.

Jason had never been able to develop the close attachment with his mother through which he could learn to regulate and express his feelings. Instead he had closed off and lived in his own world. Too 'shy' and withdrawn to feel comfortable in the company of other people, the tensions caused by the impingement of the outside world remained locked in his body where they caused a succession of illnesses.[15] Physiological studies revealed a marked reduction in the secretion of cortisol, as suggested by his lack of emotional responsiveness, while his rapid pulse and clammy hands betrayed a high level of sympathetic nervous tension. This combination enhances the activity of the immune system and may well have triggered the onset of his Crohn's Disease (see p. 68).

Recent discoveries in the neurobiology of emotional development suggest that a positive interaction between parents and infants stimulates the production of corticotrophin releasing hormone (CRH) from the hypothalamus, the structure at the base of the brain that is responsible for regulating eating, sleeping, sexual activity and many fundamental behaviours and bodily functions. This hormone directly stimulates the sympathetic nervous system and it also encourages the release of endorphines, the body's personal supply of narcotics, from the pituitary gland. Endorphines are a 'feelgood factor'. The neurobiologist Jaak Panksepp has demonstrated by an elegant series of experiments that beta endorphine is released by grooming and the company of others, and suppressed by separation.[16] But endorphines not only convey feelings of pleasure; in infancy they also stimulate the maturation of that region of frontal cortex that comes to assume executive control over the sympathetic nervous system.[17] As soon as that neural control is established, infants can generate feelings of excitement and well-being for themselves by matching a situation with the feeling encoded in a particular facial expression. They are now equipped to learn without the intervention of their parents. With their own personal supply of opiates, they are less dependent on their mothers to feel good and so, driven by curiosity, they start to explore their environment.

By the time children begin to walk, their curiosity and exploration, boosted by high levels of stimulation, are beginning to get out of control. Their capabilities know no bounds. They are in the condition that Freud called 'primary narcissism'. The world revolves around His or Her Majesty the Baby, and other people are just there to look after them exclusively. Some people never quite grow out of that stage, but for most, things are about to change. Their Royal Highnesses are about to come down to earth with a bump!

The stage is thus set for conflicts and tantrums as wilful and increasingly mobile children come face to face with the reality that although they are special, they are definitely not the only pebbles on the beach. So by the second year of life, parents usually begin to rein in their infants in accordance with the requirements for socialisation. It is said that the mother of an eleven- to seventeen-month-old toddler issues a prohibition every nine minutes. So instead of the encouraging smiling response that promotes curiosity and learning, infants experience frowns of disapproval, which curb their activity through humiliation and shame.[18] Shame bursts a child's pretty balloon, inducing a sense of deflation. It is associated with an acute sense of exposure, an awareness of the body and its functions. For example, it is not unusual for toddlers to play with their faeces at this time and want to give them to their parents as presents. This gift is not, however, received with gratitude, but is more likely to be greeted by the pinched-nose, open-mouthed, tongue-protruding facial expression of disgust, which produces a strong experience of rejection in the child. This message is quickly internalised as neurones in the orbitofrontal cortex are programmed to become acutely sensitive to odours of faeces and urine. As the child grows, feelings of disgust and nausea can be recruited as expressions of rejection. If we are 'fed up' with somebody, we may tell them that we are 'disgusted' by their behaviour, or that they 'make us sick'.

'No' is probably the most important word any of us ever hear. It inculcates us in society, encouraging us to curb our personal impulses, to go without, to share, to take one's turn, to wait, to be careful, to work together and to help one another. It represents a change from excitement to reflection, a switch from the high-arousal sympathetic state to a low-arousal state, which is brought about by the para-sympathetic loop and associated with blushing of the face, slowing of the heart and stimulation of the peristaltic activity of the intestines. This surge of parasympathetic activity decreases the production of endorphins, causing more CRH to be diverted to the production and release of cortisol, which facilitates the neural connections that give the growing infant control over parasympathetic functions.[19] It is perhaps not surprising that this is the time when infants learn to feed themselves and gain control over their bowels.

Some parents find it difficult to say no and would rather let their children get away with naughtiness than risk the loss of their love. As a result, their little darlings grow up excitable and precocious and are apt to react with rage, tantrums and dramatic 'sympathetic' symptoms when others attempt to curb their more antisocial and dangerous urges. In the past, we might have tended to call such children spoiled – hence the saying, 'spare the rod and spoil the child'.

Paul suffers from dreadful headaches. They begin as a terrible tension in the muscles around the base of his skull and a feeling of extreme pressure. These feelings then give way to a pounding sick headache that can go on for days. He hates taking painkillers because these often upset his stomach and make him very sick. Brain scans haven't revealed any abnormality and although his blood pressure is often raised when his headaches are developing, for the rest of the time it is quite normal. Paul told me that he has always had a tendency to have headaches and they were often brought on by arguments. It is not surprising, therefore, that they have got much worse since he separated from his wife and was debarred access to his children because of his violent rages. Paul cannot control the feelings of fury that occur when people reject him.

Paul's mother died in a car accident shortly before his first birthday. He never knew his father. So he was brought up by his grandmother. From the beginning Paul was difficult. If his grandmother tried to make him eat his supper, he would pick up the plate and throw it on the floor, so she would give him some chocolate instead. And if she sent him to his room, he would scream and kick until she let him out to watch the television. By the age of ten, she had had enough. Paul had started stealing from the shops and was getting into trouble with the police. So she asked Social Services to step in and he was taken into care. Slowly, and with the help of the warden of his care home, he began to curb his behaviour. At the age of sixteen, he trained as a garage mechanic and got a steady job. Then, at twenty, he met Denise, and when she became pregnant, they got married. Theirs was a passionate relationship from the start; she had a similarly volatile temperament. Within a year there was trouble. After a night out, he accused Denise of flirting with one of the lads who worked at the garage. She shouted at him and he lost control and beat her up. He was mortified and pleaded forgiveness; she took him back. He went to see a counsellor for anger management and succeeded in controlling his temper by, as he put it, 'capping his feelings', like firefighters cap an oil well that's caught fire. It was when he was struggling to keep things under control that he would get his headaches. The lid finally came off when he came home to find Denise in bed with another man.

Paul never learnt how to regulate his own feelings when he was very small. His mother had died and his grandmother tended to let him have his own way for a quiet life. So the tantrums that should have been challenged and worked through in the first few years of life persisted into adulthood, causing considerable difficulties in his relationships and, when he tried to suppress them, problems with his health.

If insufficient prohibition early in life can cause unrestrained emotional expression, too much prohibition, by contrast, can incur the risk of downward spiral into hopelessness and despair. Under most circumstances, parents will recognise their infants' genuine distress and rescue them with a cuddle, re-establishing their earlier joyous attachment and creating a focus of resilience and self-confidence. If, however, such repair is not effected, children may 'take on board' the idea that their emotional needs are unacceptable and shameful, that they are unacceptable. This can come to colour all subjective experience with a parasympathetic sense of humiliation, abandonment and despair that may lead to depression and other illnesses in later life.

Theresa could not understand why she was so tired. She was only forty, but she felt like an old woman. She just didn't seem to have the energy to carry on. She wasn't eating very much and frequently felt sick. Her husband, Anish, didn't understand and criticised her for not looking after their five children enough. She felt she was letting everybody down and just hated herself. She concluded that she must have some serious disease, but the doctor said there was nothing physically wrong with her and suggested she go on antidepressants. The total responsibility for each of her five children, her elderly mother and all the meals and the housework was more than enough to make anybody tired, but Theresa's tiredness was not the normal exhaustion from working too hard, it was more like a spiritual depletion. The light that kept her going had been snuffed out. When I suggested that, she looked down at her hands and quietly began to weep.

The trouble had started last year ever since Anish's mother had come over from India. She had told Anish that he should never have married Theresa, that she was too weak and didn't do him any credit. From that time, Anish had been saying that he was going to return to India to find another wife who would look after him better. Theresa felt devastated. It rekindled her worst fears.

Theresa had been brought up in a strict Catholic family that had come to England from Poland after the war. Her father had died when she was still a baby and her mother had to go out to work in a factory to keep the two girls. From the beginning, Theresa was made to feel that she was responsible for her mother's unhappiness. As she grew she tried in every way she could to make her mother happy, but nothing was ever good enough. Her mother only noticed the things that she had done wrong – the polish she spilt on the carpet, the soup that was too salty, her muddy shoes – and then the shouting would start: 'You have been nothing but trouble from the day you were born. Thank God your father didn't live to see you now. It would have broken his heart.' That made her feel sick and so tired that she would have to go to her room and lie down.

Theresa had met Anish at university; he had come to England to do a Masters degree and she was bowled over by how kind and appreciative he was. For the first time in her life she was really happy. They were married within the year and she was pregnant the year after. She didn't object when Anish suggested she give up her course; she just wanted to make him happy and pleased with her. But as the years went by and more children arrived, Anish started to become critical and Theresa felt ill. Then his mother came over.

We might conclude from this tragic tale that Theresa was programmed from early childhood to the fate that befell her. Like a modern-day Cinderella, she could never do anything right and would always feel ashamed and inadequate; she had to accept but could never quite understand her personal burden of 'original sin'. True, she was eventually rescued by Prince Charming, but Theresa was so subservient that he tired of her. The glass slipper no longer fitted and she faded away as a person.

These case histories are not unusual. There is now abundant evidence to show that deficiencies in parenting predispose to physical and mental illness in adulthood. Children whose parents separated and divorced early in life, those whose mothers were too busy to care and spend time with them, and those who were treated with indifference and cruelty suffer more psychological disorders and physical ailments later in life.[20] But equally, over-protective parents can predispose to illness by stifling the capacity for self-regulation.[21]

Psychological studies have shown that by the second year of life, toddlers respond in recognisably different ways to a parent's absence.[22] Some, the more balanced children, may cry a little to begin with. They then play quite happily and greet their mother with joy when she returns. Others cry as soon as they are left alone, continue to cry noisily while their mother is away and are difficult to pacify when she returns. And some seem quite detached and withdrawn into themselves. They are unaffected by their mother's absence and quite disinterested when she returns. Research from a variety of sources suggests that these patterns of behaviour are associated with quite different physiological responses.[23] Infants that respond to their mother's absence with despair tend to have rather anxious mothers and show the highest cortisol levels, while those that become withdrawn and disinterested have a more distant relationship with their parents and the lowest cortisol levels. But these observations are experimental snapshots. The maternal relationships that impair self-regulation are more complex, but there is some intriguing clinical material that suggests that particular types of relationship can impair physiological regulation in ways that may lead to specific patterns of illness.[24]

For example, the case histories of adults with binge eating disorder and unexplained diarrhoea often indicate a degree of emotional deprivation (see Janice, pp. 148–9) which may be brought about, not by parents who were cruel or wilfully neglectful, but by otherwise loving parents who were too preoccupied or busy to provide their growing children with the care and attention that they need to acquire a robust capacity for self-regulation. So when requests to play are ignored and children are distracted with television and more toys, when distress is pacified with treats and food instead of human contact, then the loneliness and uncontained despair that such infants must to some extent suffer may be expressed in uncontained symptoms and behaviours such as crying, diarrhoea and compulsive consumption of food.

On the other hand, case histories of patients with anorexia nervosa or severe constipation or chronic fatigue often reveal a family background that appears controlling and over-intrusive (see Reena, pp. 150–1). Anxious parents who rely on the relationship with their infants to satisfy their own need for love and attention can tend to smother them with attention and not allow them the space to learn how to regulate their own feelings and so gain self-confidence. As the psychoanalyst Eric Brenman explained: 'The ambivalent and diffident parent tries to protect her infant from the harsh realities of separation and provides herself as an external love object to avoid catastrophe.'[25] With every attempt at self-expression taken over, children may learn to express their frustration by disrupting those aspects of behaviour that cause most anxiety, particularly eating and defecation. As the child grows this pattern may often lead to illnesses and behaviours that seem to undermine self-expression, success and enjoyment, such as anorexia nervosa, chronic fatigue, under-achievement and depression.

Finally, the case histories of some patients with alternating symptoms of diarrhoea and constipation (irritable bowel syndrome) or binge eating and vomiting (bulimia nervosa) can reveal an ambivalence in emotional development and training. Parents who oscillate between excitement and gratification on the one hand and deprivation and frustration on the other, letting their children get away with behaviour that should be contained and then clamping down hard for some relatively minor offence, can be sowing the seeds of insecurity. Children brought up in this way exist in a world of division and danger, caught in a no man's land between feeling controlled and being rejected, unable to trust anybody and always sensitive to disapproval. It is not surprising that the children of such parents may grow up lacking trust in themselves and others and fluctuating between attitudes of need and rejection. These attitudes may be reflected in their symptoms.

Carla was referred to me for advice regarding her irritable bowel syndrome. Her bowels, she told me, were all over the place. 'Sometimes they can be right out of control and I have the most awful diarrhoea and then after a few days they go the other way and I'm bunged up. Then the cycle repeats itself.' I wondered if this cycling was related to the tablets she was taking to control her bowels, but she said she wasn't taking any. Then she added, 'It does seem to be related to how I eat. When I have diarrhoea, I feel very hungry and excited and tend to binge, but during constipated phases I often feel low and don't feel like eating at all.' Strange to relate, this emotional and bodily ambivalence bore a strong connection with her relationship with her parents. When she was a teenager living at home, Carla had to be the peacemaker, mediating between her hedonistic father, who would allow her more freedom than she really wanted, and her controlling mother, whom she described as 'silent and deadly'. As she grew up and left home, both polarities were represented in her own personality. The aspect of her identity that was more closely identified with her father encourages her to have a good time but makes her feel out of control, whereas her maternal part keeps her safe but gives her constipation. So she oscillates between the two as she tries to discover how to be.

Encouraging children to develop the self-confidence to lead independent lives is the least selfish and for many the most difficult aspect of parenthood, but it is vital for their future health and happiness. This starts very early in childhood. By gradually increasing the time she is absent, mothers condition their infants to tolerate her absences. Her obvious pleasure when she is reunited strengthens the intensity of their bond and reinforces her infant's willingness to tolerate the separation. So even if she isn't there, infants know that she is not far away. They only have to cry out and she will come and see what the matter is, change their nappy, and feed and comfort them. So through the allocation of bearable separations and predictable reunions, mothers inculcate in their infants the necessary sense of trust and self-confidence to create this safe environment for themselves, dealing with her absences and comforting themselves, at first with toys but later by the use of mental representations.

Toys are important to the emotional development of the child because they reassure and allow infants to practise the relationships they will eventually have as an adult. The paediatrician and psychoanalyst Donald Winnicott called them transitional objects, bridging the gap between regulation by mother and self-regulation.[26] When my two-year-old daughter Emily was feeling insecure, she would hide in the wardrobe sucking her thumb with her face against the satin lining of one of my wife's coats. Other objects, such as the model action heroes, the Barbie dolls, the football posters and the designer trainers may be used to represent and reinforce a child's identity. We never really do without such objects. In an adult world, alcohol, drugs, cigarettes, certain foods, remedies, our garden, books, music and relaxing videos may serve as comfort objects that allow us to cope, while our car, the house we live in, the job we do, our new kitchen, our top-of-the-range hi-fi system, even the kind of holiday we go on, may be thought of as self-objects that represent and reinforce our identity. But possessions can all too easily become lost or broken. Thus our ability to deal confidently with the ups and downs of life without getting ill must ultimately depend on the ability to think how things might be.

The creation of mental representations requires the space to develop the imagination. This does not only mean a physical separation from mother but an emotional one as well. Father, of course, has a pivotal role in the development of his child. Not only can he supply a different point of view, but through him, toddlers discover that their mothers are not just 'there for them', but have relationships with other people. Thus, although the toddlers are still attached to their mothers and will remain so for many years, they come to form nurturing relationships with both parents and with others in the family orbit.[27] Thus socialisation is associated with the development of a sense of self. This allows the growing child to develop the capacity for independent thought, judgement and decision-making. It is accompanied by a rapid increase in language, a more abstract and less dependent mode of communication, and a 'reconfiguration' of the emotional brain.[28]

As children begin to communicate more complex ideas through language, their parents help them process the raw emotions of fear, rage and despair which can make them 'feel' bad, by transforming paranoid ideas into more acceptable explanations. In essence they teach them to think about what is happening.[29] So when toddlers cry out at night because they are afraid of the dark, parents will turn the light on, explain that their room is still the same, that Teddy is there to comfort them and that Daddy and Mummy are in the next room. By communication with confident parents, children gradually learn to 'desomatise' experience – taking it from the body, where it can't be talked about, into the mind, where it can.

So 'good enough' parents not only enable the infants to withstand absences through the imprinting of consistent mental representations, they also allow them the space to modify those mental representations in the light of experience and so make them their own. In essence, they teach their children to use their imagination to create a safe environment for themselves when they are not there. If children do not have the opportunity to do this, then the terrors may remain and the tension may be expressed as illness, or as the psychoanalyst Joyce McDougall so eloquently expressed it: 'Rudimentary fantasies are trapped in a closed mind–body circuit and are not available for further mental processing.'[30]

By the third year of life, children have acquired all the neural equipment they will need for self-regulation. The emotional centres in the front part of their brains have become so connected with other brain structures that the infant is able to create internal models of social situations. These representations, tagged by their physiological signature, are stored in an extensive database of 'emotional' experience, catalogued in terms of feeling and meaning. So situations that cause frustration may come to be associated by repetition with feelings of tension in the middle of the chest and a tightness around the throat, while situations that induce fear may be linked with a tightening of the muscles of the neck and back and a pounding in the chest, and sad events are accompanied by a lump in the throat and a heaviness in the chest. This experiential resource helps us appraise situations and guides our response to them, directing qualities such as judgement, empathy and decisiveness.[31]

At the same time, the acquisition of language helps to create a symbolic database in the frontal lobes, mainly on the left side of the brain. When this is linked with our intuitive and emotional faculties, this forms the cognitive buffer that allows us to think about what has happened, discuss it with others, weigh up the possible outcomes of situations, construct an appropriate response and plan future events in ways that take into account various contingencies.

I am not implying that three-year-olds are adept at emotional regulation. Far from it; they require much more life experience and opportunity to practise before they can function in the company of others. Childhood may be thought of as a process of socialisation. With sufficient space to learn, and a containing social environment, healthy children gradually gain confidence in managing situations themselves. This is what builds a strong sense of identity. Every situation that is successfully managed reinforces our developing attitudes and beliefs, while outcomes that are not so successful do not necessarily destroy confidence but may cause us to change direction. The bodily distress induced by loss and failure etches the memory onto our brains, and by continually updating our cognitive and emotional databases, we learn from our experience so we can adapt to a changing world without becoming ill.

Adolescence is the time when emotional regulation is put to the test. It is only when children begin to think of leaving home that they find out whether their socialisation has been adequate. Many young people manage with hardly a backward glance. The few years from leaving home to starting a family of their own can be the 'time of their lives'. They may be separated from their parents but they soon gain associations with people from diverse backgrounds. With knowledge of the wider world, their horizons are expanded, revealing all kinds of new opportunities.

The situation is very different for children whose parenting did not allow them to develop self-regulation early in life. These individuals can be easily overwhelmed by life's inevitable challenges. A few may suffer frequent illness throughout childhood and find it very difficult to leave home. A greater proportion, particularly those with somewhat over-protective parents, function reasonably well until adolescence, but problems arise when their burgeoning desire for independence conflicts with their fears of assuming responsibility for themselves. Some teenagers may find escape from adult responsibility in alcohol, drugs and generally having a wild time. Insecure in their identity, some may use sex and a few may even become pregnant in order to obtain someone to love and be loved by. Others attack the needy, dependent part of their personality that ties them to their parents, by under-achieving or indulging in antisocial activities. And an ever-increasing number become ill. Depression and functional illness, especially anorexia nervosa, chronic fatigue syndrome, food intolerances, irritable bowel syndrome and constipation, often start around the time that children leave home. Such illnesses can seem a particularly appropriate means of expressing the adolescent protest; they assert an alternative identity while at the same time ensuring the continuation of care and attention. In a broader context, hunger strikes and sit-down strikes would not serve their political purpose if society took no notice.

Emma came to see me because she felt tired all the time, was not eating and had lost weight. Her mother was beside herself with worry. She had taken Emma to see several specialists, but none could find anything wrong. Her illness had come on shortly before she was due to go to university and had been so severe that she had had to defer her studies until the following year. 'The timing was perfect,' Emma's mother commented with undisguised irony. So Emma stayed at home, spending most of her time in her bedroom listening to records. It wasn't just that she was ill, she seemed to have lost the motivation to do anything.

I was struck by the contrast between Emma and her mother, who sat on the edge of the chair and answered all the questions I addressed to Emma with an air of desperation. Emma, by contrast, seemed bored by the whole procedure and slouched in the chair, looking down at her feet and picking at her nose when she thought I was not looking.

Up to six months previously, her mother said, Emma had everything going for her. She had done 'ever so well' at school and had secured a place in university to study English. She had a steady relationship with a 'nice' boy from home, who had already started university. She had been popular with her friends and was forever gossiping on the phone with them. Then, three weeks to the day before she was due to leave home, she got ill.

'I had taken her stuff up to her flat, made sure she had all the pots and pans she needed and got her a good supply of bedding and some new clothes. I had sorted out a deposit on the rent, and I had arranged to do her washing every week when she came back home. I was really excited, but Emma seemed cross and bored. That night she didn't want anything to eat and strangely for her, didn't want to see her friends. Over the course of the next few weeks, she became increasingly weak. She felt tired all the time, she lost weight and she just wanted to stay in her bedroom. That was when we decided it would be best to defer. At first her friends visited her, but Emma didn't want to go out and they soon stopped coming. Her boyfriend came down to see her every week, but after a while she told him not to bother any more. Now she does nothing. I prepare her favourite meals, but she's never hungry. She just picks at the food and then pushes her plate away and goes up to her bedroom.'

I asked about Emma's father. This provoked a snort from her mother. 'Oh, he's exactly the same as Emma. He's in his own world; never so happy as when he is out fishing. Emma used to go with him, but she's not bothered now.

I suspected that Emma was depressed, and although her mood might be lifted by antidepressants, drugs were not going to help solve the conflict over dependency that was making her ill. Between a somewhat detached father and an over-solicitous mother, Emma had received neither the training nor the space to enable her to deal with the challenges of leaving home. She desperately wanted to be independent, but when the crunch time came, she felt paralysed by fears of isolation and so she withdrew into herself and became ill. This solved the problem by providing the reason for deferring her departure.[32]

I gently suggested to Emma's mother that she might be making things worse by being so worried. She had to give herself and Emma some space. I also arranged to meet Emma weekly over the next few months. To begin with, it wasn't easy. Emma was not keen to talk and did not seem to have any thoughts and ideas about anything. Then Al Qaeda terrorists crashed two airliners into the twin towers in New York, and Emma told me she understood how angry the Arab nations must feel over America's intrusive foreign policy. This allowed her to express her own anger with her mother's intrusions, and frustration at her own passivity and dependency. She described her illness as pathetic, but I suggested that by attacking the sensitive, emotional aspect of herself so much, she was never going to feel confident enough to leave home. As she began to feel more comfortable with me, Emma admitted that she didn't want to go to university yet. She didn't feel ready. She wanted to travel, get some work for a time, find out about life. I wondered if she had thought of taking a gap year, perhaps working abroad. She seemed to like the idea, then added, 'But Mum wouldn't let me.' 'Try her,' I said. Emma only saw me for about three months and then went off to Australia. A year later, I happened to see her mother in town. I asked her how Emma was getting on. She said, 'Oh she's fine. Only since she has come back from Australia, she won't let me do her washing any more. It's so hard when they grow up, isn't it?'

Emma was lucky. She was able to compensate for the lack of personal space in her childhood by finding, in the Australian outback, a sense of self-reliance that will hopefully sustain her through times of change. Others are not so fortunate. They are the children who have never quite been able to grow up, and they lack the self-confidence to cope with adult responsibilities. And so they tend to react to life's inevitable trials with fear, anger and despair, which, with the impaired self-regulation can render them disposed to a range of emotional and functional illness.

Not surprisingly, relationships can be particularly problematic for such people. They desperately need the recognition and endorsement of other people just to prove they exist, but they attack their need as a weakness and fear intimacy as a dangerous intrusion on their fragile sense of self. Some may flirt outrageously, enticing others to demonstrate their admiration by falling in love, only to reject them when things get too serious. Others are 'sleeping beauties'; only a true prince can penetrate their thicket of thorns. But when their prince comes along, they discover that even the most charming person has his own weaknesses and irritating personal habits, and may not be able to give them the attention they crave. So differences that were just niggles to begin with grow into major issues for conflict. And if the differences cannot be resolved, the relationship is pickled in strong vinegar, which corrodes any enjoyment in life and undermines health, while the grievance becomes a totem to their martyrdom, the cross they have to bear. When vulnerable people cannot construct their identity around good relationships, they reinforce it like a bastion against the bad ones.

But relationships with other people are but projections of the relationship a person has with himself.[33] Lonely people often have nobody close enough to blame for what they see as their deficiencies and weaknesses, so they turn the attack on themselves.

Kate, an intelligent, well-educated woman of twenty-five, asked to see me because she was frightened about the amount of weight she had lost and how tired and ill she felt. As I got to know her, it became clear that she was engaged in a struggle over how she should be. For her every achievement there was an equal and opposite criticism. She was good at her research, but she was so self-critical she would 'over-egg the omelette' and under-perform. She was very pretty, but dressed in old-fashioned clothes and her hair was never properly styled. She enjoyed eating, but restricted her food intake, lost weight and made herself ill. She found a sense of peace and companionship in running, but was often too tired to do it. It was as if she could not commit to a way of being or take responsibility for who she was. So there had to be a struggle in everything she did. It made life difficult.

So why couldn't she let go of the struggle? I wondered. She replied that she needed it, rather like people who undertake extreme sports; it made her feel almost heroic! Our relationship became incorporated into the struggle and I would often emerge from a session exhausted and troubled. About three months into therapy, I asked Kate what she thought it would take to give up the struggle. She was quiet for a long, long while and then looked me straight in the eye and said in a low voice, 'Trust.'

Brought up by one parent who gave her unconditional praise and another who was distant and disapproving, Kate did not know how to trust. She did not have a close relationship with anybody and found it so difficult to regulate the bodily expressions of loneliness and despair.

People who do not trust others can lead such lonely lives. Unable to love and be loved, friendship can be little more than an exercise in power politics. Some of them may work all hours to develop the special talent or achievement that will assure them of the admiration they need. Others may make themselves desirable by enhancing the appearance of their bodies. And of course, deep down, many are desperate to become famous and attract love on a grand scale.

An insecure childhood and a fragile sense of identity can motivate some people to achieve great success. Anybody who has listened to Professor Anthony Clare's radio programme, *In the Psychiatrist's Chair*, will readily appreciate that many of our most talented and successful citizens are, behind all the fame and fortune, sensitive and vulnerable people with a fragile sense of their own identity.[34] Only people with special talents and incredible determination can be a concert pianist, a bestselling author, a famous actor, a sports star, a successful mountaineer or a round-the-world yachtsman. Their accomplishments prove to the world that they are special and serve to ward off the awful feeling that nothing really matters. As one of my colleagues, a successful author, once said to me, 'I am more of a verb than a noun. If I am not doing something special, I feel I don't exist.'

Some people feel compelled to go to the very extremes of human endurance and endeavour to find that unique and special identity. When Edward Mallory was asked why he risked his life to reach the summit of Mount Everest, he famously replied, 'Because it's there!' What he may have meant is: 'It proves that *I* am there, that *I* exist.' One might speculate that for Mallory, the process of socialisation had been insufficient to provide a strong sense of identity in the company of other people. He had to do something really special to earn their and his own regard. Few insecure but creative people could acknowledge that. So it was with real insight that the Antarctic explorer, Dr Mike Stroud wrote, 'Who but an idiot would think it macho to endure frostbite, hypoglycaemia and freezing temperatures to cross a wasteland. But this is not the most difficult thing. The most difficult thing in life is human relationships.'[35]

It could be argued that the only reason man has been so successful is because he is so neurotic and insecure. But not everybody can compensate for their fears of annihilation by becoming famous. It takes much more talent, dedication and self-belief than most people possess. The majority of us have to find other ways of creating a special sense of identity. Some do this through their employment. For priests, lawyers, politicians, scientists, writers and doctors, their sense of vocation imbues a special moral status that can shield them from the ordinary considerations of everyday life. But for every person who can successfully compensate for their feelings of inadequacy in this way, there are many more who cannot. And even for those who, by sheer dedication and industry, achieve great success and even fame, there is always the possibility that their fragile confidence may encourage them, like the mythological Icarus, to fly too close to the sun. With no admiring peer group to endorse their special status and no energy left for their own reconstruction, they can so easily slump into depression and illness. According to what is presented in our newspapers and magazines, it would seem that the decline and fall of so many of our modern leaders and celebrities is a source of unending fascination to those of us who are not so well known.

Nobody can manage without friends and family for very long. The lack of real companionship can leave people exposed to their own fears and loathing, generating irreconcilable tensions that culminate in illness.

Alistair is a theatre director. He is very successful, often brilliantly so, but he also suffers from spasms of self-doubt, during which his bowels tie themselves in knots. If he is not coming up with the brilliant, groundbreaking ideas that put him light years ahead of everybody else, then he feels utterly worthless. He just cannot seem to find the middle ground, where his skills and way of seeing things can complement those of his colleagues, allowing them to create something together. He is unable to trust anybody else enough to work with them. Other people never see things the same way and anything they produce together is impure, contaminated, just a pale reflection of the true essence of his vision. He has to be the one to do it all, to have all the ideas. 'If I have to discuss things, to negotiate, then I quickly get bored,' he told me. 'I just want to do my own thing. I guess I am a maverick, an individual. The problem is that there are times when I feel so desperately lonely. And that's when my guts seem to play up.'

In psychiatric terms, Alistair has a narcissistic personality.[36] In more human terms, he suffers from a disturbance in socialisation. His eccentric and rather distant parents did not enable him to feel he belonged to society. So he tends to flit from one group to another like a cocktail party hostess, influencing each but never staying long enough to be assimilated. He cannot tolerate notions of obligation, allegiance, fidelity and responsibility. In some ways, his situation might be seen as desirable, even enviable. His lack of cultural identity makes him a free individual, his own person, but it can also leave him feeling lonely, scared and susceptible to extremes of tension and illness when things go wrong.

So, if much of the illness in today's Western societies is narcissistic in nature and related to deficiencies in socialisation, is it all our parents' fault? This is, in my opinion, an unfair conclusion.

Firstly, children are not just passive lumps of clay, waiting to be moulded by their parents. They are a part of the relationship and, as many parents comment, some are, for whatever reason, more troublesome than others. A number may learn how to manipulate their mothers to get their undivided attention; others may encourage rejection by their persistent demands.

Secondly, the establishment of the individual as an autonomous member of society is an ongoing process. Although Mum and Dad may give us a good start, hopefully setting a pattern for future relationships, we continually need to reinforce our own ability to regulate our physiological and emotional responses. Life throws up new and unexpected challenges to self-regulation. Even people with the best experience of parenting get ill if the world as they know it falls apart; if they are imprisoned, betrayed, lose their livelihood, or if they are subjected to a sustained campaign of criticism and abuse from their spouse.

And finally, to blame parents for the health of their children is rather like blaming the drivers for the fact that so many of our trains are running late. It may not be that Mum and Dad have necessarily got it wrong. It could be that our narcissistic culture has so compromised the process of socialisation and emotional regulation that it is very difficult for any of us to get it right. This is the topic of the next chapter.

5

Why modern life is making us ill

Despite the upheavals of two world wars, the majority of British families living in the 1950s inhabited a much more certain world than we do now. Like as not, Dad worked in the office from Monday to Friday and supper was always on the table when he came home. He had a drink in the pub with his friends on Wednesdays and Fridays and attended Union meetings on Thursdays. Mum organised the home with military efficiency, washing on Monday, ironing on Tuesday, cleaning on Wednesday and shopping on a Friday. The whole family went out to town on Saturday afternoon and the pictures on Saturday night, and repented their transgressions in church on Sunday morning, before tucking into the weekly roast and two veg for lunch. Grandparents, uncles and aunties lived close by, and friends were always popping in for tea and cake. Every Christmas, the whole family gathered together for a feast, each August, they went on holiday to the same hotel in Bournemouth, and on 5 November, they lit a bonfire with the neighbours and let off fireworks. Dad would stay in the same job all his life and was presented with a barometer when he retired at sixty-five. Mum would dream of going to Spain. From our current perspective, this may not seem like a lot of fun, but nobody expected very much else and there was a stability about it, a sense of belonging.

Then, within a generation, it all changed. After years of post-war austerity, Britons 'had never had it so good'. The ambitious rebuilding programme, the expansion of industry, full employment, the introduction of the Welfare State and the National Health Service, and the possibility of university education regardless of income and class meant greater opportunities for everybody. People were more affluent; they equipped their houses with electric cookers, washing machines, vacuum cleaners, refrigerators and, of course, televisions. Few people owned a television before 1950. My parents bought one in a smart walnut cabinet to watch the coronation of Queen Elizabeth in 1953 and invited as many neighbours and friends as could fit in our small sitting room to watch it with us. Ten years later, nearly every family in the land owned one. Cinemas closed by the thousands and more and more people stayed at home to be entertained. By the 1970s, the friendly corner shop was threatened as supermarkets sprang up in every community, undercutting costs and adding convenience and variety. Within a decade, pre-cooked frozen meals offered a whole new range of dietary experience from all corners of the world. Only one in four families owned a car in the 1950s, but ten years later, nearly every family in the land was a car owner, and by the 1990s most families owned two cars. Throughout the last half of the twentieth century, people became much more mobile as the companies that employed them became national, then multinational, and people were expected to move with their jobs. Air travel became faster, safer and cheaper. Gone was the annual visit to the family-run hotel in Bournemouth. People jetted off to Spain, Greece and Italy for their annual holidays, and it was even possible to take a trip to America. The world had become a smaller place.

Women experienced a particular sense of freedom. The oral contraceptive pill liberated sex from the responsibilities of pregnancy while domestic labour-saving devices freed them from the drudgery of housework. Although it may still take many years before women have truly equal opportunities in all sectors of employment, from the 1960s onwards, increasing numbers could find work, go to university and plan their lives independently. This was to have enormous consequences for the family and society as a whole.

In most respects, life in Western countries today is much better than it was during the early part of the last century. Not only have we been little affected by wars, but there is less prejudice against people of different race, gender, class or sexual orientation, and less poverty and social injustice. Cities are safer and we have unprecedented freedom of choice. We no longer need to spend so much time on everyday necessities; we have more money and more time to enjoy ourselves. We can buy anything we desire, go where we want, eat what we like, choose our entertainment at a push of a button, and find out about any topic from our personal computer. We can even use drugs to alter the shape and appearance of our bodies, spice up our sex life, lift us when we are down and help us have fun.

So why, in the midst of so much excitement and opportunity, has life satisfaction declined so much over the last four decades? Why is depression the commonest illness in the Western world? And why, when most serious infectious diseases have been conquered and rates of heart attacks and strokes have been reduced, do so many people report that they are feeling ill? What is going on? What is it about our modern way of life that is making so many of us lonely, depressed and unwell?

Epidemics of ill health always seem to occur at times of particularly rapid change. In his book *The Third Wave*, Alvin Toffler asserts that human civilisation has gone through three major cataclysmic shifts, or waves, each on a larger scale and more concentrated than the one that preceded it.[1] The first wave was the agricultural revolution, the move from a nomadic tribal existence to larger stable communities based on agriculture. The second wave was the industrial revolution, which took place in England in the eighteenth and nineteenth centuries. The third wave started about fifty years ago and is gathering a terrible momentum. This is the shift from an industrial culture to a globalised society, linked by electronic media. Once again, old values are being questioned, social structures are being dismantled and Western populations are again experiencing a crisis of identity.

Each wave has been associated with ill health. Epidemics of illness commenced with the shift from nomadic to stable agricultural communities. Many of these were due to a limited seasonal diet, crop failure, contamination of food stores and infections brought about by the need to live in close proximity with animals and larger numbers of people, followed by the inevitable contamination of stored food and water.[2] And during the industrial revolution, the enormous migration of people from rural villages to the vast industrial cities led to overcrowding, malnutrition, lack of hygiene and horrifying epidemics of infectious illness among the poor working class. But not all the illness of the time was caused by poverty, overcrowding and infections. This was also the time when the so-called neuroses – hysteria, hypochondria, the spleen or the vapours – were so common among the middle classes that nobody seemed healthy (see also p. 19). As Athena Vrettos succinctly expressed it, 'Fictions of the nerves were used to act out cultural and intellectual upheavals on the immediate and palpable terrain of the body. The instability of the outer world was mirrored by a fragility of the self as diffuse and chaotic social issues were displaced onto more immediate questions of physiology.'[3] The population lost faith in the medical profession and sought help from a variety of alternative healers. And now, with the latest great wave of change, the illnesses that were so common in middle-class England in the late-eighteenth century have become common again, but under new names and across all social strata, and a disillusion with orthodox medicine is again causing many people to seek cures from alternative treatments.

If, as I have argued, most human illness is caused by failure to adapt to social change, then in order to understand how modern life is making us ill, we need to consider three premises. The first is that people living in modern Western societies are exposed as never before to novel situations, which create uncertainty and challenge their self-confidence. The second is that our modern way of life has depleted the social and emotional resources that would normally enable us to cope with what happens. And the third is that the dramatic social changes that have occurred over the last fifty years have compromised the socialisation of our children and their ability to cope with change.

Over a period of little more than a single human generation, the lives of people living in Western countries have changed quite radically. Like refugees in a foreign land, many of us are having to come to terms with a way of life so fundamentally different to the one we were brought up in that it constitutes a major challenge to our identity, a state of 'culture shock'.

We construct our identity from our experience – the place we were brought up in, the school we went to, the job we do, our family, our friends, the person we marry. These influences create the attitudes and beliefs that make us who we are. In the past, the social environment was more predictable. People knew their place in the world and could be pretty sure it would remain much the same. Now things are much more transient. Take the 'concrete' example of our towns and cities. During the last fifty years, many of these have been drastically redeveloped, often several times. In the market town where I grew up, the chapel is now an arts and design centre, the Odeon cinema is an apartment block, the beautiful, red-stone Victorian library is a pub, the swimming pool has been demolished to make way for a multi-storey car park and even the coffee bar we used to hang out in has become a computer store. These may have been just bricks and mortar, but their disappearance feels like losing a part of *me.*

In recent years, the reliability of the judiciary, the medical profession, universities and schools, city councils, public transport, the Church and even the Royal Family has been called into question. These institutions embody certain constant social attributes such as loyalty, justice, fairness, altruism, dependability, support, diligence and dedication. Just as children need consistent role models to provide them with a secure base, so as adults we have to be able to rely on our institutions that have authority over us. We need to know that our system of law will protect us if something goes wrong, that the trains will arrive on time and that our health service will patch us up if we are ill. If we lose respect and trust in our institutions, then our world has little security and meaning, and the uncertainty will contribute to the feelings of grievance and hopelessness that can make us ill.[4]

In the past our concepts of time and space were linked through a sense of place. An earlier generation could travel from London to Bristol by stagecoach in twelve hours and knew all the landmarks and stopping places on the way. Now we can travel to the other side of the world in the same time. And we can communicate with somebody on the opposite side of the globe within fractions of a second. This has compressed time and space, disembedding social relationships from specific locations and generating a sense of disorientation. We can at the same time exist everywhere and nowhere.

Being so well informed of what is happening anywhere in the world can mean that we are constantly threatened by global catastrophe – climate change, terrorist attack, contamination of the food supply, untreatable epidemics, depletion of the ozone layer, the weakening of the earth's magnetic field, collapse of the stock market, massive power supply failures, a virus that shuts down half the world's computer networks, a global conflict make us painfully aware of the fragility of the planet we inhabit.[5] But do so many people spend their time worrying about such apocalyptic scenarios? For most of us they are but a remote backdrop to our everyday existence and ignored like the dramatic death messages on cigarette packets. Perhaps the fragile state of the planet world provides an acceptable focus of projection for those of us who are really worn down by more personal insecurities. Rodney, a character in the sitcom *Only Fools and Horses*, put it all into perspective. When asked what was bothering him, he replied breezily, 'Oh you know, the ice caps are melting, the rainforest is being cut down, millions are starving in Africa, and Cassandra hasn't spoken to me for weeks.' So although our remote and general fears about the state of the world may create a climate of insecurity, we are probably more upset by our personal moral dilemmas, which have been conditioned by the fundamental changes in social attitudes.

To give just a few examples, in the 1950s, sex before marriage was frowned upon. By the 1960s, it was all right as long as you were in love. By the 1970s, it was still necessary to pretend you and your partner were married if you were staying together in a hotel. Now sex can be enjoyed openly for fun alone and there need be no commitment whatsoever.

In the 1950s, if a girl got pregnant, she was expected to get married. Unmarried mothers were condemned as immoral and being born illegitimate was a severe social stigma. By the 1960s, medical abortion was possible but only on medical or psychological grounds, and even then with society's disapproval. By the 1980s, abortion on demand was available in most European states. Now, an unattached woman who opts to go through with a pregnancy may even find herself accused of acting irresponsibly.

In the early half of the nineteenth century, people took their wedding vows seriously and expected to stay together for life. By the 1980s, couples tried to stay together until the children were nearly old enough to leave home. Now, many couples don't bother to get married and those that do stay together so long as it works for them. The proportion of UK families headed by a single parent has tripled since the 1970s.

Even a person's relationship with their God has changed dramatically. In the 1960s, few Britons admitted that they did not believe in God; now it seems as if Christianity has become a minority cult, and admitting to being a Christian can mark a person out as a little strange.

It is not my intention to imply that the social changes that have taken place over the last half-century are necessarily bad. Many of them, such as the reduction of social injustice, the erosion of prejudice on the grounds of race, gender and sexuality, and the greater choice, affluence and opportunities for all are very positive. I am simply drawing attention to the enormous change that has taken place within a single lifespan. Such fundamental shifts in attitude, occurring within such a remarkably short time, tear at the moral fabric of society, creating insecurity and separating children from their parents, husbands from wives, friends from friends, students from their teachers, and individuals from the way they were brought up. These shifts challenge the way a person thinks and behaves, creating conflict between what we want to do and what we feel we *ought* to do.

Illness tends to occur at times of social dissonance, when a person's expectations, based on previous experience, are threatened by external reality, generating a crisis of identity that cannot be resolved. So it occurs in the betrayal that accompanies separation and divorce, the grievance that is felt when other people fail to act according to our own inbred standards of fair play, and the guilt of behaving in a manner that runs counter to the way we were brought up. 'It's not fair', 'People just don't care any more', 'It's every man for himself', 'I can't get used to it', 'They just don't understand how I feel', 'I can never be what they want', and 'I can't stand it' are all common expressions of social dissonance.

Cultures across the globe attempt to regulate emotional expression by establishing codes of behaviour. In so doing, they create the conditions under which grievance, envy and fear can occur, and set moral standards for guilt and shame, limiting opportunities for redemption. By these means, they determine the amount of unre-solved tension and therefore the degree of unhappiness and illness in society. For example, the enforcement of strict moral codes can generate an existential conflict between personal desire and social restriction; on the other hand a permissive society can threaten our personal sense of containment. So the dissonance an individual feels and expresses in the form of an illness may well mirror a wider dissonance within society. Or as the eminent medical sociologist Bryan Turner expressed it, 'What is happening in society is played out in physiology.'[6]

If culture still serves to limit emotional expression, then it stands to reason that it will restrict those members of society that are more 'emotional'. The fact that societies have always sought to regulate women's emotionality and sexuality, even in our modern age, may help to explain the preponderance of functional illness in women. Although the feminist revolution has given women control of their own sexuality and equal property rights in marriage, and brought about a dramatic shift towards equal opportunities in employment, it has made life much more complicated.[7] A married woman may be able to work in parity with men, but many do more than their fair share of child care and domestic management. And those who stay at home to care for the family can be left isolated and unsupported by a husband who is away from seven o'clock in the morning until ten o'clock at night, by her own family who may live hundreds of miles away and by friends who are struggling themselves. Fewer women are choosing to get married and only half of today's marriages will survive until the children leave home. Thus, since the children tend to stay with their mother, it is usually women who have to bear the brunt of increasingly complex family arrangements and also the guilt when things go wrong. So it seems that for some women, the increased freedom and opportunity that their parents and grandparents voted for may perversely have created a whole new set of responsibilities and restrictions.

Lesley was always a very bright girl. Near the top of her class and bursting with enthusiasm and curiosity, she could not fail to do well. A generation previously, she would have made someone a good wife; that had been the limit of her mother's own ambitions. But Lesley was brought up in the 1970s when there were less barriers to prevent her making her own way in life. So she went to university to study molecular biology, got her Ph.D. and now works as a senior research scientist at a multinational pharmaceutical company. To all intents and purposes she is doing well, but she is not entirely happy. The annual round of grant applications, papers and conferences has become so much part of her life that if she stops she just doesn't feel right.

It was during one of these episodes, when she had given herself permission to step off the treadmill, that Lesley came to see me. She had been feeling exhausted and suffering from bad headaches, for which the doctor could not find any cause. But there was more to it than that. At forty-three, she had begun to feel disillusioned with it all. It seemed that no matter how hard she tried, her work never achieved the recognition she felt it deserved. She had once had the temerity to challenge one of the senior management team and felt she was being overlooked for political reasons. And her personal life had not quite worked out. She had married twenty years ago to her childhood sweetheart, but it didn't last. She had desperately wanted to escape from Burnley and everything it represented for him, but Alan was quite happy working with his father in their hardware store. In the end she left.

She then decided that it was not worth getting married; her career was much too important. She nevertheless enjoyed a number of casual relationships. It did not matter that most of the men she had had relationships with were married. She was a modern woman; the last thing she wanted was commitment and she enjoyed the frisson of excitement and feeling of being 'special'. Then she got pregnant. She could not bear the idea of abortion, and her daughter, Grace, has been brought up by a sequence of babysitters and childminders. Now Grace is fourteen, but looks much older. She goes out most nights and often does not return until very late, if at all. Lesley worries that she might be getting into a bad crowd and taking drugs, but is so busy that she can never seem to get the time to talk to Grace properly. And she has no close friends she can talk to about it. 'Where am I going?' she asked me in desperation. 'Soon Grace will have left home, I am fed up with my work, and I have nothing. And the sickness and the headaches just make it ten times worse.'

By promoting the expectation that women can 'have it all' (but still be left 'holding the baby'), Western culture has also created the conditions under which they might succumb to insoluble feelings of guilt and disappointment, and become ill.

People need time to adjust to the events that take place in their lives. They require space to reflect and think and talk things through with others, otherwise nothing gets resolved, the tension remains and their health may suffer. The pace of life has accelerated so much in recent years that we never get used to one change before the next comes along. As a result, many of us live our lives almost permanently off balance. We suffer from 'hurry sickness'.[8]

I could feel the pressure in Gordon as soon as he came into the room. My pulse quickened and I felt a tension across my lower chest. Although our appointment was scheduled for an hour, he summarised his problem in two minutes and expected me to write a quick prescription so that he could get back to the office. He had been getting pains in his stomach and feeling sick for about a month. The pains seemed to come on between meals and at night and were relieved by eating, but he never felt like eating very much. He had taken tablets for indigestion from the chemist and his GP had prescribed some acid-blockers, but the pains had continued. They were stopping him sleeping and he was exhausted with it all. He fell silent and I asked if there was anything else he wanted to tell me. He said that he just wanted some treatment so he could get on with his life.

I reminded him that we had an hour and a half together, and that we might as well relax and enjoy it. I saw a look of panic cross his face, but then his shoulders dropped, he slumped back in the chair and laughed until he cried. The tension just seemed to pour out of him. A few months ago, he had been offered a promotion, which meant that he had to leave his home in Aberdeen and work in Leeds during the week. He and his wife had not been getting on too well and he thought it would be good to have some time apart. In addition, he wanted to develop his relationship with Elaine, who lived in Yorkshire. So he rented a flat in Leeds and worked hard all day and into the evening and then went to meet Elaine. Late on Friday night he drove 250 miles back to Aberdeen, caught up on all the domestic activities with his children over the weekend and repeated the journey back in the early hours of Monday morning. There had been no time in his busy schedule to think about the deterioration in his relationship with his wife and the true reason for his pain.

The free market economy, the entry of large numbers of women into middle management and the intense competition for jobs has meant that businessmen and women are being called upon to work harder and longer if they want to keep their jobs and the lifestyles that go with them. People dare not step off the treadmill because there are plenty more people willing to take their place. In fact, management deliberately emphasises the threat of redundancy by devices such as continuous staff appraisals, productivity reviews and strategic plans. As Anthony Giddens observed, 'these are the cultural underpinnings of the exhausting lifestyles described by sufferers of chronic fatigue syndrome'.[9]

Life for many busy people has become more of a case of keeping out of trouble by clearing the stuff that keeps landing on their desks than on thinking creatively and developing a more rewarding pattern of work. As one of my colleagues recently commented, 'I get 400 e-mails a week, four papers to review, three official reports to scan, five meetings to go to, and still I am expected to look after my patients, supervise my research students, edit the journal and write my book. It's just a crazy world.'

Many people seem to live their lives in a near constant state of emotional tension. Everything has to be done yesterday. Even the weekend and public holidays provide no respite because the work they bring home with them has to compete with the fence that needs repairing, the shopping, the gardening, the children's activities and visits from relatives. With so much pace and pressure, there seems to be little time and space to appreciate the good things in life, to enjoy an evening with friends, to sit down to dinner as a family and to find the space to talk about the important things. A century ago, we suffered from an external environment that was overcrowded and polluted. Now it is our emotional environment that is overcrowded and polluted.

There was a time, and not so long ago, when most human activity went on during the daytime, when people slept at nights, worked from Monday to Friday, shopped or played on Saturday and took a day of rest on Sundays. These rhythms of life would ensure adequate periods of conversation and rest. Now we are a 24/7 society. Shops, clubs, bars and airports are open through the night. People can work, watch television and surf the internet at any hour of the day and night, seven days a week. They can travel across continents overnight. They can go out clubbing at eleven o'clock in the evening returning home at dawn, just in time to drink a strong cup of coffee and go to work. Time ceases to have any real meaning in terms of regulating their activity; they carry on until they fall asleep from sheer exhaustion and grab something quick to eat when they feel hungry.

Such severe disruptions in people's physiological rhythms with little opportunity to recuperate cannot fail to leave them exposed to illness. And busy people with no time to rest and think have little space to connect with others. Distanced from the support of their community and even the solace of their family, they run round their wheel until they drop from exhaustion and illness. But it's not just the pace of life that compromises our health; some people thrive on it. It's more the sense of social isolation that accompanies a busy life. As Max Ehrman wrote in his poem, 'Desiderata', 'Many fears are born of fatigue and loneliness.'

Human beings are social animals. Biological evolution equipped men and women for a communal existence, hunting and foraging in tribes of between twenty and forty people. We could never have survived this ecological niche by ourselves. We don't have the strength, the speed or the agility of other animals, we can't see so well in the dark, and we don't have a great sense of smell or even hearing. We would soon become a tasty meal for a hungry tiger. But we do have language. We can communicate with others and we are bright enough to collaborate for purposes of hunting, collecting food, defence and building shelters.

A tribal group would work as a team, assigning to each member a role according to their character and skills.

Thousands of years of history and social development have taken us further and further away from this natural niche. By successfully evading the biological controls on our population growth, we have created an artificial environment to which we are poorly adapted. Just as over-abundance of high-energy foods may have contributed to the epidemic of obesity and heart attacks, and overcrowding has encouraged the spread of infection, lack of social cohesion, I would argue, has predisposed to the current epidemic of emotional and functional illnesses.[10] But this is a recent development. Even in the large industrial cities of the Victorian era, people continued to organise themselves into tribe-sized groups: the extended family; people living in the same street; colleagues working in the office; the members of a working men's club; the regulars in the pub; bridge groups; local professional organisations. Their group identity provided an essential emotional resource of support, recognition and personal affirmation.

The society of our fellow human beings is so important. We can achieve so much more if we are working with other people and we have much more satisfaction doing it. We need the companionship of others to share joy, sadness, love and hate – in short, to feel alive. We all need the support of friends to help us get things in perspective so they don't prey on our minds and make us ill. We need to be sure of their love and respect in order to experience feelings of self-esteem. Friends modulate the excesses, they are there for you when you hit rock bottom and they can rescue you from vanity.[11] Social ties impart a collective identity, a sense of belonging, and trust in the company of others. These are the factors that make us feel safe and well. According to Professor Robert Putnam, author of the groundbreaking *Bowling Alone*, joining a club is equivalent in terms of 'social capital' to doubling a person's income, while getting married quadruples it.[12] The more integrated people are in their society, the more free they are and the less likely they are to experience depression and physical illness.

About fifty years ago medical researchers first noticed that people living in the town of Roseto, Pennsylvania, had less than half the heart attack rate of people in neighbouring towns.[13] This remarkable observation could not be explained by the obvious differences in diet, exercise, smoking, weight or genetic predisposition, but it did seem to relate to the town's social dynamics. Roseto was a tightly knit community that had been founded by immigrants from the same village in southern Italy at the end of the nineteenth century. They worked together to create a mutual aid society, churches, sports clubs, a labour union, a newspaper, scout troops and social clubs. They scorned conspicuous displays of wealth and endorsed family values. So it seemed that social capital was the key to Roseto's healthy hearts. That was in the 1950s. As a younger, more socially mobile generation of Rosetans grew up, the heart attack rate began to rise, until by the 1980s it was above that of nearby towns. In Roseto, as elsewhere, the institutions that kept the community intact slowly eroded. Increased social mobility and ease of communication meant that people no longer needed to live and work together. This distances individuals from a coherent sense of culture, challenging their sense of identity and predisposing them to increased rates of illness.

Professor Putnam's research indicates that the number of people who regularly attend public meetings, belong to a trades union or go to church has dropped by at least a half since the 1960s. It also shows that Americans are also much less likely to go to parent–teacher meetings or social clubs, or even nightclubs and bars. Instead they are more likely to stay at home by themselves and watch the television. During the same period of time, entertaining at home or going to friends for the evening dropped by nearly 40 per cent. A similar decline in socialisation has occurred in Britain, Scandinavia, Germany and many other Western countries. People, it seems, do not mix with their friends and neighbours so much. There is nothing, it seems, more lonely that a suburban street in Wilmslow, Cheshire or Denver, Colorado on a sunny Sunday afternoon, unless it's a country pub in Somerset on a wet Tuesday night. Isolated in anonymous suburbs without the support of grandparents, aunts, uncles and friends, the family is ailing.[14] It is said that a family that eats together stays together, but between 1976 and 1997, the percentage of American families with young children that had a regular evening meal together fell from 75 to 37 per cent, while in the cities, lonely singles lock themselves in their apartments, watch television and wait for the phone to ring. The percentage of British people living alone doubled between 1971 and 2004 and is estimated to go up to 40 per cent by 2010.

The same trend is occurring in the workplace. Our modern multinational corporations, global fast food chains and public services no longer depend so much on the personal loyalty of their employees and customers; the human factor has been downgraded in the interests of efficiency and profit.[15] So universities measure their success, not in the quality of their teaching, but in the numbers of students enrolled and research grants obtained. Hospitals tend to process their patients rather than care for them and are rated according to the brevity of waiting lists rather than the quality of care. As organisations have become larger and more complex, employees have to be regulated with guidelines, focus groups, strategy documents and policy statements, and monitored by audit, peer review, periodic assessment and quality control.[16] Emotional concepts of trust, faith, loyalty and identity, which maintained the well-being of employees and held smaller organisations together in the past, now seem outmoded. How can you have loyalty to an organisation that does not acknowledge your existence? How can you trust a multinational corporation? As much as advertisers and public relations personnel try to portray the human face of the company, few are fooled. Behind the bright eyes and gleaming smiles, and the brisk, stereotyped friendliness of the call centres, lurks the Orwellian spectre of Big Brother.

Living in our modern Western culture can confront us all with the awful reality of our own insignificance. So when Mrs Thatcher famously said, 'There is no such thing as society' she was perhaps responding to the notion that the population of the Western world has lost its social identity. It was suffering from loneliness. This, however, is not the same as being alone. People who have survived alone in the wilderness, embarked on long-distance solitary voyages or endured solitary confinement are not necessarily lonely. They have a strong sense of society and identity, and are sustained by their love for their family, their friends or their God as well as their relationships with animals, their guards or even inanimate objects.[17] Loneliness is a painful state of personal meaninglessness and desolation, a feeling that nothing matters and nobody cares, a state of disconnection and isolation from society – in short, a fundamental loss of identity.

In the past, people created stories, proverbs, parables and myths as templates to help them know who they were and negotiate the moral dilemmas of social life. From the sagas of the Vikings and the fables of ancient Greece to the religious dogmas of more recent times, these timeless cultural narratives were the collective conscience that glued societies together, inculcating principles of trust, altruism, loyalty, community care and collective responsibility. Now, it seems, we have lost these myths and with them our faith, not just in our gods, but also in ourselves. Depleted of suitable receptacles for our hopes and fears, and lacking acceptable reasons for the tragedies and disappointments of life, we are expected to muddle through the moral maze with just the doubt of scientific doctrine, the propaganda of political comment and the dramatics of soap operas for guidance.

So many of my patients tell me that they don't know who they are. It always seems to me such a chilling statement. Without a strong sense of their place and role in society, they lack the social support and cognitive template that would help them regulate bodily tensions induced by the challenges in their lives. Lonely people tend to suffer more tiredness, bowel upsets, muscular aches and pains, colds, heart attacks, strokes, cancer and depression. They tend to overeat and to visit their doctors more frequently. And there is evidence that they have impaired stress responses that can be rectified only if they have more social contact.[18] Loneliness may well be the most important public health risk of our time, greater than the effects of either smoking or overeating, but it is rarely considered, probably because the very idea is too threatening to society.

But what has brought about this increase in social isolation and loneliness? Is it the vast increases in populations or the high levels of unemployment in some Western countries, the building of suburbs many miles from the centres of cities, the increase in personal mobility through the ownership of cars, the entry of women into the labour market or even the erosion of faith? All of these factors have contributed to the redundancy of traditional community structure, but perhaps the greatest single influence is the introduction of the electronic media and instant mass communication and entertainment. If television has not actually caused the collapse of community, it has certainly facilitated it and filled the vacuum with a virtual society with problems that we cannot resolve. Throughout the Western world, the decline in community involvement and the rise in functional illness have paralleled the ownership of television sets.

Beamed into our homes twenty-four hours a day with a never-ending diet of news, social and political commentary and entertainment, television not only subsumes the time in which we might otherwise communicate productively with others, it is the most pervasive influence on how we feel and react to situations. In a world where there is a widespread erosion of the authority of our institutions and a decline in social interaction, it is television and the mass media that directs attitudes and sets standards of social behaviour. The most popular television programmes are the soap operas. About a quarter of the UK population watch *Coronation Street* three to four times every week, and viewing figures for *EastEnders* and *Emmerdale* are around 7 to 10 million. Although the plots of these programmes cover a wide variety of social issues, the main characters are scripted to react to life situations in the most dysfunctional ways. They encourage us to seek fun rather than act responsibly, to confront rather than negotiate, to protest rather than understand, to demand our rights rather than find ways of living together, and to fret about minor issues rather than view things in perspective. Thus, television mirrors the distorted perceptions of a narcissistic society, in which image takes priority over community values. It has to. The confrontation and passion generated by revenge and grievance are exciting to television audiences and attract high viewing figures and advertising revenue. We obtain a vicarious thrill from the dilemmas of the characters we see on the screen, and are encouraged to mimic their confrontational attitudes. Over the last twenty-five years, scientific studies have clearly shown that childhood exposure to media violence and identification with aggressive TV characters predicts aggressive behaviour in young adults and therefore may at least partly account for the rise in violent crime in Western society.[19]

The intrusive nature of the media means that events thousands of miles away, which have little direct relevance to our lives, can be experienced in all their dramatic intensity in our own living rooms. There is rarely any good news. Television journalists are not paid to inform, instruct and reassure us, but to excite us and dramatise events. So while distant events like the killing of hostages in Iraq and the murder of two ten-year-old girls in Soham may not generate a deep personal grief reaction, they stir up the topsoil of insecurity, which cannot but fail to make the lonely and vulnerable anxious and unwell. Vicarious exposure to emotional trauma is rather like the nutritional concept of empty calories, it may get us going but we can't engage with it, resolve it, learn from it and grow.[20]

Television carries mixed messages. While news bulletins and soap operas depict how fragile the world is, chat shows, consumer programmes and advertisements seduce us into believing we can all be famous and live in a fantasy land of happiness and comfort. So we may be able to have it all for a while, but it can be quickly snatched away, leaving us with nothing. With everything seeming so transient and unreliable, how can we build up a healthy sense of confidence and trust?

But surely, you might exclaim, we don't have to be affected by what we see on television? That's true, of course, but television is such a hypnotic medium. Television audiences peak in the early evening when we have finished the day's work, eaten an evening meal, perhaps had a drink or two and are settled in an armchair. This relaxed but focused state of mind is highly receptive to the evocative images and strong attitudes portrayed on the screen in front of us. So when we feel tired and lonely, the powerfully emotive images cannot fail to influence the way we feel and think, directing our attitudes, conditioning our beliefs, creating aspirations, destroying reputations, determining fashion and setting trends. It is not the rhetoric of our politicians that convinces us to vote in a particular way, but the way the television commentators interpret what they say. It is not the quality of a new product that makes us buy it, but the advertiser's skill in persuading us that we need it. And it is not always our physical symptoms that make us go to the doctor, but the fear of what health documentaries tell us it might be.

So is television bad for our health? Well, if the theme of this book is correct and much human illness is related to emotional tension which cannot be resolved, then the answer is yes. Television 'soaps' portray conflict with no clear means of resolution. Lifestyle programmes create expectations with little chance of satisfaction. News bulletins and current affairs programmes seem to offer a never-ending sequence of threats without the personal resolution that can put them into perspective. And every day, or so it seems, we hear of some new threat to our health. Media scares give form to symptoms and are eagerly consumed by vulnerable and impressionable people desperate to have some tangible cause for their illness.[21]

It may be no coincidence that the rise in medically unexplained illnesses has paralleled the development of electronic mass media.[22] For example, disordered eating was almost unknown in regional areas in Fiji before the introduction of Western television. Within a few years, dieting and self-induced vomiting had become commonplace among young Fijian women. A similar phenomenon occurred in Czechoslovakia and the previous Soviet republic of Georgia. And in Africa, irritable bowel syndrome is quite common among middle-class city-dwellers who own television sets, although it is virtually unheard of in rural communities. And tellingly, the close-knit Amish community, which forbids the use of television in their houses, has been spared the depression epidemic.

Television tends to be watched more by children than their parents. The average American teenager typically spends more time alone in front of the television and Playstation than with family and friends. And in Britain children watch at least three hours of television every day. This is not so much a training for life as an escape into fantasy. Parents who both go out to work just do not have the time to help their children understand and deal with their everyday dramas. Childcare tends to be compressed into just a few hours a day at a time when the parents are exhausted and the children are over-excited. Just as lion cubs reared by hand in a zoo will starve if released into the wild, so children deprived of social interaction will find it difficult to cope with the complex emotional dilemmas of adult life without becoming ill.

Children need a consistent and containing family and social background in order to establish the strong sense of cultural identity and self-confidence which will protect them from social illness. Unfortunately, modern family dynamics can tend to compromise the emotional development of children. Most marriages end in separation and divorce while the children are still growing up, and many modern 'families' are complicated by step-parents, 'uncles' and 'aunties', and half-siblings. Most kids have to go through the upheavals of moving house and changing school at least once during their childhood. In the UK, 30 per cent of mothers are bringing up their children alone and 70 per cent of young married mothers go out to work. Research suggests that not only do orphans and children of divorced parents find it more difficult to regulate the emotional responses to loss and separation, but also many infants looked after by informal or unpaid childminders from the first year of life.[23] Moreover, the erosion of family and community can tend to mean that many parents have little instruction and help in bringing up their children and try to muddle through with the help of manuals, leaflets from the doctor's surgery and television documentaries. People now need to be taught what in previous generations might have been acquired naturally from friends and family.

The current epidemic of depression and functional illness predominantly affects the young, but it hasn't always been so. Surveys in the 1940s and 1950s found that younger people were happier and suffered less 'malaise' than older people. Since then the situation has reversed.[24] Depression among the young has gone up an astounding sevenfold, and the percentage of young people under thirty who reported feeling ill most of the time has more than doubled.[25] Each generation since the 1950s has been less trusting, less sociable, more materialistic, more individualistic, but also more depressed and ill. Without a firm grounding in a stable society, children can reach physical maturity lacking a social sense of who they are and where they belong. These are the lost generations, the children who never grew up.

Lacking a strong sense of social identity, young people can seem to be engaged in a restless quest for authenticity. The competitive trade in smart remarks and sterile anecdotes in crowded bistros and the displays of athleticism in noisy nightclubs are more about exhibitionism than communication. And if the night's efforts culminate in sexual intimacy, that too may be a kind of performance art.[26] Love, to say nothing of commitment, have little place in this, and by the cold light of morning, it can all seem so meaningless. Young Britons increasingly prefer to have a number of sexual relationships than get married. But does that mean greater happiness? The high rates of depression and dissatisfaction among the young would suggest that it doesn't.

Cast adrift in a whirling social landscape, young people struggle to reinvent themselves to keep pace with fashion. This reconstruction is often expressed in the language of the body. So they adopt different hairstyles, spend fortunes on clothes and cosmetics, pierce different parts of their body with rings and studs, decorate their skin with tattoos, go on crash diets, and even change the shape of their nose, their breasts, their chin or their bottom with plastic surgery.[27] In the past such personal reconstruction was restricted to the upper strata of society, but now they affect nearly everybody. Young people are much more affluent, more aware of changing fashions, and the solutions for transformation are legion. They can even escape the limitations of our own biology by the use of designer drugs. Mood-enhancing drugs like Ecstasy and antidepressants like Prozac offer freedom from the painful realities of life, Viagra provides men the miracle of unlimited stress-free potency, and new drugs for obesity offer the possibility to transform body shape without the pain of dieting. But however much young people may attempt to reconstruct the self by reconstructing the body, they are creating an artificial identity that is insubstantial and transient.[28]

Brought up in an environment of commercialism and advertising, young people are encouraged to express their identity through the ownership of modern lifestyle accessories, such as video-phones, Ipods, digital cameras and personal organisers. Nowadays it is these status symbols that define a person's social identity, rather than the community in which they live. They create a virtual sense of 'belonging', but no real expression of their individuality. They feed the ephemeral excitement of spoiled children, who, deprived of the emotional engagement they so desperately need, have been given treats and presents to console and pacify them.

And the images that we see every night on television depict a kind of never-never-land, enticingly within the reach of all of us. We are living in an age when a personable but otherwise quite ordinary young couple, he with a boyish face and a cultured right boot, and she with a cute hairstyle, an enviably slim physique and a passable singing voice, can achieve the status of royalty. So it seems that any of us can earn a fortune, live a Hollywood lifestyle, visit exotic locations, have a wonderful sex life, and be loved by millions. Unfortunately, real life is never really like that. Anything that is worth having has to be worked for, often endlessly and with great sacrifice, even right boots.

A narcissistic society that encourages such great expectations is bound to induce great disappointments. For every one person who achieves celebrity, there are 10,000 disappointed wannabees. The streets of Manchester or even Chingford are not paved with gold. Too much personal investment in commodities can leave an individual vulnerable to depletion of their identity. So the loss of a necklace, the breakage of a favourite ornament, damage to the car, the hotel that did not live up to expectations and the match that was lost can leave us feeling so deprived and angry that we may become physically ill. The recent increase in illness has paralleled a rise in materialism. People who put all their faith in their dreams of celebrity and success and the lifestyle that goes with it are going to find it very difficult to cope with inevitable disappointment.

At just thirty-three, Adrian was remarkably successful. He was an executive in a public relations company and had the lifestyle to go with it. He drove a top-of-the-range Mercedes and travelled to America for meetings by private jet. He had wooed and married Sally, a television actress. They had two boys, whom they sent to an exclusive public school in Scotland, they owned a house worth

£750,000 and they took their holidays in the Seychelles. Adrian had a charmed life, so different from his very ordinary upbringing in Liverpool. He had an abiding memory of having to go across a yard to a cold outside toilet and vowed he would never live like that ever again.

Adrian's materialism helped but did not compensate for the shame of his background. And his success was not achieved without a punishing work schedule. He regularly worked an eleven-hour day and thought little of staying up overnight to meet an urgent deadline. The difficulty came when the company relocated to London. Sally did not want to move and stayed in their luxury home in the Yorkshire Dales. So Adrian lived in a mews flat in Kensington and travelled north every weekend. Then, with economic recession, the company's profits took a tumble. There just wasn't the work around and they had to lay off some staff. Adrian redoubled *his* work effort, but was over-stretched and over-tired and seemed to lose his golden touch. Then he found out that Sally had renewed her relationship with a previous lover, another actor. She was lonely and Adrian was always so tired and tense. Overnight, his world quite literally fell apart.

Sally stayed in the family house with the boys. Adrian moved to a smaller apartment. The company was sold to a larger concern and Adrian had to take a drop in salary. It was around this time that Adrian came to see me. He was quick and nervous, found it difficult to sit still and was suffering from persistent stomach pain, diarrhoea and dreadful tiredness that seemed to sap all his energy and initiative. He had seen other doctors. Apart from some mild gastric inflammation, his tests were all negative. He was reluctant to accept my suggestion that he should have some time off to take stock of his life.

According to the writer and philosopher Alain de Botton, people like Adrian are suffering from loss of status.[29] He had invested so much of his pride and sense of worth in escaping from the shame and poverty of his childhood and becoming somebody that when his dream collapsed, he became ill, not so much with an unfortunate bout of stomach inflammation, but more from a serious wound to his self-esteem and challenge to his identity. Brought up to respond to the conditional love of his parents by working hard, he was at the mercy of the highly conditional attentions of other people. So long as he was successful, he received love and approbation, but as soon as he failed, these were withdrawn and he became ill.

People may be happy with little in life when that is all they have come to expect, but great expectations can lead to great disappointment if they are removed or not realised. De Botton claims that an affluent lifestyle and equality of opportunity has created a population

that suffers great anxiety over their importance, achievement, income
and possessions. People are constantly comparing the house they live
in, the car they drive, the clothes they wear and the holidays they go
on with their friends and family. These are the status symbols by
which they measure their own worth, and they have to keep ahead of
the game.

We live in a society that stimulates envy. Advertisers make us covet
others' possessions. Politicians make us hate others for the advantages
they have. And the competition in the workplace, among our friends
and acquaintances and even within our family, causes us to be all too
aware of our status. 'What about me?' seems to be the catchphrase of
our time. Envy diminishes a person.[30] So when our lover abandons us
for somebody richer or more attractive, when our erstwhile friends
overlook us, when others get the recognition and promotion we fail to
get, when the children tell Mummy that Daddy is more fun, it
undermines our confidence and we feel bad. Or as the American
essayist Gore Vidal once said, 'When a friend of mine is successful,
something inside me dies.'

   We can save ourselves from our own self-criticism if we can blame
somebody else for our misfortune and unhappiness. Within our
narcissistic culture, people have lots of individual rights and few
collective responsibilities. Thus when something goes wrong, few of us
can just shrug our shoulders and admit we misjudged the situation.
Somebody must be to blame.

   Grievance is most likely to be expressed within the context of a
marriage. Once the passion evaporates and the idealisation of love is
exposed to the reality test of partnership and collaboration, those witty
one-liners become intensely annoying, the relaxed laidback attitude
feckless and irresponsible, the self-confidence bossy and controlling,
and the seductive manner a source of considerable suspicion.
Accusations are flung across the breakfast table while the children
cower behind the cereal packets. And as the relationship deteriorates,
instead of trying to understand what is going on and repair the
damage, too many aggrieved partners turn to lawyers to justify their
viewpoint. For them, it is much more important to be right than to be
together. And when the divorce is settled, the final loss of a partner, in
whom there was so much emotional investment, cannot be accepted;
neither can one's role in the breakdown of the relationship. And so, all
too often, the traumatised self is buttressed by self-righteousness while

the relationship is kept alive in a grievance that gnaws at the soul and undermines the health.

If we cannot relinquish our personal investment in what we have lost, eventually our impotent anger is turned in on ourselves and expressed in mental and physical illness. Depression is probably the commonest illness in the Western world, but few of us bring ourselves to acknowledge we might be depressed. Instead of being something we can learn from, it carries the stigma of moral weakness and mental instability. So in our 'have-a-happy-day' culture, depression with its negative connotations of anger, disappointment, shame and guilt are denied and repackaged as irritable bowels, chronic back pain, heartburn and persistent headaches, and treated with tablets.

But such illnesses are not meaningless, impersonal bodily expressions of disharmony; they carry the memory and express the meaning of what has happened in a way that defies scientific logic. But this is encrypted communication that is not even obvious to those of us who suffer. If it were, there would be little point in the physical symptoms. So apparently disconnected from what has upset us, they come to take over our lives, justifying why we cannot go to work, or go out and enjoy ourselves, or eat appetising foods or enjoy intimacy. They protect our vulnerable sense of self from intolerable reality, eliciting the support and sympathy of our family and friends and recruiting the care and attention of the doctor. The ways in which this can occur is the topic of the next chapter.

6

The meaning of illness and the purpose

Rachel was slightly built and had a bright elfin face, framed by straight, ash-blonde hair. I was asked to see her because she was suffering attacks of nausea, abdominal pain, cold bones, nasal stuffiness, sore eyes and deafness that occurred most days in the late afternoon. She had been referred to a variety of specialists and endured many invasive investigations that were often painful and always embarrassing. All to no avail. The symptoms just seemed to have got worse and Rachel was desperate. She particularly needed to know what to take for her 'cold bones'.

After listening carefully, I explained to her that this strange combination of symptoms did not fit with any medical diagnosis that I knew about, but I wondered if they reminded her of anything. She looked disappointed but thought about my question. After a long while, she said that they were just the same sort of feelings she had when she was nine years old. Her parents had recently divorced and her mother was finding it hard to look after Rachel and her younger sister. She had taken a job in the morning and in the evening just to make ends meet, but she always tried to make sure she was there to give them a hot meal when they came home from school. Rachel didn't want her mother to go to work and often refused the meal her mother had cooked. Her mother would try to make her eat it, but it just gave Rachel stomachache and made her feel sick. This invariably caused her mother to lose her temper and shout at her, whereupon she would run up to her room in floods of tears, lie on her bed and put a pillow over her head to drown out the noise of her mother's voice. The same thing would happen day after day whenever her mother had to go to work.

'My illness feels just like that,' she said.

'And the cold bones?' I asked.

'Oh, that was probably because the house was always cold.'

But why, I wondered, had Rachel's symptoms come on in the last two years when this had all happened so long ago? Had anything happened two years ago? With tears in her eyes, Rachel told me that that was when her mum had died.

Rachel's symptoms seemed to play out the traumatic memory: the 'cold bones' related to the cold house and her mother's crossness; the abdominal symptoms represented her reaction to eating; and the nasal stuffiness, sore eyes and deafness seemed to connect with the notion of her weeping into her pillow. And the whole visceral memory had been evoked by the fact that her mother had left her again, this time for good.

Evaluating the current situation in the light of our previous experience, our body responses express how we 'feel' about what has happened. It is as if the brain uses the entire bodily orchestra to construct the most meaningful arrangements of symptoms with the sympathetic or parasympathetic nerves contributing the emotional key (major or minor). So the type of illness a person suffers from is not just related to the predominant style of emotional expression, either despair or resistance or detachment (see Chapter Three), the particular combination of symptoms and their associations are specific to the individual patient. This would explain why some patients express their despair in back pain, another may get diarrhoea and a third just feels exhausted.

People caught up in the same traumatic situation can react in a variety of ways (see Chapter Two), according to the particular meaning ascribed to that situation by their life experience.[1]

Links between symptom expression and meaning are more obvious when the symptoms express the bodily memory of a particular traumatic situation. Over a century ago, Joseph Breuer and Sigmund Freud concluded that 'hysterics suffer mainly from reminiscences', which are suppressed from conscious thought because their recollection is too painful and disturbing to the patient.[2] Hysteria has slipped out of fashion as a medical diagnosis. Nevertheless, when I began to explore the context of the physical illnesses my patients suffered from, I was shocked to discover just how many of them appeared to suffer from the lingering effects of emotional scenarios that had not been fully resolved. My sense of shock stemmed from the realisation that these were the same patients whose painful 'memories' I had, for most of my professional life, been attempting to subdue with antispasmodics or release with laxatives.

Sadie was brought into my clinic in a wheelchair. Her face was a mask of tragedy. She had been suffering from constipation and the most awful abdominal pain for eight years. She had been to countless consultants, had many investigations, but all had failed to reveal the cause of her pain. She looked so uncomfortable that I suggested she lie down on the couch, but as she transferred herself from her wheelchair, she did so very slowly and with great caution, bent over and holding her lower abdomen like somebody who had undergone an operation the day before. When I commented on this, she looked scared, but slowly told me that she had indeed had a hysterectomy for excessive vaginal bleeding, but that was eight years ago. I noted that this was around the time her symptoms first started and asked her what was going on in her life at that time. To my immense shock and surprise, she told me that when she was still in hospital recovering from the operation, her twin sister, Abigail, who was living in Jamaica, had gone into premature labour, suffered a torrential haemorrhage and died. Sadie could not face the thought that her sister was dead. It was another four years before she went back to Jamaica to visit the grave.

Twins have a special bond, sometimes so close that they can seem to share a common identity. When Abigail died, Sadie had to carry the traumatic memory like an open wound until she could begin to release the 'spell' by talking about it. This may sound like the stuff of mythology, but body and mind are not cut off at the neck; they are a continuum, linked together by meaning. So just as thinking about food can make the stomach secrete acid and bring on sensations of hunger, anything that evokes the memory of a traumatic event can bring back the symptoms that were present at that time.

For some of my patients, their 'somatic memory' has become so deeply embedded that aspects of living that the rest of us take for granted pose the most severe restrictions on them.

Whenever Peter went out, just the thought of having to meet people made him want to go to the toilet. He tried to prevent this by making sure he emptied his bowels before he went out, but as soon as he was halfway down the street, he would feel that he had to go again and so would go back home. If he tried to fight it, then the feeling would get worse – so much so that he could be incontinent. This caused him such humiliation that he was afraid to leave the house. He was referred to me for investigation of his bowel function, but the tests were completely normal. When I asked Peter what was happening at the time his symptoms came on, he said he thought it was around the time his foreman became ill and Peter had to take on his responsibilities. His bowels had become loose and he had had to dash to the toilet on two occasions. I wondered whether he had had any difficulties with his bowels before. At first he denied it but then he remembered an intensely embarrassing experience he had had at junior school. He was, he told me, a shy boy with a slight stammer and this had made him a target for bullying. One day, the boys behind him were flicking his ears and he had this intense urge to go to the toilet. The teacher was irritated with him and told him he had to wait until the break, but he couldn't wait and so he soiled his trousers. Peter was appalled by what had happened and from then on the teasing became merciless.

It seemed that the unexpected responsibility had triggered the same shameful gut reaction that Peter had experienced in childhood. Over fifty years ago, the psychoanalyst Felix Deutsch noted how emotional distress occurring at the time of an illness in early childhood might somehow sensitise the organ to dysfunction if faced with a similar emotional stress later in life.[3] Peter had 'forgotten' the link with his childhood experience, and so, disconnected from a context that could not be thought about, his fears had remained locked in the body as the mystery illness – what the psychoanalyst Christopher Bollas termed, 'the unthought known'[4] – until revoked by the threat of exposure. But over the course of the next three months, Peter was able to look at his childhood fears and put them into an adult perspective. Slowly he began to gain confidence and extend his activities. By the end of three months, he was able to take his daughter to football matches and even go away on holiday with his family.

Functional illnesses are not always so obviously brought on by episodes of trauma. Sometimes they may be triggered by something much more prosaic, an intolerance to food maybe, an operation, a relatively minor injury, or an infection. Chronic fatigue syndrome, for example, often seems to be instigated by an acute viral infection, and irritable bowel syndrome can be induced by an attack of gastroenteritis in about 10 per cent of cases, although most people recover from gastroenteritis within a few days. So what causes the symptoms to persist, even though the infection has long since disappeared? To answer this question, my colleague, Dr Kok-Ann Gwee, studied over 100 people admitted to hospital with acute gastroenteritis and followed them up for six months. The results showed that those in whom the symptoms persisted had suffered more anxiety or depression at the time of the acute illness and had experienced more traumatic life events during the six months prior to their gastroenteritis. Corresponding findings have been reported for chronic fatigue syndrome. In each case, it seemed as if the psychological upset that caused the illness persisted as a kind of symptom memory. To test this finding, we studied people admitted with a range of acute illnesses. Again the principle was upheld: emotional upset at the time of the acute illness predicted the persistence of the original symptoms.[5] Or to put it a different way, it appeared as if the symptoms of the acute infection had been 'recruited' to express an unresolved emotional problem.

A similar phenomenon can occur after surgical trauma or physical injury. About 10 per cent of people develop chronic pelvic pain and bowel disturbance for the first time after hysterectomy. Like Sadie, this complication is more likely if they are depressed and have experienced emotional upset around the time of the operation.[6] Other studies have shown that persistent facial pain can be instigated by toothache or dental procedures, chronic backache can be triggered by back injury, and persistent headaches can be brought on by head injury.[7] In each situation, reports suggest that people are more likely to develop chronic symptoms if they are 'upset' at the time of the original injury. The link between physical injury and emotional distress would also explain why long-term medically unexplained symptoms are particularly likely to occur after a person has been physically or sexually abused. The combination of severe emotional trauma with physical injury fixes the association between symptoms and context in the long-term memory. As the memory fades, the illness declines, but will return if rekindled by association.

Psychologists call this a *conditioned response*. In the early years of the twentieth century, the Russian physiologist Ivan Pavlov demonstrated that if the presentation of food was linked with a stimulus, such as the ringing of a bell, then the test subject (a dog) would come to associate the ringing of the bell with food and would salivate and secrete gastric acid when the bell sounded and no food was given.[8] Conditioned responses are much stronger in the presence of emotion. It seems as if emotion solders the link between symptoms and context onto the circuit boards of our long-term memory and makes it particularly difficult to extinguish.

Amanda was so in love with Rick that she chose to ignore how late he was coming home and the increasing number of nights he had to spend out of town. Times were tough for both of them and she knew that Rick was taking on extra jobs so that they could get married and start a family. So when Rick suggested that they go out for a meal because there was something he had to say to her, she felt thrilled and excited. The venue was perfect: a little fish restaurant in a village a few miles away. She thought she would wear the little black dress that Rick liked – and just for good luck she wore the expensive perfume he had bought her during their first Christmas together. Rick was attentive as usual but seemed somehow tense and sad. They chose poached salmon with prawns and Hollandaise sauce and a lovely bottle of South African Sauvignon Blanc. There was something not quite right with the sauce but Amanda felt so relaxed and happy that she ignored it. She had just finished hers when Rick announced that he had been having an affair with Margaret, who worked in his office. It had been going on for some time. He still loved her but he loved Margaret, too, and well – somehow she had got pregnant.

Amanda listened with mounting horror. How could this be happening? Suddenly she couldn't sit there any more. She rushed through the restaurant to the ladies where she was seized with the most violent spasms of retching. She didn't stop vomiting for three days. Every time she even thought of food she would be sick. That was three years ago. Rick married Margaret, but they lost the baby. Amanda took a job in another town. She could not bear the shame of meeting her friends or telling her family and so she withdrew from them. She has been out a few times with other men, but always feels sick and often makes excuses not to go out. Subsequent to the attack of gastroenteritis on that fateful evening, she has developed an allergy to fish; even the smell of it makes her violently ill. Other foods upset her as well, and she has lost a lot of weight.

It seemed that Amanda's gut reaction combined with Rick's catastrophic news had created such a strong association in her mind that anything reminding her of that fateful evening made her feel sick. Perhaps, if she had been able to talk about what happened, the emotion would have been worn away, and any food intolerance would have dissipated with it, but she was too ashamed to tell anybody, even her family. So the emotional reaction fashioned a memory loop that could be activated by the slightest association with that night.

The ability of emotion to implant associations into a person's mind may also explain how somebody can come to 'adopt' an illness they have seen on television, read about or witnessed in somebody else. This is dramatically illustrated by a case that was originally reported by

Dr Paul Joire, a family physician working in Lille in the late-nineteenth century.[9]

> Exactly eight days after having witnessed his sister's crisis ... [the patient] was taken with a similar crisis. At the beginning he too complained of pains in the right side. And he indicated the hepatic region as the seat of those pains, but it was established on palpation that the liver was not at all sensitive. His acts and his complaints were absolutely identical to those of his sister; he emitted the same cries, he grasped at his right side with the same clasping fingers, as if to tear out what was hurting him. After a certain time, this same pain seemed to radiate towards the epigastric region, the chest and the lower abdomen. He writhed on the bed eight days later in the same manner as his sister. The scene could not be more perfectly imitated, and one might indeed have believed in a true hepatic colic.

The young man's sister had suffered from acute biliary colic, and he had been so affected by her distress that he adopted her illness. In much the same way some anxious husbands appear to identify with their wife's pregnancy by developing the abdominal swelling and associated symptoms of a pseudo-pregnancy. And was it just coincidence that five out of seven members of my first therapeutic group of patients with irritable bowel syndrome had experienced the shock of losing a close relative (parent or grandparent) from colonic cancer when they were very young?

Situations that evoke strong emotion focus the attention and induce a highly receptive state in which associations are likely to be established in long-term memory. The famous French neurologist Jean-Martin Charcot called this 'choc nerveux', and compared it with a hypnotic trance, in which suggestions implanted by the therapist can continue to affect physiological sensations, reactions and behaviour long after the person has woken up. Traditional witch doctors used hypnotic chanting and rhythms to 'cast spells' on people, causing illness and even death.[10]

The focused state of receptive relaxation induced by the hypnotist is reminiscent of the state of mind of the dreamer. Indeed, I suspect that the function of dreams, with their strong emotional tone and rich allegory that ignores the constraints of reality, might be to encourage the assimilation into long-term memory of the meaning of what has happened.[11] This can even bring on symptoms. For example, the

Viennese analyst Wilhelm Stekel told the story of a banker who had recently been fired from his job and woke up one night with pain and paralysis in his leg, which lasted for several months. When he had woken up he was having a vivid dream about a chamois being shot in the leg. Four years previously, he had been on a hunt with a guide. They fired a shot at a chamois, which plunged down a ravine. The hunters climbed down and found the chamois still alive with its hip shattered. The banker was struggling to come to terms with the fact that at the height of his success he had been shot down by his colleagues. This theme was so vividly expressed by both the dream and his symptoms.[12]

Like it or not, we are all suggestible. If I lecture to my students about a patient with a stiff neck, many of my audience will instinctively start to rub their neck. And just like the character in Stanley Holloway's recitation, 'My word, you do look queer,' if somebody tells us that we don't look very well today, then indeed we can start to feel unwell.[13]

Entrained through years of social experience and constantly refined by change and circumstance, our bodies respond unconsciously to the associations and meaning of particular situations and ideas. Every significant life experience has the potential to change the way we feel and our bodies react. Events that cannot be acknowledged and resolved are encapsulated in our minds as illness memories, which may be rekindled by contextual association – an anniversary maybe, or a particular place, food, perfume, or meeting an old friend. It is therefore like other aspects of our personality, a learnt and predictable response to certain cues, which fashions our body as a unique expression of our identity.

With the passage of time, our experience becomes etched on our faces, and the way we hold our bodies, elaborated and refined through countless social interactions, becomes a predictable and eloquent expression of how confident or nervous we feel, and how much we are weighed down by life experience. The neurologist Oliver Sacks expressed this succinctly when he wrote that 'walking, at its most elementary, is a spinal reflex, but it is elaborated at higher and higher levels until finally we can recognise a man by the way he walks . . . by *his* walk'.[14] So when somebody enters my consulting room, I am curious to see how they carry themselves, how they sit down, what their face expresses. I observe the tragic mask, the challenging stare, the averted gaze, the slumped shoulders and the way they collapse into the chair or perch on the edge of it, twisting a handkerchief in their hands. The major emotional themes of their life stories are eloquently portrayed before each patient speaks, and are often confirmed in the first few words that they say. This gives me clues as to the cause of their illness. But it is not just therapists who can read bodily language. Two years ago, I was visited by a Romany fortune-teller who read my face and posture so perceptively that she could recount the essence of my life story without me saying a thing. I was so shocked I gave her £50!

Similarly, the choices we make in life – the person we marry, the house we live in, the kind of food we eat – are rarely the result of careful objective analysis; they are based on how our life experience has caused us to feel about those things. Meaning is implicit in the way we react to every aspect of our existence. And so even the illness people get can convey in symbolic form the most difficult issues or themes in their lives. George Groddeck, psychoanalyst and corre- spondent of Freud, even suggested that such illnesses are unique expressions of the personality:

> Whoever sees in illness a vital expression of the organism will no longer see it as an enemy. In the moment I realise that the disease is a creation of the patient, it becomes the same sort of thing to me as his manner of walking, his mode of speech, his facial expression, the house he has built, the business he has settled or the way his thoughts go – a significant symbol of the powers that rule him.[15]

Thus it seems likely that many expressions of functional illness are bodily representations of what has happened to us. Generated by a particular context, they convey a specific meaning, which our emotional brain has translated into the intimate and personal metaphor of our bodily feelings and physiological reactions. This is an encrypted communication; its meaning is encoded by the life narrative of the individual and can only be deciphered through detailed insight into the patient's experience and cultural background. It is, as Freud indicated, 'disease at the level of the idea'.

James was a successful solicitor in a fashionable Derbyshire spa town and was highly respected in his local community. He had always conducted his business with authority and self-confidence, but in recent years that confidence had been undermined by rumblings in his guts. These often came on in meetings with clients and were so bad he would need to excuse himself and leave. They had commenced when he had been on traction for an injured back caused by a car accident. He had hated being so dependent on people for everything, even to have his bowels open. It reminded him of his early relationship with his mother, who had always had a rather obsessional interest in his bowels. James recovered from his accident, but not from the noises in his guts, and his distress seemed out of all proportion to the nature of the symptoms. I listened with a sense of incredulity and told him, perhaps rather insensitively, that we all get rumblings in our gut and perhaps, if we stopped talking, we could hear our intestines rumbling away in unison. Jim looked cross and retorted, 'But you don't understand. These symptoms are *so bad*!' The stress on the words 'so bad' sounded to me as if James was making a moral judgement. As I said this, James looked shocked and upset. Slowly it all came out: the dubious deals with local businessmen; the forged accounts; his clandestine sexual relationship with the social secretary of his golf club.

From early childhood, James had struggled to keep his bowel function secret from his mother's intrusions. His determination to be self-sufficient had made him very successful. One could say that he had become rich trading in secrets. His accident literally meant that everybody seemed to know his business and so the movements of his intestines represented the threat of exposure.

Wendy was sent to me because for the previous three years she had been suffering from a disfiguring rash on one side of her face, over her cheek and left ear and involving the left corner of her mouth. The dermatologists had diagnosed eczema, but the rash just didn't respond to the usual creams. Even steroids had failed to resolve it, and she could not conceal it with make-up. It was particularly embarrassing because Wendy worked as a beautician in the cosmetics department of a big store. Her employers had been understanding for a while, but she eventually lost her job.

I asked what was happening in her life when her symptoms first came on. Wendy looked down in embarrassment and told me that they had started around the time her sixteen-year-old daughter, Jane, became pregnant. Wendy had felt angry and deeply ashamed, and Jane had left home to live in her boyfriend's flat. To Wendy this was history repeating itself. She had become pregnant with Jane at around the same age. Her mother had been furious when she had found out and had slapped her so hard across her cheek, the mark did not go for months. This was the first time her mother had ever hit her. It was, she said, the sign of

her shame. At the time, she and her brother were living with their mother in quite deprived circumstances. Their father had left home to live with another woman and had refused to pay any maintenance. They had very little money and Wendy told me of how deeply ashamed she was at having to dress in worn-out, second-hand clothes. And then she fell pregnant.

Wendy had never been able to resolve the humiliating sense of shame and anger she had felt when her mother slapped her. Instead, the memory of the slap and her shame were buried, but continued to function as an undercover agent, influencing her decision to train as a beautician and work in cosmetics and her assiduous protection of Jane. Eventually, however, her worst fears were realised; Jane became pregnant and Wendy's crushing shame was there for all to see in the rash on her face, the slap that could not be healed. Over the course of the next five months, Wendy was able to talk not only about her embarrassment over Jane's and her own pregnancy, but also the deep sense of anger she felt over her father's adulterous relationships. Slowly, with no treatment, her rash faded and she was able to return to work.

The symptoms of medically unexplained illnesses are often not so much indicators of the damage or irritation of specific organs, but a kind of language that conveys the otherwise hidden meaning of what has happened. James and Wendy are just two of my patients whose symptoms were an appropriate metaphor for the major themes in their lives. There are many, many others: Jessie, whose 'burning mouth' represented what she wanted to say to her mother but couldn't; Agnes, whose vaginal irritation spoke of her loss of trust for her husband; Roy, whose cardiac arrhythmia betrayed his fears of imminent disaster if his wife ever found out about his affair; Alan, whose backache expressed his overwhelming burden of responsibility; and Jean, whose persistent and noisy cough announced her anger at not being heard and acknowledged. In each case, decoding the symptom meant the underlying issue could be discussed and resolved.

Illnesses 'at the level of the idea' have a purpose as well as a meaning. We have all used the excuse of bodily discomfort at one time or another to avoid facing up to difficult social situations, when we have a headache before a difficult meeting, when we feel sick before an exam or even when we leave a tiresome party guest to go to the toilet. Occasionally, this is a fabrication, but more often than not the symptoms are real, almost like the fulfilment of a wish. The most striking example of how illness can rescue a person from a situation they find painfully embarrassing was relayed to me by a young man called Mark. This is how he explained it:

I met this girl down the pub and she gave me her number and asked me to phone her some time. Well, I started to worry about it. I didn't have any money. Where would I take her? What would I talk to her about? She was bound to think I was a right idiot. Well, I worried and worried and after a few days the pain started and it took it out of my mind. The pain just took over so I phoned her up and said, 'Sorry, love, I'm not feeling very well.' She said, 'Oh well, just forget about it, then.' And you know, it felt like I had won the lottery. I felt so happy. I was so relieved. And over the next few hours, the pain disappeared.

Mark's pain offered him an acceptable means of finding relief from the social obligations that scared him so much. His stomach-ache took his mind off his fears and gave him something concrete to focus on. Mark didn't need tests and painkillers to get over his illness; he required help to enable him to understand the source of his painful embarrassment.

Illness has a way of excluding all external considerations. It just takes over, like an obsession, narrowing the perspective, so that the painful reality of the outside world becomes out of focus and our whole attention is concentrated on the illness. So when I have a migraine, it is impossible to engage in any meaningful conversation or do any work. I just have to go home and lie down in a dark room, shutting the world out.[16] Illness removes us from the situations that are causing intolerable tension. And the rest and inactivity create the optimal conditions for the body to heal itself and also to allow the necessary reflection to get things into perspective. But some situations cannot be easily dealt with: the fearful entrapment of an abusive marriage, for example; the guilt of a secret love affair; the grinding demoralisation of poverty; the shame of unemployment; and the disappointment that one's expectations never worked out. Then only the illness may provide respite from the emotional pressure.

One of the most obvious social purposes of illness is to prevent us from dealing with difficult moral dilemmas. Illness can be the excuse that leaves us stuck in the unresolved situation, sometimes for years.

Sarah has been seeing Tom for five years now. Tom is single and wants to marry her, but Sarah is already married to William who is a chartered

accountant. They have two teenage children and live in a comfortable house in the country, but William is away a lot and their relationship has become very distant. By contrast, Sarah loves Tom, and their intimacy gives her more joy than she has ever known. She has promised Tom on many occasions that she would leave William and live with him, but whenever she gets close to making a move, she realises what she would be giving up: her comfortable home and the lifestyle that goes with it, her freedom and perhaps even the children. William would surely fight her for them. And then there is the complication of her illness.

Over the last five years, she has suffered from attacks of breathlessness, palpitations and severe abdominal pain that make her feel sick and stop her from eating. At first the attacks came on when she was under stress, like when she feared that one of the boys had discovered her secret and told William, or the time that Tom had gone out with somebody else. The attacks were so bad, she felt as though she was going to die. Now, as the boys are growing up and applying for university and Tom is again trying to impose deadlines, the attacks are more or less continuous. She has lost 2 stone in weight over the last year and has been vomiting quite frequently. She has been to the doctor many times. He has examined her, carried out blood tests, X-rays and an ECG, but apart from a very rapid heartrate during the attacks, nothing specific had been found.

But although Sarah wants to get better, somehow her illness has focused her mind. As she said to Tom recently, 'I can't possibly leave William now, but I promise you, as soon as I am better, it will all be different.' And so the symptoms continue, ruling her life and the lives of everybody else, turning her into a passive invalid, dependent on the doctors to validate her excuse to keep things the way they are.

Sarah is stuck. She does not want to give Tom up – that would kill her emotionally – but she cannot relinquish the comfort and security of her life with William and the children. So, caught between safety and desire, her illness provides a reason to opt out. It conveniently freezes her dilemma.

So if the situation cannot be thought about, the disconnected tension, the risk of devastation and the feelings of hopelessness are converted into the unexplained illness, which the doctor finds impossible to cure. As such, it is no longer the result of outrageous fortune, but in a curious emotional *volte face*, becomes the cause of it. As Freud neatly described in his paper, 'Inhibitions, Symptoms and Anxiety': 'The symptom may have originally had a function, but the original reason for it has long gone, so it continues to function like an outlaw, a foreign body which keeps up a constant succession of stimuli and reactions in the tissue in which it is embedded.' Illnesses that are generated as a result of unresolved emotional tension can appear to organise the patient's life around themselves, attracting attention, providing a good reason for them to avoid occupational or domestic responsibilities, and social obligations, eliciting sympathy, care and assistance from family and friends, and if that is not forthcoming, creating a focus for the expression of grievance. As Freud commented: 'The ego appears to recognise that the symptom has come to stay and makes the best of it, drawing as much advantage from the situation as possible. It exploits the situation, like somebody with a disability getting a pension.'[17] But for this to be effective, the illness needs to be recognised and validated through the conferment of a diagnosis and the prescription of treatment. So people with severe unexplained illnesses will often undergo the most humiliating tests and debilitating treatments – even surgical operations – in order to validate an illness identity.

When the writer Alice James, who had suffered with lassitude and abdominal pain for years, was finally diagnosed with cancer, she felt that she had achieved the public recognition as a person who deserved to suffer. Her illness, however dreadful, gave her an identity, 'lifting her out of the formless vague and setting her within the very heart of the sustaining concrete':

> To him who waits all things come! My aspirations may have been eccentric, but I cannot complain now, that they have not been brilliantly fulfilled. Ever since I have been ill, I've longed and longed for some palpable disease, no matter how conventionally dreadful a label it might have, but I was always driven back to stagger along under the monstrous mass of subjective sensations, which that sympathetic being, the 'medical man', had no higher aspiration than to assure me I was personally responsible for, washing his hands of me with a graceful complacency.[18]

Chronic illness can so easily take over a patient's identity, becoming a sick sense of self that can act to prevent engagement with the difficult underlying emotional issues. The last thing patients need for an illness that protects them from intolerable reality is that it is cured, because then there would be nothing between them and despair. This, I believe, is why the powerful treatments for long-standing functional illness rarely seem to work.

Trying to cure people whose identity is protected by their illness can be like offering a hermit a room in the Holiday Inn or sending a priest to a dating agency. The role of the doctor in such illnesses is not so much to find the cause and give an effective treatment, but more to validate the individual, sanction the illness behaviour and work with him to find some way of resolving the situation that has caused the illness. As Freud commented in 'Inhibitions, Symptoms and Anxiety': 'The symptom is like a ball thrown between patient and doctor; the doctor is expected to play the game.' While the doctor attempts to treat the illness with all the science at his disposal, the patient seems to counter all his moves by evading the cure. So to extend Freud's metaphor, the game often goes into extra time, there are many replays but never a result and 'sudden death' is not an option.

But I do not for a moment believe that patients with functional illness are deliberately thwarting their doctors' efforts. Of course they want to get better, but not at the expense of continued emotional torment. It is as if the unconscious mind has decided that the illness is better than being overwhelmed with shame, consumed with rage and torn apart by self-doubt and criticism. This may also explain why the intrusions, flashbacks, mood disturbances and nightmares that so torment the victim after severe trauma often give way to a chronic illness that shields him from reality and allows the personality to function, albeit with a recognisable handicap. Seen from this perspective, illness is a desperate bid for preservation of the self. So if the illness is to be cured, a person has to be able to confront and tame their demons, but not go mad in the process. It can be a difficult thing to do.

Illness does not just serve the purpose of protecting the individual from intolerable reality, it can also have more active, even aggressive functions of punishing other people or manipulating the social environment.

Take the hunger strike of the anorexic, for example. Resentful of parental control but fearful of striking out alone, anorexic youths stage a revolt by refusing to eat. Chronic fatigue, under-achievement, drug abuse and antisocial behaviour are other ways in which adolescents may unconsciously attack their dependency on their parents or other authority figures. But at any stage in life, illness can be a powerful weapon for expressing a grievance and exacting revenge.

Judy was cross. 'You've left all the dishes in the dishwasher again. I asked you to mop the kitchen floor yesterday and it is still filthy. And why is there no milk in the fridge? I told you we were going to run out. You can't get the simplest thing right, can you? I suppose you expect me to do it all with my bad back. You just never think.'

'Oh, you can be such a pain at times,' John snaps but immediately regrets it. 'I'm sorry, love. I am trying my best.'

'But your best isn't good enough,' she retorts.

Judy is so crippled with pains in her back, her legs and her shoulders that she spends much of the time in a wheelchair and has to be taken to the shops. She also sleeps poorly and is constantly exhausted. She suffers severe headaches when she and John have 'words'. And everything that he cooks for her seems to upset her stomach. She is always down at the doctors' surgery, but they cannot find out what is wrong with her and she is sure they have stopped trying. She has written a letter of complaint to the health authority. Why should she have to suffer so much with so little help?

It wasn't always like that. When they got married, she was such a happy-go-lucky person, in love with John and lively and energetic. That was before John was posted abroad, before he got involved with gambling and before he met Ginny. But, like the trooper that she was, she worked hard, bore the loneliness, blocked out all the suspicions in her mind and brought up the children. The change came when John announced that he wanted to buy an apartment in Germany so that he could move in with Ginny. She was so angry with him that she smashed all his records, threw all of his clothes out of the bedroom window and drank the best part of a bottle of whisky. John left her to it and went for a drink with his friends. When he returned Judy was lying crumpled up, semi-conscious, at the bottom of the stairs. There was a gash on her forehead. Stricken with guilt, John called the ambulance and Judy was rushed to hospital. Fortunately, she had not sustained any serious injury, just cuts and bruises, but she never really recovered from the shock of it all, and continued to suffer severe back pains and headaches after the accident. John never left. He now works from home and spends most of his time caring for Judy.

It seems that Judy's illness has reorganised her life so as to keep John at home where she can keep an eye on him and make sure he cares for her. I don't think this is a conscious strategy, and Judy has reacted with anger when I have drawn her attention to that possibility. John's relationship with Ginny has, of course, finished and neither of them has ever talked about it again.

John is right. Judy *can* be a real pain. Her illness is an envious attack, an expression of grievance and a punishment for John's infidelity. And so, by force of projection, her pain is his pain and he has to suffer as well. We might well conclude that he deserved it, but that is not the point. It seems that Judy's illness has trapped both of them.

But illness is not only deployed to attack other people. It is often used to attack oneself. Rather like the scourges of medieval penitents, illness can punish the body for some sin that is so alien to a person's sense of self it cannot be acknowledged or forgiven. But however bad the pain may be, it is better than being exposed to the devastating reality of what has happened.

Yvonne came to see me with a combination of headaches, vomiting and abdominal pain, for which there was no obvious medical explanation and which didn't respond to any treatment. Over the course of the following weeks, her story came out.

Yvonne was an only child who had been brought up by elderly parents in their house in the country. She went to the local school, enjoyed riding her horse and going to town on Saturday afternoon with her friends. By the age of sixteen, she was desperate to leave home and experience 'life'. Unfortunately, she got more life than she was prepared for. During her first year at university, she met and fell in love with Jim, a likeable lad who was so much more streetwise than she was. Within a few months she was pregnant. Jim tried to persuade her to have an abortion, but Yvonne could not bear to think about that, and she could not tell her parents about what had happened. She tried to forget about her pregnancy and carry on with her college work, but she couldn't sleep and suffered from frequent and severe headaches. Jim became impatient and left her. She was desperate. She was not keeping up with her college work, she was pregnant, she felt ill, her boyfriend was going out with somebody else and there was nobody she could talk to about it. One night she swallowed a handful of the tablets the doctor had given her to help her sleep and washed it down with a bottle of vodka. She woke up ten hours later with a blinding headache, was very sick and had severe abdominal pain. She was rushed to hospital where she went into labour. Her baby, a little girl, was nearly three months premature and did not survive more than a few hours.

Yvonne was numb. She did not return to her studies, but spent days wandering along the riverbank in a dazed state, contemplating suicide. She felt she had killed her baby girl and deserved to be punished. She was rescued by her landlady, who rang her parents and asked them to come down and collect her.

Yvonne's parents never discovered what had gone wrong and Yvonne almost succeeded in blotting the whole episode from her mind. Her sick headaches and bouts of abdominal cramping commenced shortly after she had returned home and started to pull herself together. They not only kept her at home and stopped her moving on, but became her punishment, essentially putting her in prison. As she explained to me, 'I have done such a terrible thing, I just don't deserve to get better.' Eventually she did tell her parents and although they were shocked they did not judge her.

The turning point came when Yvonne realised that she was not the only person who had done something to be ashamed of. She began to ask herself why she was so special, why she needed to make her parents suffer so much, why she couldn't take responsibility for her own life. Slowly she began to forgive herself and let go, and as she did, so her headaches and abdominal symptoms abated and she felt well enough to go out. Several years later I received a letter from Yvonne. She had just given birth to her daughter, and she and her husband, Mike, were very happy.

Yvonne's symptoms not only exacted a fearful punishment for her perceived sins, but they protected her from the reality of what had happened and the unbearable emotional torment.

In the same way, when somebody is depressed, physical symptoms can often hide the shame and guilt that diminishes them and project their unhappiness onto much more acceptable external causes. What is played out in the individual is also represented at a cultural level. Western societies have sought to deny emotional causes for unexplained physical symptoms and have provided a variety of definitive causes. It is little wonder that people with functional illness hold on to these fixed attributions with a fierce tenacity. For them, the food allergies, the candidiasis, the mercury poisoning, the immune dysfunction can seem like a life raft thrown to a drowning man.

I do, of course, realise how offensive the protective or adaptive notion of functional illness will be to the many people who believe there is a definite physical cause for their illness, but let me emphasise one important point: in the whole of my medical career, I have yet to meet anybody I thought was imagining their symptoms or making them up, but I *have* met thousands upon thousands of ill people who are struggling desperately to protect themselves from the potentially mind-shattering effects of unbearable life situations. These people don't deserve to be dismissed with a diagnosis that cannot be treated. Their illness needs to be understood as a state of disharmony involving the whole person – mind, body and spirit – within their particular social environment. And they need to be helped to uncover its meaning and to find an appropriate resolution for what caused it.

Illnesses that have no basis in pathology can only really be understood in the context of specific events in a person's life. Only if the doctor can hear the illness 'narrative' and understand the plot can they help their patient write their own happy ending. Unfortunately, in Western countries, doctors are scientists, not storytellers. This can lead to a mismatch of expectations, resulting in a grievance and in some cases litigation.

In the beginning the patient may feel that the doctor is the only one who can understand and help them: 'You are my last chance. I have been to so many specialists, but nobody has been able to find out what's wrong. But I know you will be able to help me.' The problem with being put on a pedestal is that when the idealised person falls from grace, as they must, they come down with a bump. So the insistent quality of the symptom, the demand to be heard, the elusive diagnosis and the failure of treatment frustrate the doctor, who retreats behind logical explanation and bland reassurance. The complaints become more insistent and the doctor ultimately reacts with rejection, recapitulating the patient's life experience and intensifying the grievance.

Surgery is particularly fraught with danger for such patients and their medical carers.

Jason was fine until he had the laparoscopy; at least, that's what he told me. The doctor was sure that there was nothing seriously wrong, but his pain was so insistent and Jason was so distressed that he asked Mr Thompson, the surgeon, to see him. But it wasn't the consultant who conducted the procedure, it was Mr Hasim, his trainee registrar. Jason was disappointed and irritated by this but couldn't explain to Mr Hasim how he felt. Unfortunately during the procedure the bowel was perforated and an operation was required to repair the tear in the colon. He woke up four hours later in much more pain and with a wound across his abdomen. When his drowsiness wore off, he was very angry. Nobody, he asserted, had told him this could happen. Although the repair was successful, Jason's pain continued and over the course of the next few months, it spread to other parts of his abdomen and even into his back. He found walking difficult, became quite constipated and even experienced episodes of urinary incontinence and leakage. Jason was quite unable to go to work and Simone his wife had to take on extra hours at the call centre where she worked. Jason declared that the surgeon had wrecked his life.

As I got to know Jason better, it became clear that his pain had started after an argument, during which he had accused Simone of not caring for him and flirting with Andy, his best friend. But what started as an expression of grievance against Simone had been transferred to the hospital and doctors who didn't care. With no opportunity for any reasonable discussion with the hospital, he started litigation proceedings. The most important thing for Jason was to be proved right, even though this meant he could not let go of his grievance and his illness. He could not acknowledge that the grievance against the surgeon was the latest in a sequence of grievances against Simone for ignoring him, his mother who was always too ill to have time for him and – the big one – his father who had abandoned him and left home. But none of this came out in court. In fact, the hospital settled out of court for a six-figure sum. The symptoms improved, but not to the extent that Simone had to stop looking after him.

Although Jason had undoubtedly received an injury, due to the inexperience of a trainee who had not explained the possible complications of laparoscopy, and deserved some compensation, it was clear that his treatment by the hospital tapped into a pre-existing deep well of grievance, for which he demanded revenge.

Litigation against employers, the health service and national corporations has risen exponentially in the last thirty years and professional indemnity for doctors in the UK has increased fivefold since 1980.

From the religious martyrs of antiquity to the political hunger strikers of the late twentieth century, illness can be employed as an eloquent expression of social discontent. As the medical anthropologist Arthur Kleinman wrote: 'Physical symptoms are the weapons of the weak, and they can be skilfully deployed to gain attention, attenuate injustice, apply leverage, express grievance, secure compensation and otherwise undermine otherwise unassailable power holders.' For example, the epidemic of neurasthenia in the decades following the Chinese Cultural Revolution eloquently symbolised the way in which the revolution had affected the population. According to Kleinman: 'The exhaustion expressed how recent history had deprived society of "Qi" or vital energy, the complaints of pain connoted painful social relationships, dizziness represented alienation from the local social context and from the political process. When seen in context, neurasthenia created a channel for expressing sanctioned criticism against the state in coded form.'[19]

So what occurs at the level of society is played out in the physiology of the individual. If the culture denotes the meaning of events (how we feel about them) and meaning is expressed in the body, it must play a major role in configuring illness and determining the conditions which lead to its expression. That is the topic of the next chapter.

7

Cultural ailments

My brother, Simon, is an artist who uses photography to investigate the notion that any image is not only a record of the particular event, but also a product of a chosen medium and specific circumstance. He once built a hand-driven panoramic camera, which, when used on a mobile platform, would document the particular conditions of making the picture. With this camera mounted in the bows of his workboat, the North Sea swell turned the Suffolk coastal horizon into an exotic squiggle, complete with prosaic details such as beach huts and shingle.[1] So just as a photographic image can be governed by the characteristics of a camera, the way we perceive our world and the meaning it has for us is determined by the particular conditions of our culture. Culture is a perceptual filter that conditions the ways we interpret and respond to life situations, regulating our feelings and directing our behaviour.

As we began to explore in Chapter Four, children are entrained by their parents and mentors to 'take on board' the attitudes, beliefs and customs of their culture. It is these cultural mores, as expressed in the behaviour of their parents, that direct the way the emotional brain develops and thus the way children feel and think, and the way their bodies react. This nascent process of socialisation, underpinned by neuronal growth and destruction, is further conditioned during childhood and adolescence by interactions with the extended family, friends, teachers and mentors, and informed by cultural narratives in the form of historic events, fables, myths, religion, beliefs, lives of famous people, and, in our current age, newspaper comment, television drama and documentary. And throughout the life cycle, changes in the culture are incorporated into the personality, directing the life of an individual through predilection and prejudice. Cultural attitudes influence every aspect of our emotional lives, from the most sophisticated aspects of personal engagement to the way we dress and eat, right down to the most basic bodily function.[2] In his book, *The Body and Society*, the sociologist Bryan S. Turner wrote: 'As a vehicle for emotional expression, the passionate body, its secretions, its sexuality, the activity of its guts, all of its unruly behaviour and irrational functions come under the control of the culture.'[3]

Thus, there is a hot line between society and physiology that can link religion to eating behaviour, education to asthma and maybe even politics to bowel function. I am not trying to suggest that all Roman Catholics have a tendency to anorexia or that members of the British Conservative Party are prone to constipation, but the possibilities are intriguing.

In the last chapter, I described how functional illness may be configured according to the meaning it conveys for the patient. But meaning is conditioned by the attitudes, beliefs and customs of the culture. So the illness comes to embody the experience of the individual as perceived through a cultural filter. In other words, the sorts of illness that are prevalent in a particular culture could be said to represent the sickness of the society at large. Or, as Athena Vrettos elegantly expressed it, 'If human bodies can register signs of cultural distress – then the interpretation of illness becomes an important form of social cartography.'[4]

There is one illness that has survived for over two and half thousand years of Western civilisation. Its transformations offer fascinating insights into the influence of changing cultural attitudes on the expression and attribution of illness. That illness is 'hysteria'. Ilza Veith wrote a scholarly and fascinating monograph on the subject:

> Hysteria is an extraordinarily interesting disease, and a strange one. It is encountered in the earliest pages of recorded medicine and is dealt with in current psychiatric literature. Throughout all the intervening years it has been known and accepted as though it were a readily recognisable entity. And yet, except for the fact that it is a functional disorder, without concomitant organic pathological change, it defies definition and any attempt to portray it concretely. Like a globule of mercury it escapes the grasp. Whenever it appears, it takes on the colours of the ambient culture and mores; and thus through the ages it presents itself

as a shifting, changing, mist-enshrouded phenomenon that must, nevertheless, be dealt with as if it were definite and tangible.[5]

Hysteria, derived from the Greek work for 'womb', was first used to describe a variety of unexplained feminine illnesses that were thought to be associated with barrenness and absence of sexual relations. Plato (427–347 BC) provided the most graphic contemporary description in his dialogue, *Timaeus*:

> The womb is an animal which longs to generate children. When it remains barren too long after puberty, it is distressed and sorely disturbed and, straying about in the body and cutting off the passages of the breath, it impedes respiration and brings the sufferer into the extremest anguish and provokes all manner of diseases besides. This disturbance continues until the womb is appeased by passion and love. Such is the nature of women and all that is female.

For the ancients, barrenness was a social stigma and caused great anxiety. But observing that unmarried women or widows were more likely to suffer such symptoms than those who enjoyed a normal married life, the ancient physicians – all, of course, male – assumed that if a womb was deprived of its regular infusions of semen it would shrivel and migrate around the body in search of moisture and sustenance, attaching itself to other organs in its restless journey and causing all kinds of symptoms. The notion of the wandering womb offered a convenient explanation for the various expressions of female illness. For example, if the womb came to rest under the ribcage it caused spasms and convulsions; if it rose towards the chest, it cut off the respiration and caused shortness of breath; if it attached itself to the heart, it caused anxiety and oppression and could induce vomiting; and if it fastened itself to the liver, the patient lost her voice, gritted her teeth and her complexion turned ashen. When it lodged in the loins, it could be felt as a hard ball or lump in her sides. When it rose into the neck, it caused suffocation and could be felt as 'a lump in the throat'.[6] When it reached the head, it caused pains around the eyes and the nose, the head felt heavy and drowsiness and lethargy set in. Observing that young women suffered more illness than old women, the physicians of the time assumed it was because their womb was more erratic.

But not all the ancient medical philosophers believed in the wandering womb. Galen of Pergamon (AD 129–99), whose anatomical insights were refined after his appointment as physician to the gladiators, was scornful of the notion. Instead, he came up with another womb-based theory, that the retention of menstrual blood and semen could poison the body, causing a variety of dramatic symptoms. This explanation neatly overcame the awkward fact that expressions of hysterical illness, in particular indigestion, could be observed in men, particularly those who were sexually continent. Galen's ideas were to endure for another 1,800 years and were a popular explanation for the toxic 'vapours' that women suffered from in eighteenth-century Europe.

In medieval England, hysteria was much more likely to be equated with sin. Taking the words of Saint Augustine as their source of inspiration – 'there are no diseases that do not arise from witchery and hence from the mind' – a defensive Christian Church attributed the expression of otherwise unexplained physical illness to diabolic possession and witchcraft.[7] This changed the expression of hysteria from the more familiar aches and pains to a theatrical portrayal of demonic possession. And so people who were troubled in spirit for the sins they feared they had committed often 'presented with' dramatic symptoms, including refusal to eat, muteness, crying, shouting, swearing, disrespectful behaviour, visual hallucinations, delusions, fits as well as such bodily symptoms as pains, sores, itching, abdominal distension, loss of hearing and sight, a sensation of a ball in the throat. These symptoms became the punishments, people suffering from guilt and shame felt they deserved, and the means of their redemption.

By the late Georgian and early Victorian eras in England, hysterical illness had taken the form of an epidemic of paralyses, faintness, weakness and weight loss, more in tune with contemporary discoveries in the nervous system. These curious neurological ailments primarily affected young upper-middle-class women.

Accomplished, highly educated but not allowed to work, women of society were expected to marry well, love their husbands, run the marital home and bear children. Thus, when they reached marriage-able age, they were often confined to the family home and were chaperoned if they went out, lest they ruin themselves and their families by falling in love with a charming man with no prospects. Their only hope of freedom was in marriage, but marriage was often arranged as a contract between the parents of the betrothed. So what value freedom if they could neither lead their own lives nor marry the man they loved? Caught between the restrictive tedium of family life and the oppression of an unfortunate marriage, 'spinal irritation' was a peculiarly apt diagnosis. It expressed in dramatic form the sense of powerlessness or inability to 'move'. As Dr Walter Johnson expressed it: 'Many a young maiden stretched herself upon the bed or sofa and vegetated many a weary month in slothful languor or was sent away to the spas of Europe for the water cure.'

The famous Victorian traveller, Isabella Bird (1831–1904), suffered from an undiagnosed spinal complaint, insomnia, aches and pains and depression. When her husband died she took herself off to India, Persia, China, Australia and Hawaii, and all her ailments mysteriously disappeared. 'I am well as long as I live on horseback, go to bed at eight, sleep out of doors or in a log cabin, and lead in all respects an unconventional life,' she said. Every time she became 'civilised' she went downhill again.[8]

'Spinal irritation' not only acted out the dilemma that young women found themselves in, it also provided an acceptable if somewhat dysfunctional solution for it. How could young women commit themselves to a marriage if they were too weak to walk? Popular romantic novels of the Georgian and Victorian eras contributed to the epidemic of 'nervous illness' of the time by offering templates that young women could identify with. As Athena Vrettos commented: 'Heroines embodied sentiment, they were able to swoon at length and weep at will, take to their couches and waste away from disappointment.'[9]

So, by the nineteenth century, the feminine ailments that were originally attributed to the clumsiness of the 'wandering' womb or to the toxic degradation products of retained blood or semen, were ascribed to nervous reflexes triggered by the 'irritable' womb or ovary. Nowadays these womb-based theories of hysteria have echoes in the multifarious symptoms associated with premenstrual syndrome or the menopause, but are more likely to be explained by disturbances in the secretion of the reproductive hormones, oestrogen and progesterone.

As the hypnotic cures popularised by the Parisian neurologist Jean-Martin Charcot became fashionable, hysteria took on increasingly theatrical dissociations and paralyses. But when neurological diagnosis became more refined in the early years of the twentieth century, the florid neurological expressions faded away to be replaced by sensory symptoms of pain, fatigue and pins and needles, which were more difficult to disprove. But as Dr Henri Schaeffer, a Paris physician, indicated, 'the neuroses never disappear. Old as the world, they will vanish only with humanity itself. Hysteria is much the same: really just a manner of speaking. Its symptoms have changed in form . . . because the times and the culture have changed. The patients we see nowadays no longer present the stigmata of old-style hysteria because they have not had the same conditioning.'[10]

Hysteria was not the only historical concept to account for unexplained illness. Throughout history, people have needed to find an explanation for their illness that was compatible with contemporary beliefs. Moreover, the shape that illness adopted reflected those beliefs.

For example, young men of education and learning living in London towards the end of the sixteenth century were said to suffer from a strange kind of malaise. The predominant symptoms were lassitude and a lack of ambition and purpose best characterised by the French term '*ennui*', but they also included faintness, abdominal pain, bloating, constipation and heartburn. At the time, the disorder was attributed to 'melancholia', a surfeit of black bile, but medical historian Lindsay Knights suggested that this Elizabethan malady reflected a state of cultural dissonance, the effect of being lost in a changing world.[11] Young upper-class men living in London in the late-sixteenth century were better educated than their forebears, but far from providing opportunities for advancement, their education created expectations that could not be realised. The old system of patronage for educated men with literary, musical and artistic talents was in decline and few could find support. Life seemed pointless, and they literally became bored sick.

Boredom was rarely the problem for people living in the overcrowded communities of Victorian cities. Many felt afflicted by the sheer pace of life, and often complained of their 'nerves'.[12]

William Griesinger, erstwhile Professor of Psychiatry in Berlin, explained what was happening by evoking the scientific concept of 'irritable weakness':

> The more excited or irritated that the brain becomes, the less effectively it executes its functions. In individuals born with a nervous constitution, irritable weakness amplifies sensory impressions into great agitation. On the motor side irritable weakness means that the motor nerves are hallmarked by a decrease in power; there is easy exhaustibility, a tendency to quicker and more widespread but simultaneously less

energetic movements and a heightened tendency to convulsions [and] ... greater psychical sensitivity, an easier susceptibility to psychic pain, the condition wherein every thought causes some emotional agitation. This in turn causes a rapid and unopposed change in self-image and mood, also weakness and lack of consequence of the will, a lack of energy in all affairs combined with rapidly alternating desires.[13]

But it was George Beard's concept of nervous exhaustion or neurasthenia that really captured the public imagination (see p. 21). By 1906, neurasthenia was six times as common as hysteria in the city of London.

In non-Western cultures, there is not the distinction between body and mind that Descartes has bequeathed to Western medicine. So what we call depression in the West manifests in Eastern cultures as somatic symptoms, especially weakness, bowel consciousness, exaggerated fear of a heart attack and concern over the health of genital organs.[14] The Korean syndrome, *hwa byung*, is a distinctive physical illness that is easily recognised by members of the same culture. Bodily symptoms include feelings of heaviness, burning or a lump in the region of the lower chest and upper abdomen, headaches, muscular aches and pains, dry mouth, insomnia, palpitations and indigestion. But *hwa byung* also incorporates sadness, loss of interest, feelings of regret, guilt, anxiety, irritability, tendency to lose one's temper and absent-mindedness. It is thought to be associated with difficulties in adapting to social change. Among Korean immigrants to the United States, *hwa byung* is found predominantly among middle-aged married men and women of lower socio-economic status. Separated from their culture and disadvantaged by their background, their sense of injustice cannot be expressed verbally for cultural reasons and its suppression leads to the bodily expression of resentment and despair.

Throughout the Middle East, references to the heart are commonly understood as natural metaphors for a range of emotions. *Naharatiye qalb*, which literally means 'my heart is uneasy' afflicts the Maragheh people in Iran and combines symptoms of trembling, fluttering and pounding of the heart with feelings of anxiety, unhappiness and anger. More frequent among women, it often follows quarrels or conflicts within the family. The medical anthropologist Byron Good described it as a culturally prescribed way of expressing a number of personal and social concerns primarily related to loss and grief, but also to recent conflicts over the use of the contraceptive pill. In the Punjabi people, *dir ghirda hai*, or the sinking heart, is associated with profound fear of social failure, loss of honour (*izzat*) and low self-esteem. Men with *dir ghirda hai* fret about not being able to carry out their social and moral obligations, and particularly their inability to control the sexual behaviour of their wives, sisters or daughters. It is a powerful expression of shame.

And in Southern Asia, many physical and psychological symptoms are attributed to the loss of vital essence through semen. In India, this is called *dhat*; in Pakistan, *jiryan*. Patients often feel shame over masturbation and express great concern about nocturnal emissions and turbid urine. The same concerns were expressed in Victorian England. Compulsive masturbation, or so it was believed, did much more than ruin the eyesight of Victorian males; it was thought to cause increased appetite, parched skin, loss of hair, stammering, deafness, blindness, shyness, suspicion and fear, dread, suicidal impulses and heart palpitations. General weakness was a most common result, followed by headache, backache, acne, indigestion, blindness, deafness, epilepsy and finally death.[15] But it wasn't necessarily masturbation as such that made men feel so awful, it was feeling so disempowered and lonely that compelled them to find relief through masturbation.

So patients with cultural illnesses do not so much need doctors to carry out diagnostic tests, they need interpreters to help them understand the allegory of illness and support their return to health. In South Africa, the traditional healers, called Sangoma, are not only knowledgeable in herbs and spices and simple surgical procedures, they are also storytellers. They are able to frame the illness in a narrative that the patient can identify with and use to get well. Traditional folk medicine survives alongside Western scientific medicine in Africa, China and many other parts of the world. People go to their traditional healers for illnesses that need interpretation and to the Western doctors for more obvious manifestations of organic disease, like tuberculosis.

Just as historical and traditional illnesses have been shaped by the cultures in which they are found, so modern illnesses are configured by the particular fears and concerns of our contemporary culture. So when prolonged feelings of guilt, shame or grievance disturb the harmony of the body, then the illnesses that ensue embody the dilemmas of our age and culture. If, as I have suggested in Chapter

Five, people are struggling to find some meaning in their lives, then illness not only conveys that sense of disruption, it also becomes a vehicle for conformity.

The medical sociologist Bryan S. Turner coined the term 'the Somatic Society' to express the idea that the major political and personal problems of our age are expressed through the body, especially in areas of sexuality, eating behaviour, bowel function and illness. So concerns over food safety may be represented as increases in reports of food intolerance or allergy,[16] fears of pollution as rising rates of asthma and hay fever, and fears of disempowerment as sexual impotence. This connection between society and physiology might also explain why allergies have been noted to increase (and skirt lengths fall) at times of economic instability, and how medicalised fatigue can be an acceptable way of opting out of the ever-increasing demands of modern society. Displacement of more abstract and distant threats onto the more tangible areas of the body allows us to discern what they mean for us – literally, how we feel about them – and how they can be resolved.

There can be no clearer example of cultural influence on physiological function than in disturbances in eating behaviour. Obesity, for example, may be thought of as a personal state of overconsumption within a consumer society.

Madonna proclaimed that because we are living in a material world, so she is a material girl. The culture insists on it. We are a population of consumers. The belief that particular products will make us feel good about ourselves is reinforced everywhere; it shouts at us in the street from giant advertising hoardings, it slips in through the letterbox, and it captures and seduces us in our living room through the television screen. Every pause in the scheduled programmes is filled with advertisements with images of happy, healthy, beautiful people exhorting us to buy, buy, buy if we want to be like them. The jingles and catchphrases become so much part of us that we find ourselves passing them on, promoting the message in our daily conversations – just because, according to the L'Oréal advert, we're worth it! Buying things, eating and drinking might be regarded as personal therapy. They fulfil our needs, they plug the emotional gap – for a while.

In the last fifty years, not only have we become increasingly isolated from the emotional support and comfort of family and community, we have become increasingly exposed to the seductions of television advertising. So people who struggle to find their place in the world obtain a surrogate for the love they so desire and the companionship they crave, by eating special rich foods, drinking the alcopop with a kick, and going out shopping.[17] And the more we consume the better we feel. So it is not surprising that diseases of overconsumption have increased dramatically over the last twenty to thirty years.

Janice is 5 ft, 4 in, weighs nearly 13 stone and works as a receptionist for a local dentist. She has always struggled with her weight. She knows she eats too much but she can't seem to stop herself. When she feels insecure, she binges on chocolate, biscuits and breakfast cereals. She just can't stop. She hates herself for what she is doing but the more she hates herself the more lonely she feels and the more she needs to eat. She can eat a whole packet of cereal with milk and sugar plus several bars of chocolate until she makes herself sick. Then she starts all over again. Eating seems to relax her, but only for a short time. So she has to go on eating and being sick until she falls asleep with exhaustion.

The following day is often different. Disgusted with her weak behaviour, she resolves to be better. So she has a bath, puts on clean clothes, tidies her hair, plans her day's work and becomes focused and controlled. She tries to fill her time by doing things. She takes a book into work to read whenever there is a gap between clients. She does not dare to relax, even to sleep, because it is when she cannot fill the time that she feels empty and needs something to eat. And once she has started, she says to herself, 'What the hell, I've given in now, so I'd best have as much as I want.' But it isn't just eating that relieves Janice's tension. She loves to buy new clothes and when she is on a 'binge', she cannot stop herself from spending hundreds of pounds on blouses or skirts that she doesn't really need. And if she has a drink of wine, she cannot have just one, she has to finish the bottle and start another one. When Janice talks to me, I am constantly aware of her need to 'devour' the space between us by feeding me with information. She seems so greedy for my attention.

She tells me how much she hates being fat. It makes her feel worthless. But at the same time she feels safe. As she put it, 'When I am fat, girls are not jealous of me and boys don't whistle at me.'

Janice knows that the cause of her problems is that she has no confidence. Her mum and dad split up when she was three. She and her sister lived with their mother in an isolated high-rise apartment in the centre of the city. She hated it there; people would urinate in the lifts and there were piles of rubbish at the

bottom of the stairwells. She just dreamt of when she could go and stay with her father and his wife in the pretty bedroom they had prepared for her, but that only happened very rarely. In the meantime, she had to cope with poverty and squalor. Her mother was loud and unkempt; she would drink heavily and invite male friends into the house. She just didn't seem to care. Janice was always a fussy eater, so in desperation, her mother would often give her 50p to get some snacks from the corner shop.

Deprived of love and attention and feeding herself on junk from the corner shop and images of the luxuries that were advertised on television, it is not surprising that Janice grew up with a tendency to console herself by bingeing on snack foods and buying pretty clothes. These activities compensated for the mother who couldn't look after her enough and the society that didn't care. Overeating rarely occurs by itself. It is often associated with other compulsive and consuming behaviours that calm tension and induce temporary feelings of well-being. These include heavy drinking, drug taking, compulsive sexual behaviour and, as in Janice's case, shopping, and might all be seen as strategies for finding release from the loneliness of modern life.[18]

Overconsumption and obesity can be viewed from many different perspectives: biochemical, physiological, psychological, developmental, cultural, genetic and evolutionary. But no matter from which angle we view it, a similar impression emerges: obesity appears to be a response to a sense of deprivation. For example, Professor David Barker and his colleagues from the MRC Epidemiology Unit at the University of Southampton have shown convincing evidence that infants who were born abnormally small or who weighed less than normal at the age of one, are more likely to become overweight or obese in middle age.[19] Low birth-weight and failure to thrive in the first year of life often occurs as a result of maternal stress, leading to a resetting of cortisol levels, a more conservative metabolism and a tendency to overconsume in later life.[20] Similarly psychological studies have confirmed Janice's story by showing how emotional deprivation in childhood may predispose to binge eating and obesity.[21] And most surprisingly, it seems from an evolutionary perspective that the societies that are more at risk of obesity are those who have lived in an inhospitable environment and become adapted to a very low level of food intake. These include the Pima Indians of Arizona and Northern Mexico, and the nomads of the Arabian peninsula. Only those endowed with the genetic configuration favouring the most conservative metabolism would have been able to survive and breed in such a harsh environment. But when the culture changes and food is available in abundance, these same people would tend to put on a lot of weight.[22] And from a cultural perspective, the current epidemic of obesity might be seen as a reaction to the loneliness of living in our modern narcissistic society where everybody is preoccupied with their own problems and nobody really cares. So a society that has grown too large and impersonal to provide a nurturing environment is also a society where the population is likely to suffer from illnesses of need and overconsumption. Viewed from this perspective, bingeing is a desperate cry to be looked after.

So if cultural change is responsible for the epidemic of over-consumption and obesity, how is it that so many young women are starving themselves? Anorexia nervosa is a wasting illness that affects about 600,000 young women in the UK, but if we add the vast numbers of girls who put themselves on strict diets in order to achieve the slim physique so envied by our culture, this figure is multiplied tenfold. Anorexia nervosa tends predominantly to affect girls who have only recently gone through puberty. What may start as dietary restriction caused by a concern about weight can quickly develop into a profound suppression of eating behaviour resulting in an alarming and often dangerous loss of weight, a reversal of adult body shape and suppression of menstruation. In mainstream medicine, anorexia accompanies infections, cancers and inflammatory disease, but ano-rexia nervosa is a functional illness. As such, it has a social context, a cultural identification and a political purpose. So what does anorexia nervosa mean for the person who suffers from it, the family and for society as a whole? Is it just a reaction to the ideas of a consumer society – or is it much more complicated?

Reena came from an ambitious Asian family. Both parents were health professionals and Reena was expected to go to medical school and become a doctor. Her mother would make sure that she did four hours of homework every night as well as help her with the housework and cooking. Theirs was a traditional Asian family. They ate Asian food and wore Asian clothes. Reena embodied the family culture until the age of sixteen; she worked hard and passed puberty to achieve the desired rounded feminine shape. But Reena was a spirited young woman with a mind of her own and she was determined to express it. Most of her friends were fashion-conscious girls with trim figures and a modern outlook on life. So after completing her GCSEs and achieving the expected excellent grades, she started dieting. She wanted to be perfect and, in her adopted Western culture, that meant being slim. Within six months her weight had gone down from 10 stone to less than 6 stone. She felt wonderful; so powerful and invincible. She was totally in charge of her life and her parents could not do a damned thing about it. She didn't need anyone or anything. It was as if her feelings were numbed; she had no regrets, no worries, no desires, nothing. She described this as feeling 'innocent'. During her first year in the sixth form, she worked very hard, but by the time she was in the upper sixth, she was finding it difficult to concentrate and she needed to take a cushion in to sit on because the bones in her bottom hurt. Her father urged her to see a psychiatrist, but what prompted her to resume eating was when one of her close friends was admitted to hospital with extreme weight loss and nearly died.

Now the problem changed. Once she had started to eat, she couldn't stop; she became obsessed with food and her weight rebounded to 12 stone within a few months. She began making herself sick, but this was much worse than the anorexia, because it seemed so self-destructive. She hated herself. She failed to achieve the required grades to go to medical school and, much against her parents' wishes, decided to leave school and applied to study nutrition in a university 200 miles away.

Her eating disorder resolved almost as soon as she left home. She felt happy at university, stopped thinking about food and her weight stabilised at 9 stone, which was about normal for her height. When I interviewed her, another four years had gone and she had not returned to her anorexic or bingeing behaviour, though she did notice that she had a tendency to put weight on when she felt under stress.

Reena's anorexia could be seen in many ways: as a rebellion against her parents' ambitions; a reaction to a consumer society; a clash of cultural identities; an assertion of her self; and a denial of adult responsibilities. As a child she had never had the space to be herself. Her anorexia gave her that space, and while that could be a powerful, heady experience, it also made her feel frightened and vulnerable. That vulnerability was expressed by her fragile, painfully thin body. What nourished her sense of identity destroyed her body.

For the anorexic, the over-protective family is a metaphorical prison, or as Hilde Bruch described it, *The Gilded Cage*.[23] The mothers of anorexic girls are often portrayed as anxious and unable to relinquish control over the lives of their daughters, who can grow up feeling that their mother's happiness depends on them doing well. Their fathers, on the other hand, are often depicted as absent figures, either physically away a lot or busy and emotionally distant, unable to rescue their daughters from the smothering attentions of their mothers by providing another point of view. So, lacking the space to be themselves and desperate to get out, anorexics resort to extreme measures. They refuse to eat, just as they might have done when they were toddlers. What better act of rebellion against parental control? Anorexia provides the imprisoned ego with a sense of power, freedom from the obligation of having to work hard and be good. But in the very act of gaining that autonomy, the anorexic loses it by becoming ill and creating a very special identity that attracts and requires care and concern.

As a symbolic rebellion against seemingly overwhelming control and an attempt to create a purer and more powerful identity through self-denial, anorexia equates with ancient concepts of religious asceticism – the attainment of spiritual purity through mortification of the flesh. But there would be little purpose in such a strategy unless there was a fear of being corrupted and overwhelmed by society. Therefore the asceticism of diet is inevitably harnessed to the hedonism and dependency of consumption.

Post-modern culture offers so many temptations for unbridled hedonism that people who are able to avoid being taken over by its corrupting influence are respected and envied, even if this means half starving themselves in the process. Of course, not all dieting leads to the clinical picture of anorexia nervosa, but both are part of the same process. A culture that predisposes to dieting as a means of gaining self-esteem will also create the template for anorexia. Many young women can only feel good in their own eyes and in the eyes of others by avoiding temptation. But such a strategy needs some focus of identification to sustain it.

In modern Western societies, slimness is culturally equated with personal control and social acceptability. For the last fifty years, contemporary representations of feminine style and beauty have been slim. Starting with 'Twiggy' in the 1960s, thin personalities such as Princess Diana, Elle ('the Body') MacPherson and Victoria Beckham have become cultural icons for millions of young women. They embody the notion that a woman who can control her weight can also control her emotions and be successful, powerful and attractive. But although slimming establishes a body that conforms to contemporary ideas, it also discourages the dangers of sexual attention by its immaturity and fragility. A century ago, women with tuberculosis were portrayed as tragically romantic figures with a fragile and ethereal beauty that protected them from more earthbound relationships. And for fashionable Victorian ladies, the corset offered respectability and attractiveness while denying desire. So by keeping the body 'strait-laced', and 'uptight' and 'in shape', it also kept the self together.[24]

Feminist writers such as Susie Orbach portray the cultural phenomenon of anorexia nervosa in women as a rebellion against male dominance. This notion is embodied in the suppression of both eating and sexuality in anorexics, both activities that encourage emotional dependency. The idea rings true to a point and is certainly fashionable, but anorexia nervosa might also be seen as a reaction to the sexual and emotional liberation of women. With liberation comes greater expectations. Not only are women expected to compete for jobs with men, there is also peer group pressure to behave in a more sexually adventurous and assertive manner as well as to be a caring and responsible mother. This places great demands on the modern woman. As never before, she is expected to do it all and while she may be less dominated by men, she is perhaps less protected by them. No wonder many adolescent girls approach adult responsibilities with trepidation and back away into illness.

Although modern society places great emphasis on the demands of the self over the needs of the community, it provides mixed messages. In the workplace, it promotes a collective, corporate responsibility, while at home and in personal lives, it encourages people to exercise choice. From a historical and cultural perspective, this might be seen as a transitional state from the work ethic of manufacture to the freedoms of consumerism – from asceticism to hedonism. This cultural contradiction has been mirrored in the regulation of the self and the symptoms people suffer from,[25] although nowadays we might view it as a dialectic between autonomy 'implying control' and need 'implying dependence'. Unable to deal with and resolve situations that challenge their notion of who they are, insecure personalities can either withdraw and close up, keeping their behaviour tightly controlled, or escape into consuming behaviours such as eating, alcohol and drug abuse, gambling, spending and sex in order to relieve their bodily tensions. This lack of balance is also played out in fluctuating bodily symptoms, most obviously in areas of eating behaviour and bowel function.

Tanya is tall with raven-black hair, laughing eyes and a ready smile. She works for a high-profile public relations company and seems to be a young woman who likes to enjoy life. Appearances can be deceptive.

Tanya was referred to me with a strange constellation of symptoms: burning stomach; sore throat; sore eyes; hot head, hands and feet; and bowel upsets. They reminded her of the feelings she would have if she had drunk too much. And as she told me more about herself, it became increasingly clear that her pattern of symptoms bore a striking relationship with her personality and ambivalent way of life.

Tanya is popular and can be the life and soul of any party. She is amusing, flamboyant and extrovert. When she feels happy, she enjoys eating rich and spicy foods and drinking red wine. She frequently drinks too much, takes recreational drugs and may spend the rest of the night in bed with somebody she has only just met. But after such a night out, she would invariably feel awful; she would have a bad headache, get diarrhoea and bloating, and feel sick. She would also feel dirty, out of control and deeply ashamed of herself, and determined to get her life together. So, for the next few days, she would refuse invitations, stay in, eat sensible foods, such as scrambled eggs, soup, custard, milk, toast, baby foods, salads, bran and vegetables, avoid alcohol, go to the gym and take frequent showers. Her bowel habit would change to constipation and she would begin to feel tired and depressed. So after a week or two she would tell herself to get a life. So she would go to the next party and the cycle would repeat itself. Tanya has never really been able to establish a long-term relationship with a partner.

Isolated from family and close relationships and unsure of how 'to be', Tanya oscillates between hedonism and restraint, and each is played out in her body. Neither seems to satisfy what she really needs – a consistent, loving relationship – but unfortunately she cannot trust other people or indeed herself.

The erosion of social ties and the replacement of them by consumerism and celebrity as means of personal gratification has coincided with 'epidemics' of bulimia nervosa and irritable bowel syndrome. It is as if the instability of modern society is represented in physiology as expressed through alternating activity in the sympathetic and parasympathetic nerves. The ambivalence in the regulation of bodily intake and expulsion expresses what post-modernism means to the individual – 'hunting' for a place to be. So the contemporary epidemic of bulimia nervosa might express a cultural ambivalence between neediness, as represented by bingeing, and disgust and the assertion of the self, as represented by vomiting and restricted eating. And irritable bowel syndrome is characterised by constipation – restraint and self-preservation – and diarrhoea – emotional incontinence and lack of control.

Of course there is another personal strategy to cope with the contradictions and complexities of contemporary life and that is to give up the struggle altogether. Chronic fatigue syndrome, otherwise known as ME or 'yuppie flu', is a state of sheer exhaustion, apathy and inertia, like somebody has pulled the plug and drained out the very essence of life. This enervating fatigue is often associated with aches and pains in muscles and a multiplicity of other symptoms, such as headaches, ringing in the ears and bowel upsets. The symptoms are very similar to those of 'flu' and in many cases are preceded by an infectious illness. While there is very strong support among patient advocacy groups for a biological cause for the condition – perhaps a chronic low-grade infection, a disorder of the immune system, a deficiency of essential vitamins or minerals, or the effects of environmental poisons and contaminants – the scientific evidence for any of these factors does not amount to a convincing case. Instead, the data would seem to suggest that psychological and social factors play a major role in the cause of chronic fatigue syndrome. Therefore, like anorexia nervosa, CFS might be seen as a cultural illness, not unlike the epidemic of neurasthenia a century earlier.

Before their illness commenced, histories from sufferers reveal that many have led extraordinarily busy, driven lives. The medical anthropologist Arthur Kleinman described it in the following way:

> Believing in the value of hard work, those who were employed, devoted sixty, seventy or even eighty hours a week to their jobs. Employment was combined with major responsibilities in other domains, such as child-rearing, graduate study and/or attending the needs of an ageing or ill parent. A desire for accomplishment and success, underwritten by exacting standards for personal performance impelled these individuals always to try harder, go further, in an attempt to meet the expectations they had set for themselves at work, at home and at school. The result was an overextended, overcommitted lifestyle that left them feeling breathless – fragmented by competing demands, straining towards achievement and perfection, constantly pressed for time.[26]

According to this description, it would seem that the kind of people who are likely to succumb to chronic fatigue are the supermen or more often the superwomen, who have struggled to conform to the cultural imperative to 'do it all'.[27] Such people often sleep poorly and seem quite literally to work themselves to a standstill, but instead of being able to negotiate some help or relief in some of their roles, they let the illness do the negotiation for them.

But why do some people feel the need to push themselves so hard? And what is it about our Western culture that gives shape to this illness?

Some described Jack as an enthusiast. Others just dismissed him as a workaholic. He had always felt uneasy in social relationships, but living in a culture that encouraged and rewarded industry and achievement, he found that he could obtain recognition and approval, even admiration, by working harder than anybody else. He had always felt that way. His parents – intelligent people who never had the chance to go to university – had always been very ambitious for him, and were bitterly disappointed on the rare occasions that he failed. But Jack was intelligent and talented, and soon became a molecular scientist of some repute. Driven by the excitement of discovery and fame, he would stay in the laboratory long after everybody had gone home, testing his latest hypothesis. He would rarely refuse invitations to conferences, often preparing his talk on the journey there. The more papers he published, the more he was invited to do. He just couldn't say no. When his family complained that they rarely saw him, he would whisk them all off on action holidays, which left them feeling bewildered and exhausted. His colleagues told him to slow down, but he couldn't. He seemed to need the buzz that the recognition gave him.

Then one day, out of the blue – according to Jack – Susan, his wife, announced that she could not take it any more and was leaving him, taking the children with her. Jack was confused and shocked. Hadn't he always worked hard for them? Hadn't he been successful? Hadn't he been a good dad? What was all the struggle for if not for them? What indeed.

After Susan left, Jack still could not slow down. In fact, he seemed to work even harder. Jack's work literally became a matter of life or death; if he didn't work, he felt that he was disappearing, losing his identity. His desperation was tinged with a dawning realisation that all his success was a fabrication; it didn't count for much. In life, he had failed. So he worked even harder just to block out those depressing ideas.

Jack had never slept well, but now it got ever worse and he would stay awake until four or five o'clock in the morning, gloomily ruminating on the futility of it

all. Far from being innovative and creative, he had become an instrument of the system and the powerful multinational corporations that supported it. He began to lose confidence and question the validity of his research. But what was he to do? It was the only thing he knew. He was on a treadmill and he just had to keep going. One by one his grants ran out, his research staff left and his students complained that his ideas now seemed flaky and even subversive. He was so tired of it all. He would sit in his office trying to write, but just couldn't think straight. He felt confused, exhausted, his ears seemed to ring with alarm bells, his eyes hurt and his shoulders ached so much, and he had pins and needles in his hands whenever he tried to work on his computer. Every nerve in his body was crying out for him to have a rest, but the fear of not being known and not existing was terrifying.

It is only when we can understand the whole narrative of Jack's life that we can see how his tiredness fits in. His illness is unlikely to be diagnosed by sophisticated immunological tests for rare infections or allergies. What Jack is suffering from is a depletion of hope and meaning. He had worked all his life to compensate for the feeling that he was never good enough, but in so doing he created a false sense of self that had no real meaning. Confronted with that dreadful realisation, he suffered a physical, emotional and spiritual collapse.

Kleinman has suggested that chronic fatigue syndrome may signal discontent with an ethos in which core cultural values – hard work, success – have become inflated to the detriment of personal relationships. No longer encouraging people to work for the collective good, our narcissistic culture impels us to compete with others to become special, more intelligent, more capable, more attractive, richer and more powerful. We are seduced by television images of the good life to live beyond our means in order to achieve the trappings of celebrity – the expensive house, the private schools, the exotic holidays, the new car. But we have to work unreasonably long hours if we want to achieve the privileged status which is our right and expectation, and also afford the mortgage or school fees. And academics like Jack have to keep getting the grants, publishing the papers, staying one step ahead of the rest of the world. Otherwise they die! Jack's despair reflects the meaninglessness of that notion.

So chronic fatigue syndrome is more than exhaustion; it is more a state of despair, a depletion of the will. The psychiatrist Peter Henningsen described it as an intentional defect, a 'disorder of vitality' in relation to obligations and responsibilities, about which the sufferer has come to feel deeply ambivalent.[28] This may explain why fatigue has become the most common chronic symptom affecting teenagers, especially those who are made to feel they have to fulfil their parents' obligations. We recently conducted a survey of 200 first-year university students and found that no fewer than 60 per cent said they felt tired all the time. You might think this was just purely due to late nights and not enough sleep, but that was not necessarily the case. Neither was it due to medical causes like anaemia or high blood pressure. Among the comments that were most frequently expressed were: 'There is too much pressure'; 'My parents expect too much'; 'I'm afraid I'm not good enough'; and 'I just want to do my own thing'. But when asked what their own thing was, they didn't know. So contracting chronic fatigue syndrome may be seen as a valid (albeit unconscious) excuse for opting out of cultural pressures and avoiding responsibility for their own future.

This chapter has described how, when people in a narcissistic culture become ill, the cultural dilemmas are expressed in the nature of the symptoms. So binge eating might represent the shoring-up of an insecure sense of self by overeating, anorexia a desperate attempt to establish an independent sense of identity against cultural intrusion, tiredness the desire to opt out, and backache the burden of modern life. But the manner in which an illness is configured does not just express the meaning of cultural changes, it also confers validity on the patient's distress by being constructed in a way that is compatible with contemporary medical notions. How the practice of medicine shapes the expression of illness is the subject of the next chapter.

8

The medicalisation of illness

As a young doctor, I was given a spotless white coat and lectured on the importance of clinical detachment. The message was clear. Under no circumstances was I to get 'involved' with my patients. My job was to make a provisional diagnosis through a combination of a focused clinical history and an informed clinical examination, to confirm my suspicions using blood tests and X-rays, and to apply a specific treatment. I could not afford to let my mind become cluttered with the possible wider meanings of the illnesses that my patients had. Trained in the application of medical science, I viewed my patients through the microscope of my 'indoctrination'. My white coat protected me from all the messy emotions.[1] Even if the illness had no pathological basis and was clearly related to what was happening in my patients' lives, I had to treat it objectively with diet and drugs. That was thirty-five years ago, but the trend has continued apace. Boosted by its spectacular success and encouraged by a powerful pharmaceutical industry, Western medicine is increasingly turning its attention to everyday human ailments and transforming them into disease.

It was the French philosopher René Descartes who severed the mechanics of medicine from its religious meanings and freed it to develop along scientific lines. And as medicine became more scientific and objective, so the configuration of illness kept pace with contemporary notions of illness. Doctors created the template of what it was to be ill, and their patients readily adopted the idea.

The discovery of the nervous reflex by the Edinburgh physiologist Robert Whytt (1714–66) may have instigated this trend. Whytt conducted experiments in a variety of animals to demonstrate how stimulation of one organ could lead to symptoms in another by means of nervous reflexes centred upon the spinal cord, a nervous connection he called 'sympathy', from the Greek meaning 'suffering together'. In his book on nervous diseases,[2] he sought to explain contemporary notions of illness such as hypochondria, hysteria, the spleen, melancholy and the vapours by invoking an uncommon delicacy or a natural sensibility of 'the nerves', that encouraged 'sympathetic illness' in various organs throughout the body. Patients suspected of 'spinal irritation' (see also p. 143) commonly complained of backache (probably caused by wearing a tight corset), plus weakness, fits, anaesthesia, paralysis and a host of other symptoms. Since all nervous connections went through the spinal cord, spinal irritation could explain almost any manifestation of illness.[3] The diagnosis would be confirmed by the pressing on each of the vertebrae of the spinal cord in turn and scalding them with a hot sponge. If the patient winced, the physician would then exclaim with a triumphant air, 'A-ha, there it is!' If the doctor did not succeed in finding the sensitive spot at first, he would persevere until he did. People quickly learnt that to be treated as an invalid they needed to exhibit symptoms that could be attributed to spinal irritation. Then they could be diagnosed, ordered to rest and treated in the spas by jets of hot and cold water directed against the spine.

Spinal irritation offered such a strong focus of identification that within a very short time 'health spas and sea bathing places of resort were crowded by hundreds of young women, who were confined to a horizontal or semi-recumbent posture for years, were excluded from society, debarred their education, restricted in their natural food and compelled to adopt the miserable substitute of a medicated diet for years, simply because a hot sponge created a sensation of uneasiness or, if you prefer it, a pain to a given vertebra'.[4]

Thus a wonderful symbiosis was therefore established between patient and doctor. Physicians diagnosed disorders of the nerves and patients responded by developing backache, exhaustion, widespread bodily pains and muscular weakness or paralysis.

Any of these young women may have had a real paralysis. Neurological examination and diagnosis had not advanced to the degree of sophistication that exists nowadays, and tuberculosis, which was of course common at that time, was known to affect the spine. But the pattern was just not right. How could this epidemic of paralysis occur in such a large number of otherwise healthy young women? What neurological lesion could explain the sudden occurrence of blindness and paralysis of one limb? And how could neurological conditions causing such severe manifestations recover almost overnight from treatments that had no obvious scientific basis? The vast majority of the paralysis *had* to be 'functional' in nature and implanted by the medical culture of the time.

As ever, the uterus was regarded as the source of feminine woes. But this was not the deprived womb of the ancients that bumped about the abdomen, causing problems wherever it happened to lodge. Neither was it the 'suffocated' uterus, full of retained blood and poisoning the body with its noxious vapours. It was the 'sensitive' womb that irritated other organs through nervous reflexes and needed to be calmed by vaginal douches, avoidance of masturbation and, in the last resort, pelvic surgery. A surgeon from Rome, Georgia, Robert Battey, pioneered the removal of the ovaries of women for nervous symptoms.[5] To 'Batteyise' a woman quickly became popular, not only among patients but also their doctors, although not all surgeons were so convinced. Carlton C. Frederick, chief surgeon at the women's hospital in Buffalo, declared in 1895 that it was patients' neuroses that caused the backache, thigh pain, loss of sexual appetite and so forth rather than the other way round. 'These women come to us expecting us to pronounce the verdict that their uterus, tubes or ovaries in some way are the direct cause of their ails. Do not operate on them,' he urged his colleagues. His advice was largely unheeded and even to this day, millions of women are deprived of their healthy uterus, often for no more rational reason than it is perceived to be an organ that causes all sorts of pelvic mischief.

The influence of medical ideas in shaping an illness reached its zenith in the wards of Hôpital Salpêtrière in Paris under the charismatic presence of physician Jean-Martin Charcot. Charcot's reputation as a neurologist and medical scientist was second to none. By the systematic comparison of clinical findings to post-mortem pathology, he had established the origin and pathology of many neurological illnesses, including neurosyphilis, multiple sclerosis, Parkinson's disease, motor neurone disease and poliomyelitis. But by 1870 he was ready to tackle the last frontier, the illness he called the 'functional neuroses', which were, he asserted, inherited disorders of the brain.

Charcot suggested that many of his patients with otherwise

unexplained neurological symptoms were suffering from *la grande hystérie* (or major hysteria). This was characterised by patches of anaesthesia, pins and needles, pain and tenderness in the left lower part of the abdomen over the site of the ovary, visual disturbances, writhing movements, and the bizarre lapses of consciousness and strange behaviours of 'hysterical fits', which could be stopped (or started) by firm pressure on the ovaries.[6] A vivid description of this phenomenon was provided by a predecessor, Professor Pierre-Adolphe Piorry:

> Very commonly during fits a woman will grasp her throat with her hands as if to tear it open ... The hysteric woman strikes out at the things around her and even at the back of the bed, in which she seems to be bouncing up and down ... There is a close analogy between these pathological movements and the movements a woman makes during a venereal orgasm or while giving birth ... You might see a slender young woman, her limbs rigid, holding her own against a number of strong men trying to pin her down. She sobs, cries out, screams, cuts off her words, rages angrily about things that have vexed her or about the man she loves.[7]

The public demonstrations at the Salpêtrière came to resemble the stage performances of modern-day hypnotists. The visiting Swedish doctor Axel Munthe, who had come to study under Charcot, wrote how, under the instructions of *le patron*, the patients barked like dogs, flapped their arms when told they were a pigeon and shrieked in terror when a glove was thrown at their feet with the suggestion it was a snake.[8] In this way, Charcot defined the rules for *la grande hystérie*, and his patients complied with his suggestions. The detailed reports in the popular press amounted to an instruction manual for ill and suggestible people, who achieved a kind of celebrity by being good patients. Charcot, with his heavy brow and serious demeanour, possessed the necessary gravitas and authority to implant suggestions, but he was singularly reluctant to acknowledge the notion that the illness itself might be shaped by this high degree of suggestibility. Instead, he suggested to clinicians that the symptoms of hysteria resembled organic disease so closely that they must search tirelessly for the cause. His legacy might in part explain the tendency for patients with severe functional illness today to be subjected to such exhaustive investigations to rule out the possibility of treatable pathology.

Within ten years of Charcot's death, *la grande hystérie* disappeared from the wards of Salpêtrière. His successor, Dr Jules-Joseph Dejerine, told his house staff not to talk about hysteria in front of his patients because it encouraged new symptoms, and he was prepared to be quite ruthless when any of them developed a classic hysterical crisis.[9]

Gradually, anything that resembled hysteria became tainted with simulation and play acting, and became less a diagnosis and more a term of abuse. Faced with disbelief and rejection, the expression of illness changed from the dramatic paralyses and fits of Charcot's time to pain and fatigue, which were less easy to disprove. Records from the Cery Hospital in Lausanne from 1910 to 1929 reveal that 81 per cent of all hysterical patients displayed muscular spasms; by 1970–80, only 27 per cent did so. Over the same period, fainting declined from 47 per cent to 31 per cent, amnesia from 32 to 18 per cent. By contrast, fatigue rose from 4 to 13 per cent, and indigestion and bowel upsets from 8 to 22 per cent.[10] The medical culture had turned against the more florid manifestations of hysteria, and the patients had obligingly complied.

Throughout the twentieth century, the dramatic discoveries in medical science have identified the causes and mechanisms of diseases that had plagued the lives of people for centuries. This has meant that the number of listed diseases has gone up from about two hundred at the end of the nineteenth century to around five thousand at the end of the twentieth, and generated a massive expansion in the range and complexity of diagnostic procedures and therapeutic possibilities. Indeed, a general doctor can no longer hope to remain familiar with the latest advances in the diagnosis and treatment of every single disease. So a whole generation of 'ologists' has been spawned: urologists, gastroenterologists, oncologists, rheumatologists, cardiologists, neurologists and otorhinolaryngologists. But it doesn't stop there. Many of these specialists have an extra-special focus of interest, such as the middle chamber of the ear, the surgery of the knee, the motility of the oesophagus, or motor neurone disease, and as they become well known their case load consists predominantly of patients with illnesses that fall within their special interest.[11]

Specialists are not trained to see the whole picture. Each applies the diagnostic algorithms they have developed for the symptoms that fall within their remit and when these symptoms indicate no known disease, they create a new one. Each speciality has its own collection of functional illnesses. For example, neurologists recognise several categories of headache, many of which have no obvious cause, and they still see patients with fits or attacks that do not conform to classic epilepsy. Over 50 per cent of a gastroenterologist's case load is composed of patients with irritable bowel syndrome and functional dyspepsia. Ear, nose and throat specialists see many patients with unexplained dizziness and ringing in the ears. Fibromyalgia is the second most common cause of referral to a rheumatologist.

Dr Simon Wessley, Professor of Psychological Medicine at London University, has written that the modern classification of functional illness is a product of medical specialisation.[12] Nevertheless, the symptoms that patients have are rarely confined to one particular branch of medicine. Overlap among the territories claimed by different specialists is a characteristic of functional illness. Thus it can be a lottery whether a patient is referred to a gastroenterologist, a chest physician, a psychiatrist or a neurologist, and whether they are investigated with a gastroscope or a brain scan. As one woman wrote in a recent letter to *Gut Reaction*, the organ of the IBS Network: 'Could somebody please explain how my doctor can tell me that the headaches and dizziness I get are caused by my irritable bowel?'

So people who suffer from persistent functional illness can often end up doing the rounds of specialists, each of whom carries out his or her own particular battery of investigations. And so their notes bulge with the results of negative investigations and failed treatments. This is certainly not the fault of the patient, but neither is it the fault of the specialists. After all, their job is to rule *out* the possibility that the patient might have one of the rare diseases unique to their speciality. They are not trained to 'understand the patient'. Nevertheless, many people with unexplained illnesses insist on seeing a specialist. They seem to know that for their illness to be taken seriously it needs to be presented in a way that is compatible with the specialist's sphere of expertise. And if, after investigation, the cause of their particular illness is not apparent, then there are always plenty of possibilities, such as food allergy, candidiasis, heavy metal poisoning, reactive hypoglycae-mia and fluoride toxicity that are much more difficult to disprove.

For Western medicine, the name's the thing. Patients feel much more confident if they have a diagnosis, and for the doctor, naming the illness at least provides the illusion of control. The need to name lies deep into our collective psyche. Few of us can look at a painting in an art gallery without wanting to know what it is called. And when introduced to a new person, we need to know what job they do, what town they live in, whether or not they are married or have children, in order to assign them the appropriate place in our internal catalogue. And naming is particularly important to 'tame' those things that threaten us, like illnesses. Systems of classification undoubtedly helped an earlier generation of doctors to identify the causes of different infectious illnesses and treat them with selective antibiotics. Nowadays, however, they are most likely to flourish to offer an appearance of control on those illnesses that have no pathological basis and no obvious cause. As Thomas Kuhn commented in his book, *The Structure of Scientific Revolutions*, 'Where man does not understand, he seeks to classify.'

Thus, in recent years, the medical taxonomists have turned their obsidian gaze first on the mental disorders then on the everyday aches and upsets that seem to be so much part of our contemporary human condition, such as 'rheumatic' diseases and functional disorders of the gut.[13] And so diseases that do not have an obvious pathology have been subjected to ever more elaborate diagnostic classifications, based on the patients' symptoms. And all this in the rather forlorn hope that it might facilitate the discovery of a treatable cause. But that rarely happens. In 1859, Dr William Brinton wrote:

> As advancing knowledge brings us better means of investigation and so enables us to discover and distinguish structural changes of which we can now only observe the functional results, the aggregate of maladies called dyspepsia must undergo successive subtractions, tending more or less completely to its total subdivision into special maladies, then to the removal of this term from our nosology.[14]

Well, 136 years later, despite the introduction of barium meals, fibreoptic endoscopy and the bacterial determinant of duodenal ulceration, functional dyspepsia is still there and shows no signs of disappearing. In fact, it is getting more common and now affects 40 per cent of people living in Western countries.

The classification of unexplained illness, which is by necessity purely based on symptoms, is an artifice that can obscure the true nature of the illness. In the last thirty years, a whole new cast of diagnoses have appeared on the medical stage. The recent classifications of functional gastrointestinal disorders, derived by a team of experts sitting in conclave in Rome, have identified no fewer than forty-five different diagnoses, including 'unspecified functional bowel disorder'! Each diagnosis is characterised, like other diseases, under headings of epidemiology, diagnosis, physiology and management. All that is lacking is a definitive cause and pathology. They are illnesses without any evidence of disease. As Karl Popper said: 'One might assert that the amount of worthwhile knowledge that comes out of any field of enquiry tends to be inversely proportional to the amount of discussion about the meaning of terms that goes on in it.'[15]

Classification has not brought us any closer to finding a treatable cause for any of the functional disorders; it has just offered an illusion of control in a system that is showing alarming signs of getting *out* of control. Indeed, we might wonder whether, after a glorious century of medical advance, the whole edifice of Western medicine is in danger of collapsing under the weight of its own taxonomy.[16]

It could be argued that the medicalisation of cultural ailments is adding to the burden of health care. The highest rates of illness are found in affluent societies. The United States of America is, by all objective measures, one of the most healthy places to live, yet (as highlighted in Chapter One) population surveys indicate that proportionately more Americans suffer from ill-defined illnesses than any other nation on Earth.

In his book *The Tyranny of Health*, the London GP Dr Michael Fitzpatrick argues that by highlighting all the various dangers of modern life, governments are actually creating an increased sense of vigilance about health that induces fear and dependency and this may actually make people ill.[17] We cannot enjoy the simple pleasures of life any more without a government health warning of the consequences of our actions. We can't have a drink without wondering if it will damage our liver. We can't enjoy a meal without worrying about getting fat and having a heart attack. We cannot lie in the sun for fear of getting skin cancer. We can't even enjoy sex without worrying about the dangers of AIDS. The message is clear: life is harmful to our health. But surely, you might exclaim, it is important to make people aware of these health risks? That is true, but we have to maintain a sense of proportion. Government health warnings, health screening and health awareness campaigns rarely present a balanced impression. And all too often such health concerns can be promoted by politicians and amplified by the media until they assume the status of imminent catastrophe.

Medicine used to be a matter of personal common sense. People knew when illness was the result of an upsetting life event and required rest and when the disease needed the specialist attentions of the doctor. Now, not only are we all more aware of health risks than ever before, but medicine is much more complex and most of us lack the scientific knowledge to put those risks into perspective. So we can all too easily exaggerate their significance and use them as a convenient receptacle for our own fears. Thus, if every ailment is regarded as a potential threat, it can only serve to make the anxiety and the symptoms worse.[18]

Faced with threats to our health from all sides and suffering from symptoms that have no obvious cause, people have no recourse but to rely on the mysterious technical skills of the white-coated exponents of modern scientific medicine. But doctors appear to have become too sensitive to the threat of serious disease to see illness as an adaptive response to what happens in a person's life. They are wonderful in a crisis when confident decision and action are needed, but not so effective when the cause of the illness is less obvious. Indeed, in that situation, some have the unnerving tendency to transform their patient's illness into a potential crisis that they alone can manage.

Most doctors have neither the time nor the inclination to explore the influence of grievance, anger, fear, shame and just plain unhappiness on bodily function. Such initiatives are not encouraged. Research into the emotional background of physical illness still receives only a fraction of the funding that genetic, immunological, infective and metabolic factors receive. Reports, reviews, disease management guidelines, papers and books channel ideas about illness in a direction that appears to be dictated more by medical politics than clinical reality. As the medical sociologist David Armstrong asserts in his book, *The Political Anatomy of the Body*, 'It is not just that textbooks of medicine contain representations of illness; the illnesses are also representations of the textbook as the arbiter of the medical belief system.'[19]

Medicine is more than a system of scientific ideas and practices; it is a political system that seeks to regulate the behaviour of society. As Bryan Turner has said: 'Illness is a language, the body is representation and medicine is a political practice.'[20] So in the same way that conversion to medical disease protects individuals from being overwhelmed or torn apart by the trials of their lives, the same transformation defends the state from the destabilising impact of profound social change.

The conversion of the instability of modern life to medical illness shifts the burden of society onto the individual while at the same time eroding his capacity to cope, and creating dependence on the medical system. The social narrative of illness has been marginalised. We have lost the plot. People have been encouraged to perceive their bodily feelings not so much as expressions of tension or disharmony caused by the vicissitudes of modern life but as diseases. In so doing, they shift the focus of responsibility for their illness from themselves to the doctor, who has to treat them using drugs.[21]

What religion once condemned as sins, medicine now commandeers as diseases. Gluttony and sloth have now been reconfigured as epidemics of obesity and chronic fatigue. Antisocial behaviours such as alcoholism, naughtiness, truancy, drug abuse, violence, gambling and theft have undergone a subtle shift from criminal acts deserving of punishment to psychological diseases requiring treatment.[22] And as I explained in the previous chapter, bodily expressions of grievance, shame, envy and loneliness, which might threaten the integrity of society, are now contained in medical illnesses such as irritable bowel syndrome and non-cardiac chest pain. And when soldiers, fighting real wars, succumb to illness, as they invariably do, it cannot be attributed to combinations of fear, rage, grief and shame, brought about by the most fundamental and catastrophic cultural dissonance. That would be a recipe for insubordination and mutiny. Instead, chronic illness that develops in the context of wars tends to be regarded as a mysterious physical disease and attributed to toxic combinations of inoculations, depleted uranium and biological or chemical weapons. In the Soviet Union, dangerous intellectuals and political dissidents were diagnosed as schizophrenic in order to justify their forced segregation to camps, like those described in Alexander Solzhenitsyn's *Gulag Archipelago*.[23] I am not for a minute suggesting that the free democracies of the Western world would ever dream of exiling potentially subversive elements in society on the pretext of disease. But if the current high rates of illness in Western populations are indeed the bodily expression of rapid social change, then it would be more politically expedient to frame unexplained illness as medical diseases than a social or political problem. Ring-fencing certain groups of unexplained symptoms as specific diseases, attributable to factors external to society and the self, would not only provide an illusion of control in a turbulent world but would also tend to obscure the sheer scale of the problem, keeping official figures much lower than they really are. Moreover, since only doctors treat disease, providing a massive increase in funding for health creates the illusion of care and control, and maintains confidence in the political system. So bodily expressions of grievance are treated with bran, anger with aspirin, sadness with antispasmodics, shame with antidepressants and the enormous epidemic of loneliness and need with diet and exercise.

Seen from this perspective, the political campaign to eliminate illness in affluent Western countries is about as futile and expensive as the war against terror. Like terror, illness is an elusive yet all-pervasive enemy that cannot be vanquished by concrete solutions – in this case, drugs. But, to be fair, doctors are only giving their patients what they want. If illness is an adaptive configuration which people unconsciously adopt to deal with the personal conflicts and dilemmas that are just too painful to contemplate and impossible to resolve, then they will want to avoid the source of their pain and seek resolution in drugs. As George Bernard Shaw said in *The Doctor's Dilemma*, 'What the public wants is a cheap magic charm to prevent illness and a cheap pill or potion to cure all illnesses.'

The late twentieth century witnessed a dramatic increase in the wealth and power of the pharmaceutical industry. The discovery of antibiotics and their marketing on a vast scale changed it from a collection of small, family-based concerns making tonics and vitamin pills to vast multinational corporations that hold medical services in thrall. Hard on the heels of the wartime introduction of penicillin (1941), came cortisone for treating the crippling inflammatory conditions of rheumatoid arthritis and ulcerative colitis (1949), streptomycin and para-amino-salicylic acid (PAS) for treating tuberculosis (1950), chlorpromazine for treating schizophrenia (1952), the purification of factor VIII for haemophilia (1957), the oral contraceptive pill (1960) which gave women control of their own sexuality for the first time and heralded the feminist revolution, the awakening of patients with Parkinson's disease by levodopa (1972), the treatment of ulcers with highly selective and potent inhibitors of acid secretion (1981) and the lowering of blood pressure with safe and powerful vasodilators.

Drugs have since been perfected to treat all known ills from cancer to impotence. They have prolonged the lives of vast numbers of people with chronic diseases and improved the quality of their existence.

Indeed, it is difficult to imagine what our society would be like without insulin, antibiotics, anticoagulants or drugs to treat angina, high blood pressure or cancer. There cannot be a household in the land that does not have a cabinet full of drugs to treat everything from chilblains to migraine. We have become so dependent on drugs that we use them not just to manage serious organic diseases, but to prevent us getting those diseases, to regulate the symptoms of functional illness and to have fun, to make us happy, to give us better sex. As the psychiatrist Peter Henningsen wrote, 'Prescribing a drug gives personal and cultural meaning to the patient's suffering. It changes cognitive representations of the illness, alters the attitudes of family and friends, and contributes to the ongoing configuration of medicine as a handmaiden to the pharmaceutical corporations.'[24] The prospect of a world without drugs has become a truly terrifying prospect for most people. The total volume of prescriptions in the UK rose by nearly 6 per cent per year from 2000 to 2004 and the cost of prescription drugs has increased by 8 per cent in the same period.[25] The immense revenues from drug sales have made the larger multinational pharmaceutical companies more wealthy than many nation states. For example, the Pfizer corporation is now richer than Sweden and Singapore and nearly as rich as Australia.

It goes without saying that the pharmaceutical industry has a vested interest in medicalising illness because this expands the markets for their products. Thus, most drug companies employ public relations firms to raise awareness of a certain disease, which they alone have a cure for. The first step is to set up an 'advisory board', consisting of experts who provide advice to the corporate sponsors on current medical opinion and opportunities for shaping it. This is followed by publication of best practice guidelines, written by, or with the help of authorities in the area, editorials in medical magazines, featuring opinions by members of the advisory board, and finally, patient information leaflets. Although this is presented as an education programme, it all helps to influence first medical and then public opinion, favouring the marketing of that particular product.

But the interaction between the pharmaceutical industry and the medical profession is more widespread and insidious. Drug companies directly or indirectly fund most of the 'independent' medical research that is carried out throughout the world. They sponsor nearly every international meeting, endow university chairs and underwrite the publication of nearly all of the multi-author books on specific medical conditions, and most special issues of medical journals. To be fair, the companies rarely feature their own drugs prominently in such publications, but they do not need to. In the same way that renaissance artists depended on the patronage of rich and influential benefactors, many medical opinion leaders would find it difficult to achieve prominence without the patronage of the pharmaceutical industry as gatekeeper to conferences and authorship. By creating medical reputations, increasing public awareness of new diseases and health threats, and influencing government policy, the pharmaceutical industry not only shapes the perception of illness, but also creates the corporate-sponsored medicalised environment where their products can flourish.

In recent years, pharmaceutical companies have sponsored a series of articles claiming that irritable bowel syndrome is caused by specific disturbances in the gut wall of receptors for the transmitter called serotonin. These carefully co-ordinated campaigns have coincided with the launch of new pharmacological treatments that have a specific action on those receptors.[26]

But current notions of illness are not so much determined by doctors as by newspapers, magazines, television and the internet. So, pharmaceutical companies use the media to frame conditions as being more widespread and severe than they really are. Just in the last few months, I was sincerely informed by the chief executive of a company marketing nutritional supplements that our modern diet is so depleted in essential nutrients that we must all take supplements every day of our lives! Such media scares provide a tangible focus for our fears. Vulnerable people who have lost faith in their doctors are all too ready to identify with theories of illness that are currently fashionable, and put their faith in cures for which there is little evidence. Patients have begun to move from the technical uncertainties of orthodox medicine to the dangerous convictions of media propaganda. So where they can, companies are only too willing to by-pass the doctor and advertise directly to the consumer.[27] For example, the launch of Merck's hair growth drug, Finasteride, in Australia in 1998 was accompanied by articles in leading newspapers featuring new information about the emotional trauma associated with baldness, while double-paged advertisements identifying the high frequency of male impotence in Australia were sponsored indirectly by Pfizer, the manufacturer of Viagra. Around two and a half billion dollars were spent on direct-to-consumer advertising in the USA in 2001. Americans saw more advertisements for medications on television than for any other group of products. The message is that for every ill there is a pill to treat it.

Such 'disease mongering' can turn the ailments we all experience into medical problems and potential markets. This erodes the shaky self-confidence of a society in transition by feeding unhealthy obsessions, disseminating alarm and despondency, and replacing common sense with serious medical disease. Moreover, modern drugs are not harmless sugar-coated placeboes. They are, to a lesser or greater extent, toxic. They cause significant changes in physiology and are often associated with many potential side effects. Thus, if they are given to reassure a sensitive person whose real worries cannot be acknowledged, they are more than likely to consolidate the patient's illness by the addition of pharmacological side effects, which can only be treated with more drugs. All too often, this can relegate the patient to a pharmaceutical wasteland, from which there is no escape and no resolution.[28]

But we've been here before. With regard to the health of the affluent classes, the period we call the Enlightenment in England (between about 1700 and 1800) more closely resembles the present day than perhaps any other period in history. Like today, this was a time of enormous social change. People were on the move. The Enclosure Acts had dispossessed a rural peasantry from the land and the spread of industrialisation promised a better life in the new cities. The authority of Church, Crown and Parliament was being questioned. Illnesses were rife throughout the population and were attributed, as they are now, to fashionable concerns. In his book *The English Malady* (1737), the physician George Cheyne attributed 'the frequency of these nervous distempers of late, especially among the fair sex' to the climate, the overcrowded, polluted cities and the 'encroachment of foreign and esoteric customs and products upon English life such as coffee, tea, chocolates and snuff'.[29] He also found that in London, 'the greatest, most capacious and populous city of the globe', nervous diseases were the most frequent and the symptoms most bizarre. There was a dramatic growth in the number of physicians in the late eighteenth century and a diversity of medical opinion. As the historian Roy Porter expressed it, 'By the late eighteenth century the medical profession was in bad shape, saturated from below by swarms of druggists, irregulars and itinerants, and rendered top heavy by an oligarchy of elite physicians and surgeons wielding power and making fortunes out of all proportion to their deserts.'[30] A vocal cosmopolitan society with more knowledge on health matters than ever before refused to accept the dogma of the medical professions and shopped around for quick cures.

Alternative practitioners in the late-eighteenth century offered quick solutions for busy people. These not only included cures for orthodox diseases such as scurvy, gout and the pox, but treatments for chronic distempers, the rheumatism, colic, wind and gut upsets. So-called 'quack medicines' were particularly targeted at diseases of women, from 'fits of the mother', vapours, passions or tremblings of the heart, to green sickness or chlorosis (anaemia and wasting), weakness and pains in the back, barrenness and loss of libido. Purging was often the vital operation performed by such medicines. Thus Edward Ewel's Panaseton or Humoreum Extractum, 'eradicates obstructions, flushings, windy belching, fumes, headaches, surfeits, gripings in the guts, vomitings, looseness, fainting and loss of appetite ... and leaves the stomach mightily strengthened ... purges away those salt briny, melancholy, sharp humours, which so universally indispose the body'.[31] As time went by, the traditional hydraulics of purging were slowly displaced by medicines that promised to recover vital powers and galvanise the sufferer into healthy activity, but echoes of it persist in the modern enthusiasm for colonic irrigation.

Physicians would often prescribe alternative medicines alongside more orthodox remedies. Polypharmacy – heavy dosing with mixtures of what were quite poisonous medicines – was common among those who could afford it. Many doctors actually made their own pills, and some, such as James Morrison, Thomas Hollowing and Thomas Beecham, assisted by the new pill-rolling machines, marketed them on a very large scale. Their enterprises became household names. Nowadays it is the descendants of the pill rollers, the pharmaceutical corporations, who are offering quick cures and designer drugs, facilitating polypharmacy with cocktails of toxic drugs and getting rich on the credulity of ill people and the doctors that look after them. Despite the availability of antibiotics, steroids, insulin and a range of other pharmaceutical solutions, it can still seem that as far as the largest component of human illness is concerned, medical treatment has not advanced very far beyond that practised in Georgian times. Acclaim for Dr Morrison's vegetable pills in Georgian England seems very similar to the enthusiasm for Sir Dennis Burkitt's high-fibre diet in the 1980s.[32]

And there is a modern feel about the desperation and frustration of Dr John Moore's patient in the following account.

> Failing to find a cure, he worked his way through the whole tribe. He subsequently moved on to quacks, receiving from them an appearance of sympathy which the rest of his acquaintance refuse, and they possibly relieve or palliate the costiveness [tendency to constipation], the flatulency, the acidities and other symptoms which are brought on by the anxiety attendant to this complaint. What such quacks could never achieve was the eradication of the disease, the original cause continuing in spite of all their bitters and their stomachies and their purgatives and analeptics, the same symptoms constantly recur. The wretched patient growing every hour more and more irritable, remedies hurry on the bad symptoms with double rapidity ... He returns to physicians, goes back to quacks and occasionally tries the family nostrums of many an old lady. His constitution being worn by fretfulness and drugs, he at length despairs of belief.[33]

So I wonder whether the current increasing enthusiasm for complementary and alternative medicine throughout the Western world reflects the same quest for certainty in a changing world. With more and more people getting illnesses for which there is no medical cure, complementary and alternative practitioners offer a sense of conviction and personal reassurance that conventional medicine can seem to lack.

The bedrock of our current Western practice of medicine is a scientific method that is based on the principle of doubt. Something may seem to cause a particular disease, or a particular treatment may appear to work, but unless you can prove that the effect is greater than could possibly be achieved by chance alone, then it cannot possibly be true. Scientists have to prove their hypothesis beyond any reasonable doubt, and in order to do this they have to show that it applies to many different people under differing circumstances. In an evidence-based system of medicine, the personal and individual has to yield to the collective. Our knowledge of medicine is derived from the science of epidemiology, the study of disease in populations. But while cohort studies of tens of thousands of people in South-east Asia have demonstrated that diets depleted of leafy green vegetables may be associated with colonic cancer, this doesn't mean that people who don't like cabbage are necessarily going to get cancer. Although one cannot dispute the premise that the practice of medicine has to be informed by experimentally proven biological mechanisms, epidemiological studies and properly controlled clinical trials, there is more to it than that. As we have discussed, illness depends upon the intimate blend of factors: lifestyle; inheritance; pure chance; and our personal history and circumstances. Medicine has tended to concentrate on the first three and ignore the latter. The Prince of Wales summed up this view in his address to the British Medical Association back in 1982 when he observed that for all its breathtaking success, the imposing edifice of medicine is, like the celebrated Tower of Pisa, slightly off-balance.[34] He further claimed that one of the most unfortunate consequences of this unhealthy imbalance is that the patient's individuality and his or her emotional, mental and spiritual needs are ignored.

The rapid rise in psychological and functional illnesses has contributed to a crisis of confidence in the medical profession, which is unlikely to be solved by creating diagnostic classifications and care pathways, reducing waiting times and shifting more responsibility to primary care. If, as I have argued, functional illness is the meaningful response of the individual to the trials and tribulations of modern life, we need to change the perspective. So instead of society being burdened by an ever-increasing number of chronically ill patients, who need to be treated with diets and drugs, the patients should be seen as the expression of an ailing society and the problem will only go away when we begin to address the fundamental causes of social stress and isolation. This is the topic of the last chapter of this book.

9

Breaking the mould

Annie was referred to me by a colleague, who wrote: 'I should be grateful if you could see this twenty-year-old geography student, who has been suffering with persistent diarrhoea and tiredness for the last ten months.' He then listed all the investigations he had carried out: X-rays of the small and large bowel; fibreoptic examination of the stomach and colon; blood tests to detect signs of malnutrition; and various tests for malabsorption. I worked it out. The combined cost of the investigations plus the costs of consultation came to £5,240 and the whole process had taken the best part of a year. Yet none of them had revealed any objective signs of disease. 'I have conducted trials of treatment,' continued my colleague, 'with anti-diarrhoea medication, supplements of pancreatic enzymes and even anti-inflammatory agents for colitis. She has seen a dietitian, who has recommended gluten-free, lactose-free, low-fat diets and even a rigorous exclusion diet to test for food allergy.' He concluded: 'I have been seeing this young woman for a year and despite all my efforts, her diarrhoea has remained resistant to treatment and her tiredness is becoming more of a problem. I should be grateful for your advice.'

My colleague's careful elimination of treatable diagnoses was the very model of modern medical practice. But although no diagnostic stone was left unturned, not even the smallest pebble, his patient remained ill.

Annie came to see me with her mother. She slouched in the chair and seemed faintly disinterested in the consultation. Nobody would guess that she had had such a disabling illness for the last year. By contrast, her mother was almost beside herself with worry; she was so eager to answer for Annie that I quietly asked if she would mind leaving the room so that I could speak to her daughter alone.

I asked Annie when her symptoms first started. She replied that it was just a few days after her birthday. She had been to the cinema with Mark, her boyfriend, and they had had some fish and chips on the way home. But the next morning she woke up with stomach pain and had severe diarrhoea. I asked whether Mark had had the same symptoms. Annie said that she wasn't sure, because that night he had 'dumped' her. He had explained that he just didn't love her any more and that as they were coming up to finals, they both needed to focus on their studies. I asked Annie how she had reacted and she replied that she had not given Mark the satisfaction of being upset and made out she didn't really care. In fact, they had been going out together since they were fifteen and there had never been anybody else. A few days later, she found that Mark had been seeing Sue, her best friend. I wondered how she felt about this. She was silent for a long time and just stared at her feet. When eventually she looked up, there were tears in her eyes and a catch in her voice. 'I was gutted,' she replied.

At the time, Annie just carried on as usual and tried to pretend it didn't matter. She ignored Mark and Sue, threw herself into her studies and worked at her bar job until after midnight every night. But the diarrhoea persisted. She kept on having to rush to the loo. She was also sleeping badly, often waking in the early hours with her pulse racing, and she was finding it very difficult to focus on her books.

Towards the end of our consultation, I suggested to Annie that while it was quite possible she might have got food poisoning from the fish and chips, this should have cleared up very quickly. Instead the persistence of her symptoms probably had more to do with her suppressed anger and grief at being rejected by Mark. I also told her that she was overdoing it and suggested she stop the bar job and allow herself more time to go out with her friends and talk about how she felt.

The look on Annie's face told me she wasn't convinced, but she took my advice, and for good measure I also prescribed some sachets of cholestyramine, containing a resin that bound any surplus bile acids that may have been irritating her colon. Within a few weeks her symptoms were much better and she had stopped taking the medication. During our weekly therapy sessions, she had been able to admit how much she had missed Mark and how betrayed she had felt by her relationship with Sue. She had stopped the bar job and allowed herself more space during the day to think and talk to people. And, she added, 'I've met a man.' Three months later she had moved in with her new boyfriend. I asked about the diarrhoea. 'Oh, that went weeks ago,' she replied.

Annie's diarrhoea may have been due to food poisoning, but cultures of her stools had not revealed any of the obvious culprits. Instead, there was such a clear association with the traumatic collapse of her relationship with Mark. And his affair with Sue had been a severe wound to her self-esteem, so much so that she couldn't talk about it. So she blanked it out of her mind and worked harder than ever, while her feelings were expressed in the diarrhoea she developed that same night. As time passed, Annie's illness took over her life and became the focus of her misery. It took Annie twelve months of medical investigations, numerous trials of treatment and six therapy sessions to get over Mark. Although some investigation was necessary to rule out the possibility of serious illness, the enormous number of investigations she underwent may well have distracted her from coming to terms with the real cause of her symptoms and reinforced a prolonged, non-productive pattern of illness behaviour. An hour's conversation to discover what had 'gutted' her during her very first consultation might have saved an enormous amount of time and expense.

As a young house physician, I was fortunate enough to work in the Royal United Hospital in the beautiful Georgian city of Bath. The ward I worked on was called Parry Ward, after Dr Caleb Parry, physician to that city in the late eighteenth century. Dr Parry was not only one of the first doctors to describe the symptoms of thyrotoxicosis, but also emphasised that it was as important to know 'what sort of patient has the disease' as 'what kind of disease the patient has'. Unfortunately his wise words have been somewhat overlooked in the march of medical science.

In the last hundred years, Western medicine has increasingly conformed to a deterministic scientific model that assumes that all the operations of the human body are reducible to mechanical processes, while the influence of emotion and mind on bodily illness has, until recently, been ignored. Though science demystifies, it also dehumanises, creating a detachment from real life and reducing illness to a series of remote, narrow, technical questions. So diseases tend to be seen as malfunctions and treatment has to repair or replace the damaged part in much the same way as a mechanic would mend a car. Indeed, some of the high-tech garages now use impressive equipment that seems remarkably similar in concept to the complex biochemical and radiological equipment used by medical laboratory scientists. Doctors, it seems, are often little more than technicians ordering tests, more out of fear of missing a life-threatening condition than making a positive diagnosis, and administering treatments which do not necessarily work.[1] And if the tests fail to reveal any evidence of pathology, then doctors can do little more than attempt to suppress the symptoms and reassure the patient that there is nothing seriously wrong.

It wasn't always that way. In 1956, the American physician Carl Binger wrote:

> Time was, and not so long ago, when the family doctor delivered babies and supervised their nursing, their weaning and their teething when he vaccinated them and saw them through their measles and chicken pox and whooping cough. He told the boy about the facts of life and treated the girl for her menstrual cramps. He advised about diet and rest, gave spring tonics, clipped tonsils, set a broken arm, reassured fathers who couldn't sleep because of business worries, pulled mother through a case of typhoid or double pneumonia, reprimanded the cook who was found on her day out to have a dozen empty bottles of whisky in her clothes closet, gave advice about the young man's choice of college or profession, comforted grandma who was losing her memory and becoming more and more irritable and closed grandpa's eyes in his final sleep. He went on his endless and incessant rounds leaving in his wake a faint odour of carbolic with which he disinfected his beard.

The point is that the family doctor, albeit somewhat romanticised in that passage, knew his patients and understood the context in which the illness occurred.[2]

How much things have changed. Nowadays the busy practitioner makes sure that a pregnant mother is referred the local maternity hospital for all ante-natal visits and for the birth of her child, while infant feeding and weaning are supervised by district midwives. Teething problems and immunisations are often dealt with by the practice nurse while childhood infections are much rarer thanks to immunisation. The doctor now is probably the last person a boy would talk to about the facts of life. His mother would have picked up a pamphlet at the surgery. The doctor would refer enlarged tonsils to an ENT surgeon, a broken arm to the fracture clinic, treat insomnia with sleeping tablets, arrange for serious infections to be admitted to the infectious disease unit, refer the cook to an alcoholic rehabilitation unit, send grandma for assessment to the local psychogeriatic unit and arrange for grandpa to be admitted to a hospice for terminal care. The role of modern doctors is not so much that of a health counsellor, who would understand the patients and have time to discuss their illnesses, but more that of the efficient health administrator, the gatekeeper who would refer patients on to specialist units. There is so little time to listen to the patient's narrative. There are more patients clamouring at the door waiting to be heard and there is always the six-monthly audit to prepare.

Three centuries ago, the French philosopher known as Voltaire derided doctors as men who poured drugs of which they know little to cure diseases of which they know less into human beings of whom they know nothing. This is no longer true. Doctors now have a detailed knowledge of pharmacology and have a comprehensive understanding of pathology but many have little understanding of the emotional background of many common illnesses. The most common complaint expressed angrily in the chatlines and pages of self-help organisations is that the doctor never listens: 'As soon as I come in the door, she is writing out a prescription. I never have time to explain what is wrong with me. She's already made up her mind.'

This patient's doctor is not necessarily a poor clinician. By the standards of modern medical practice, she is efficient and effective. She will have been trained in a biomedical model of medicine that is based on pathology, and supported by evidence. She will be highly skilled at identifying the most likely causes for her patient's symptoms among many different possibilities. Then, with only about six minutes to see each patient, she will have to make a diagnosis, prescribe some tablets and quickly disengage before the next patient comes in.

Blinkered by the requirement for good clinical governance and evidence-based medicine, the medical profession has lost sight of the narrative and culture of illness. This is not the fault of the doctor. Most of the doctors I know are hardworking and care deeply about their patients' welfare. It's just that there is no time to listen to the patient's story, to understand how the symptoms might represent the patient's dilemma, to discuss a different way of looking at things, or to negotiate the possibility of changing the patient's circumstances. In other words, there is no time to practise the *art* of healing. The system does not enable a proper therapeutic relationship to develop.

Despite the technological advances, the current system of medicine is a product of a time that has past. The days when populations of industrial nations were decimated by infections, and health care had to be planned as a military exercise are gone. The war against disease has been spectacularly successful. The question is, can we now tolerate the peace? In its distinguished middle age, our modern system of scientific medicine has encountered a new environment of unexplained illnesses, and the way it has reacted demonstrates a certain 'hardening of the attitudes'. The informed common sense that underpinned the art of medicine has been buried under a vast pile of scientific papers, diagnostic algorithms, care pathways, working party reports, leaving society at the mercy of an epidemic of social malaise.

The fact of the matter is that we are never going to defeat sickness, just as we are never going to defeat unhappiness. Both are part and parcel of being human. Research into genetics or neuroscience is unlikely to provide a satisfactory answer to most modern ailments. People need a true health service that helps them to cope emotionally with the isolation and demands of twenty-first-century life, not an institution that inculcates fear and dependency by treating them as if they might have an incurable disease.

For patients with functional illness, taking a clinical history is not so much a matter of fitting the pattern of symptoms to a specific disease, but more about understanding the illness 'narrative' – that is the development of the illness in the context of the person, their life situation, the events that have befallen them, their attitudes, beliefs and family history.[3] If doctors are going to help their patients get better, both need to understand not only how the illness has developed but also why. There are several important questions that can lead to this insight. Perhaps the most important is: What was going on in the patient's life when the illness first started? As I have indicated in previous chapters, it seems that the majority of functional illnesses, and probably a sizeable percentage of organic diseases, are caused by our reaction to the things that have happened to us. So if we can appreciate what instigated the illness and the meaning that event held for the patient, then we can begin to solve the illness.

Symptoms of functional illness tend to come and go, so two other important questions are: What is associated with a remission of symptoms? and What seems to bring on a relapse? In many cases a pattern emerges. For example, symptoms may change during trips abroad, at weekends, when the children are on holiday, or around Christmas, and it is always important to explore the possible reasons for those fluctuations. An acute recurrence of the illness can represent the suppressed memory of the anniversary of a tragic event, like the death of a close relative or the day your partner left home. Kath, whose case history I outlined on pp. 26–7, always became ill on Friday, even many years after her lover had taken his own life, because Friday was the day he went home. Even if patients cannot initially accept that their illness might be caused by the effect of what has happened, they will usually be able to acknowledge how their illness can fluctuate according to certain events in their everyday life and may be able to gain an understanding of what is triggering them.

Finally, since the symptoms of functional illness may rekindle the feeling of a particular traumatic situation earlier in life, it is important to explore whether the patient might have had similar symptoms in the past and what the symptoms remind the patient of.

Malcolm's severe attacks of stomach pain had caused him to have so many emergency admissions to hospital that he had lost count. Despite several exploratory operations and numerous tests, no cause had ever been found. But I was struck by the way he talked about his pain. He told me that he hated and feared the pain, but it was like an old friend. It made him feel alive. It relieved the emptiness and loneliness of his life and was in fact often worse when he felt close to people. I wondered why. He was silent for a long time and finally muttered, 'Because I then have to face the pain of my guilt and worthlessness.' The first time he experienced the pain was when his sister had died. He had promised to pick her up from a local dance, but was with his mates in the pub and didn't bother. His sister therefore accepted a ride on a friend's motorbike. She did not have a crash helmet, the bike skidded on some ice and she was killed. After that episode, he was stricken with an attack of pain that went on for three days.

Talking about the guilt he felt over his sister's death brought it back to mind and helped Malcolm decode his symptoms of pain and let go of his perverse need for punishment. For the duration of therapy, he was pain free.

The importance of being able to change the 'story' in order to heal the illness is well established in traditional medicine, where healers are also artists and storytellers (see p. 146). They bring these representational skills to provide insight into the patient's illness and change the narrative. They make people feel better. It is unfortunate that in taking over total responsibility for illness, Western medical culture seems to have lost a lot of the good stories that can help the patient understand and move on. Instead, the narrative that modern doctors and their patients so often relate is a sterile and futile quest for the mystery infection or allergen.

In Western cultures, it is often the psychotherapists that facilitate insight into the meaning of the symptoms and help people find options to resolve them. Different therapists tackle this in different ways. Psychoanalytically- or psychodynamically-oriented therapists explore the meaning of the symptoms in the context of the dynamics of key relationships, especially, but not exclusively, those which occurred within the family early in life. These relationships are crucial because they can set the template for how a person relates to other people, including the therapist. Thus the analysis of the developing relationship between client and therapist, the so-called 'transference' relationship, provides powerful insights into the suppressed feelings that may exist at the heart of the illness, and an intimate setting where the issues causing them can be worked through.

Alison could never forgive her father for abandoning her when she was ten years old and never really understood why he left. She had thought the world of him. Her mother was very bitter and needed a lot of emotional support. Alison felt trapped and resentful. It seemed that her childhood had been stolen from her. Her father had bought a house across town and the arrangement was that she should go and stay at weekends. She tried to object, but her mother insisted that she had to. In any case, Alison knew that when she wasn't there, her mother's boyfriend came to stay.

Torn apart between the two of them, furious that she was never considered and feeling somehow responsible or in the way, Alison became ill. She couldn't sleep properly and would often wake up with frightening dreams. She also felt tense during the day and was too exhausted and preoccupied to concentrate. Her school work suffered. She was plagued with indigestion and nausea. Everything she ate seemed to make her sick. She lost a lot of weight. That was ten years ago, but the cycle of sickness continued to rule her life. Although Alison was an intelligent young woman, she never went to university but found a sequence of jobs in restaurants and pubs. She had had a number of relationships with men but none of them seemed to last very long. As she explained to me, as soon as they started getting serious, she felt sick and panicky, her sleep was disrupted and the indigestion started all over again. She had been to the doctor on numerous occasions, but he could find no obvious cause for her symptoms and none of the tablets he prescribed ever seemed to work.

At first my relationship with Alison was difficult. She was wary and resentful, and rejected every interpretation I offered. But when I suggested that she could not bear to trust me because I might leave her just like her father did, Alison allowed herself to get cross. She railed at me in a way she had never been able to with her parents. It was harrowing and difficult and the sickness was awful, but she slowly began to accept the reality that her parents had not meant to reject her, but they were too preoccupied with their own unhappiness to realise how she felt. With that, all the pent-up grievance seemed to dissipate and she came to the conclusion that she didn't have to carry the burden of her parents' anger and unhappiness any more. Later she arranged to meet her father. They had gone for a long walk and talked like they had never talked before. Her father had told her how devastated and guilty he had felt over the separation and how he had tried to make contact and explain. The last time I heard from Alison was a note to tell me that she was married and expecting her first baby. Morning sickness had not been a problem.

It was when Alison had the courage to get cross with me that she could begin to re-examine her relationship with her parents and accept personal responsibility for her health and for her life. She felt dreadful for a time, but she was able to live with the anger and the sadness, talk about it and let it drift away. She had at long last relinquished her identity-in-illness and dared to expand her notion of herself to embrace other possibilities, including having her own children.

The somewhat challenging and intrusive nature of psychoanalytically-informed therapies is not suitable for everyone. Although it may be intellectually satisfying to get to the root of the problem, that may not always be in the patient's best interests. A vulnerable personality may be so held together by the mythologies around which their identity is structured that stripping these resistances away can cause a spiral down to panic and despair. An alternative approach is cognitive behavioural therapy (CBT). This is more concerned with the 'attribution' of the symptoms than the 'archaeology' of a person's relationships. It challenges the way a person interprets bodily sensations and physiological reactions by seeing them not so much as symptoms of a disease that needs to be treated but more as expressions of emotional tension that can be controlled. Thus by understanding the links between life situations and the symptoms, patients are encouraged to find different ways of managing the illness. Both CBT and psychoanalytical psychotherapies have been shown to be effective in a variety of different functional illnesses.[4]

In recent years, there has been a resurgence in the notion of body psychotherapy for working with people with functional or psychosomatic illnesses.[5] Body psychotherapists do not treat the body as an object, which doctors are trained to do, but encourage their clients to identify with their bodies, seeking to discover what their symptoms represent for them and using touch to help them modulate it. When the body is used as a dumping ground for a patient's overwhelming concerns, there is a certain logic in working with the body to resolve those.

Although purists proclaim the merits of their own psychotherapeutic approach, the path to recovery is the patients' journey and the therapist can only help them find their own way.[6] The most insightful interpretation cannot take root unless patients can take their own meaning from it. So it is not necessarily what the therapist says that brings about change; it is more the quality of the relationship that sets the scene for change to take place. Communication, trust, relaxation and time comprise the essential elements of healing. If the patient feels that it is possible to communicate with the therapist and be heard and understood, then the sense of confidence that is generated can provide the space to think and perhaps alter the way things are perceived. Memories are never fixed; every time an event is brought back to mind, it is thought about and changed, either becoming more of a threat or less, according to the emotional climate.[7] Thus, by revisiting the source of pain in an environment that is safe and contained, the therapist can help to diminish the threat to the individual and promote a more positive and creative outlook, which may enable the patient to move on while the symptoms slowly fade into the background.

Gordon was initially very suspicious of me. He said he had great difficulty with authority figures. He had worked in the university and regarded all academics as devious and manipulative, and doctors were the worst! So he attacked the therapy. He belittled my interpretations. He tried to pin me down with demands for evidence. He insisted on definitions, on facts he could hold on to and on medications that had some logical physiological action. Nevertheless, despite himself and with great reluctance, he began to recognise that his constipation represented his extreme wariness of other people, which hindered any ability to get on with his life. Literally, his whole existence was constipated! When he expressed his frustration, he discovered he could have a very satisfying bowel movement, but the fall-out from that uncontrolled 'expulsion' could cause a lot of mess, which would just reinforce his attitude of wariness. He was stuck

and the therapy became stuck. The changing point in our relationship was when I decided to share with him the knowledge that I had also had my difficulties with university politics. Slowly he began to trust me sufficiently to share more of his feelings and develop the confidence to express his feelings without getting angry. Although his bowel habit still signals danger for him, he recognises this and can use the insight to deal with the things that frustrate him in a more healthy manner.

Not everybody can use the opportunity to tell their story in order to get better. For some, the event that instigated the illness may have occurred so early in life it cannot be recalled. For others, it may be so devastating and alien to that person's sense of self that it cannot be thought about. In our otherwise liberal and enlightened society, people still tend to view emotional disturbance with shame and humiliation. It is more acceptable to be racked with pain, exhausted and to suffer bowel upsets and indigestion than to admit to being depressed or unable to cope. Physical symptoms protect the psyche from being shattered by what has happened and provide an acceptable reason for avoiding social responsibilities. And when no cause is found, the symptoms can be attributed to an allergy or undetected infection, and blamed on the incompetence of the doctor. This saves face. So it is not surprising that many patients with functional illness reject the offer of psychotherapy or counselling. Instead, they prefer to continue the quest for biological solutions which are compatible with their world view – the new drug, the special diet or a particular alternative therapy. As the Romantic poet Robert Southey wrote: 'Sickness humbles the pride of man. It forces on him a sense of his own weakness and teaches him to feel his dependance on unseen powers that therefore makes wise men devout, makes the ignorant superstitious.'[8]

People who suffer from illness 'at the level of the idea' (see p. 126), often need treatment that works at the same level. They need something to put their faith in so they can let go of the illness. In the past, healers would sell amulets or magic charms. Some people with arthritis still use copper bracelets in much the same way. In a society that seems to be losing its faith in the scientific system of modern medicine, the application of an inactive treatment that the patient believes in can be very therapeutic. Unfortunately such remedies are so associated in the medical mind with charlatanism and the exploitation of vulnerable people for financial gain that they are derided as 'placeboes'.[9] In the past, placeboes were burlesque and counterfeit medicines. Often sold at fairgrounds, they were pills containing dough, sugar and coloured water, whose effectiveness was related entirely to the charisma of the showman.

In contemporary medical culture, the healing effect of belief and expectation is downgraded by the use of placeboes as 'blanks' in randomised controlled trials of drug treatment.[10] But herein lies a problem. The effect of the placebo is often so strong in functional or mental illnesses that it can be difficult to distinguish from the effect of the active drug.[11] For example, in some trials, 60 per cent of patients with functional abdominal pain responded to placebo. And recent trials of Viagra for female sexual dysfunction were inconclusive, not because the drug didn't work. Far from it; too many women responded to the placebo – which contained the idea but not the active ingredient.[12]

Although most practitioners would be reluctant to acknowledge it, almost all complementary treatments, and most of the so-called 'active' treatments employed by orthodox medicine, probable owe much of their efficacy to the recruitment of the patient's confidence and belief. Indeed, Roy Porter has even claimed that the history of medicine is largely the history of the placebo effect. As an example of the importance of belief, an article published in the *Lancet* over 160 years ago reported that when a patient was given twenty-five drops of laudanum, thinking it was a purgative, he was disturbed all night by the need to open his bowels. In fact, laudanum contained opium, which would normally induce constipation. The patient was responding more to the expectation that his bowels would be active than the biological effect of the laudanum.[13] But treatments that recruit the patient's confidence and expectation should not necessarily be dismissed as foolish or dishonest. Both the doctor who prescribes antispasmodics and the healer who administers homeopathic remedies believe in the effectiveness of their remedy. In each case, their patients often feel better because they trust their therapist's judgement and adopt the belief. We should therefore be very cautious lest we sacrifice this essential component of healing on the high altar of the National Institute of Clinical Excellence. Instead of trying to restrict the prescription of otherwise useful remedies through the artifice of randomised controlled clinical trials, medical institutions might do better to harness the therapeutic power of the healing effect to the pharmacological properties of the drugs.

Author and behavioural psychotherapist Ian Wickramasekere has argued that successful therapy requires the appropriate combination of faith and science.[14] During the fibre revolution of the 1980s, coarse wheatbran captured the public imagination not only because it caused a more satisfying bowel evacuation, but also because it resonated with the ancient ideas about the importance of healthy bowels and more modern notions of moral fibre and a more natural way of living. The knowledge that a treatment has some biological action that the patient is aware of gives the treatment 'credibility'.[15] The doctor can prescribe it with conviction and the patient can take it with confidence. The patient, it seems, has to believe in the treatment for it to work. In contrast, a drug that has an appropriate biological action but is administered without the endorsement of the media and the prescribing physician can have disappointing results. As Theodore Rousseau is reputed to have commented as early as 1854, 'You should treat as many patients with the new drugs while they still have the power to heal.'

With healing, as with so many other things in life, it's often not what you do, but the way that you do it. A doctor who appears calm and confident and exudes a serious air of conviction and authority, who pays careful attention to the patient's history and offers an unhurried explanation of why a particular remedy can be so effective, inspires trust and is likely to obtain better results than an exasperated doctor who makes his patients feel they have not been listened to.[16]

The following scenario, described by Dr Jane Worrall, illustrates the therapeutic potential of a charismatic doctor:

The patient was very demanding and difficult to please and claimed to suffer continuous agony from her ulcer. All of the many mild to moderate analgesics were useless and I did not feel opiates were justified, so I asked the advice of my immediate superior. The superior saw the patient, discussed her pain and, with a grave face, said he wanted to try a completely different sort of treatment. She agreed. He disappeared into the office, to reappear a few minutes later, walking slowly down the ward and holding in front of him a pair of tweezers which grasped a large, white tablet. As he came closer, it became clear (to me, at least) that the tablet was none other than effervescent Vitamin C. He dropped the tablet into a glass of water, which, of course, bubbled and fizzed, and told the patient to sip the water carefully when the fizzing had subsided. It worked – the new medicine completely abolished her pain.

This doctor recruited his patient's positive response to his special treatment through his personal gravitas and a simple bit of play acting.[17] The eighteenth-century hypnotherapist Anton Mesmer carried this to extremes. He used to dress up in a cloak and pointed hat covered in moons and stars and connect his patients by metal bars to a tub full of iron filings. This created powerful theatre and tapped into contemporary ideas on electricity and cosmology. Although few contemporary healers would go as far as Mesmer, the processional ward round of the dark-suited consultant and his white-coated attendants, the theatrical conclave in the middle of the ward and the complex and bewildering scientific language conveys a similar sense of awe and authority.[18] And the clinical examination does not only elicit the abnormal sounds, reflexes, lumps and tenderness, but the 'laying on of hands' breaks down reserve and suspicion and generates confidence. Thus, to be effective, it needs to be conducted in a calm, unhurried, reverential manner that respects the privacy of the patient. This is the art of medicine.

The creation of a customised treatment, concordant with the patient's own beliefs and convictions together with special instructions for when and how the medication should be taken, reinforces its effectiveness. I often use a resin called cholestyramine to treat otherwise untreatable diarrhoea. It binds unabsorbed bile acids which can irritate the colon, but it has to be taken half an hour before meals and titrated with both the size of the meal and the patient's response. It can be remarkably effective, but its efficacy is probably based as much on the fact that I believe in it and my patients are given detailed instructions on when and how they should take it and control on how to adjust the dose to obtain an optimal response. Similarly, when injections of normal saline have been administered with authority and a convincing explanation, they have cured everything from angina to asthma and from vomiting to vertigo.[19] But it is surgical operations that have the most powerful and dramatic healing effects (and greater danger of inducing personal grievance if they go wrong). The operating theatre with its gowned and masked players, the quiet atmosphere of concentration and the intimacy of the entry into the patient's body convey an awesome impression, which cannot fail to have a powerful influence on the patient. A successful operation requires an attitude of paramount authority on the part of the surgeon and one of absolute trust on the part of the patient. No wonder people can recover as a result of the operation alone, even when nothing is found and nothing repaired or removed.[20]

All traditional and complementary systems of medicine are powerful applications of the art of healing, the process by which rituals and natural products are used to facilitate a person's own natural capabilities to re-establish a state of well-being.[21] But the sheer variety of therapies can seem so bewildering. There are acupuncture, shiatsu, reflexology, massage, aromatherapy, chiropraxy, homeopathy, relaxation therapy, faith healing, meditation, yoga, hypnotherapy, medical herbalism, iridology, the different forms of psychotherapy, biofeedback – to name but a few! Surely they cannot all be effective – or can they?

Different therapies emphasise different aspects of healing. The more physical therapies, such as massage, aromatherapy, acupuncture, reflexology and shiatsu, use touch and massage as a means of making a deep sense of communication that helps to relieve tension. Music and art therapies are said to restore a sense of balance by enhancing the emotional and creative activity of the right side of the brain. Biofeedback training allows patients to learn how to change bodily functions by altering the way they feel. It is said to work better for those who are more sceptical and require convincing.[22] The scientific appearance of homeopathy, with its resemblance to immunisation and chemotherapy, conveys a high degree of credibility and most closely resembles the practice of orthodox medicine without the toxic effects of drugs. Both meditation and hypnotherapy induce a trance-like state of relaxed and focused attention using calming mental imagery, progressive muscular relaxation and a slow, repetitive vocal cadence. While in this state, suggestions implanted by the therapy can be employed to alter bodily functions. Accordingly, hypnotherapy has been employed to slow the heart, reduce the blood pressure, alter the electrical activity of the brain, reduce pain, relax muscular tension and regulate gut function.[23]

A colleague of mine, Dr Peter Whorwell, combines his practice of gastroenterology with hypnotherapy. When his patients are deeply relaxed, he advises them to envisage their bowels as a river. If they are constipated he suggests that their river is stagnant and murky and encourages them to change it to a highland stream where the water is clear and tumbling merrily over rocks. It works – often quite dramatically. I once applied Whorwell's technique to one of my constipated patients and induced such a merry attack of diarrhoea that the patient was unable to leave the house for three days. The next week I had to let the river meander through verdant meadows.

It has to be said that the specific scientific basis of many 'alternative' or 'complementary' therapies is rather dubious. There is, to my knowledge, no anatomical basis for the body meridians which form the basis of acupuncture. There is no physiological reason, so far as I am aware, than can explain why pressure on the sole of the foot, as employed by practitioners of shiatsu and reflexology, can heal dysfunction of the liver or the heart. And it is difficult to believe that homeopathic dilutions – which would need to split the atom to retain any of the active substance – have any biological action at all. But I do not think we should worry too much about whether the specific mechanism of action can be proven scientifically. That, in my opinion, is not what makes people feel better. What matters is the skill of the therapist in recruiting the belief and self-confidence that encourages healing. Seen from that perspective, the tinctures, powders and needles are like Mesmer's tub of iron filings, stage props focusing the impact of the therapeutic drama. Thus, complementary medicine is not just a random collection of specific therapies, each of which needs to be validated by random controlled trials; it is, I believe, an alternative therapeutic approach that uses different techniques to harness the patient's own powers of healing.

Complementary therapies confer what is often missing from a modern medical consultation: the time to listen; the development of a therapeutic rapport; the reduction of emotional tension and establishment of a sense of harmony; and the space for creative possibilities to take root and grow. The specific techniques provide a positive identification around which patients can focus their own capacity for healing. Ian Wickramasekere has called this the Trojan Horse approach, conveying the idea that the active treatment (psychotherapy) is concealed inside a therapeutic symbol or idea that gains the patient's confidence. Touch can be used to reassure anxious and ill people, allowing them to feel relaxed and safe in the hands of another person.[24] Most mothers know how they can soothe away their infant's aches and pains by a cuddle. And lovers know how that combination of physical and emotional intimacy can break down their resistances and completely transform their lives. So it is not so much the specific techniques that need to be evaluated but the therapeutic approach. Therapies as diverse as massage, acupuncture, relaxation, hypnotherapy and reflexology reduce the secretion of stress hormones, rectify physiological functions and have been shown to be of great benefit to people with functional illness.[25]

The active selection and participation in an individual therapy imparts a sense of personal control and confidence that is often lacking in orthodox medicine's rushed appointments, peremptory diagnoses and reflex dispensation of pills. Add to that a specific belief structure that the patient can identify with and you have a powerful healing concoction. In our 24/7 society with its daily challenges and threats, we seem to have lost the knowledge of self-healing. Yet our bodies have a restorative capacity that is better than any tonic, supplement or symptomatic remedy. Complementary therapies can help us find this.

Our health service, like the rest of our society, appears too preoccupied with waiting lists, efficiency, accountability and audit to think about holistic aspects of health and well-being. Yet there is abundant scientific evidence that feelings of peace, contentment, relaxation, confidence and containment reduce emotional tension, restoring a healthy balance of hormones and reversing pathogenic processes. The more scientific medicine becomes, the more it seeks to deny the art of healing, which is fundamental to any therapeutic relationship. So there is little point in deriding complementary therapists because the materials they use do not stand up to scientific scrutiny. Instead, we should be encouraging health service managers to recognise the importance of the healing methods perfected by psychotherapists and complementary practitioners and seek to incorporate them into mainstream medicine. We urgently need to restore the balance between the art and science of medicine.

The scientific development of mainstream Western medicine has allowed the healing arts popular expression in psychotherapies and the variety of complementary or alternative therapies. This has led to the coexistence of two completely separate medical philosopies: the so-called orthodoxy of scientific, Western, evidence-based medicine; and a collection of heterodox healing methods. So now as many as 40 per cent of people living in Western countries seek alternative medicine often alongside orthodox medicine.

The two approaches to health care could not be more different.[26]

Where Western orthodox medicine is mechanistic and specific, complementary medicine is holistic and general. Where Western medicine is disease-oriented, complementary medicine is patient-oriented. Where Western medicine can be seen as detached, scientific and impersonal, complementary medicine is engaging, humanistic and personal. Where Western medicine dissects out the disease mechanism, complementary medicine attempts to integrate the forces that have made the person ill. While Western medicine restores and maintains the function of damaged organs by external means, complementary medicine uses the body's own resources to maintain health. And where Western medicine saves lives, complementary medicine restores health and tries to prevent those lives being put at risk in the first place.

But patients should not have to choose between competing philosophies. They need both.[27] According to Greek mythology, Asclepios, the son of Apollo and healer to the Gods and his wife Epione, the soother of pain, produced twin daughters, Hygeia and Panacea, who worked together to maintain the health of the nation. Panacea had knowledge of medicines to treat disease while Hygeia advocated living in harmony with nature to avoid illness. A proper medical service needs to combine the specific remedies of Panacea with the holistic understanding of Hygeia. This is the vision behind the notion of integrated health care.[28]

So the challenge for the twenty-first century is to integrate the scientific approach of orthodox medicine with the holistic approach of the healing therapies to produce a more balanced and effective health care system that is centred around the ill person. But integration is not just about employing an approved acupuncturist in the pain clinic, offering a weekly massage session in a GP's surgery, or sending the occasional troublesome patient for psychotherapy. Complementary medicine and psychotherapy cannot be bolted onto the monolith of medical orthodoxy as a token gesture to demonstrate that doctors are sufficiently broad-minded to embrace popular trends. Partnerships based on political expediency instead of understanding and respect are doomed to collapse. A true integration would incorporate an understanding of the patient and the philosophy of self-healing with a scientific knowledge of pathological mechanisms and the capability of medical treatments.

The realisation that doctors cannot cure most of the patients who attend their surgeries will have an enormous impact on the way we practise medicine in the future. Doctors will still need to recognise and treat infections, cancers and inflammatory diseases, but these conditions may be more realistically perceived to be at the biological end of a continuum of illness that includes a much larger component of emotional distress, functional illness and psychosomatic disease. In 1999, the Center for Advancement of Health in Washington DC recommended that medicine should recognise how intimately health is linked to people's attitudes, thoughts, feelings and behaviours, and should seek to treat the whole person – mind, body and spirit – not defects in individual organs. The pay-off, it concluded, would be healthier individuals, healthier communities and a healthier nation. This is not a new idea; it is as old as medicine itself. In Plato's *Charmides*, Socrates would prescribe no 'physick' for Charmides's headache till he had first eased his troublesome mind.

But to bring about such a shift in emphasis might mean turning our current health system on its head. Supposing, for example, we regarded illness as not so much a specific cellular malfunction that requires scientific tests to identify it and powerful chemicals to treat it, but as a reaction to what has happened to us? This might have several advantages. By understanding their patients better, doctors would only investigate those symptoms that were out of keeping with the illness narrative and may indicate a pathological process. This could save so much of the time spent on fruitless investigations, futile trials of treatments, repeat appointments, referrals to other consultants and letters of complaint. Magnified throughout the country, it could lead to more healthy and confident patients, who would be less likely to seek help for familiar illness and considerable reductions in doctors' workload. But doctors would need to spend more time getting to know their patients and gaining a clearer appreciation of when certain symptoms seem out of context and need medical investigation. Only then could they avoid the risk of missing serious disease. At present, they have neither the training nor the time to decode the illness and help their patients make the necessary adjustments to get better. As one GP said to me recently, 'If I spent half an hour listening to what every patient wanted to tell me, I would never get home before midnight.'

But would a more integrated practice necessarily be centred on the GP? Could the role of gatekeeper not be conducted by a tier of health workers, who would not have the detailed scientific training of the modern doctor but would nevertheless be skilled at understanding and dealing with ill people?[29] We already have some excellent nurse practitioners but I wonder whether in the absence of a specific training it would be feasible to recruit practitioners of integrated health from the ranks of counsellors, psychotherapists and complementary therapists. This new body of healers could be trained to recognise when the patient needs medical treatment but otherwise they would work with the ill person to help them restore a healthy state of equilibrium. And instead of focusing on a single healing technique, they would have knowledge of a variety of healing methods and would help the ill person select those that are most compatible with their attitudes and beliefs. In such a health service, the modern doctor with his or her scientific knowledge and discipline could be seen more as a diagnostician and pharmacotherapist, to be consulted when there are obvious indicators of organic disease.

But even with the involvement of nurses and complementary therapists, there would still be insufficient professional resources to cope with the burden of ill health. If utilisation of resources continues to rise at current rates, health services could be swamped by the burden of long-term illness in a matter of decades. Therefore, the British government has begun to develop initiatives to shift the responsibility for health care from the doctor to the patient. In the future, patients will be at the heart of the health service.[30] This will not only require a commitment by health professionals to share knowledge and information about treatment options, it will also mean that patients will have more choice in terms of where and how they are treated, and they will be empowered to take responsibility for the management of their illness in partnership with health and social care providers.

Experience in North America and in Britain shows that today's patients with chronic illness need not just be the recipients of care, they can become key decision-makers in the management of their condition. The British government's Expert Patient Programme has recently been piloted in primary care trusts throughout the UK.[31] Based on a model developed in Stanford University by Professor Kate Lorig for people with rheumatoid arthritis, it is specifically designed to help people with long-term medical conditions reduce the impact of their symptoms, improve confidence, resourcefulness and self-efficacy and lead to a more effective partnership with health professionals. The programme is a short course of just six modules, comprising generic instruction into the key components of self-management such as relaxation, diet and exercise, cognitive symptom management, communication with doctors, medication and pain control. These are run by patient tutors and conducted within the primary care trusts. As Dr Mike Pringle, Professor of General Practice and Chairman of the 'Joining Up Self-Care in the NHS' explained: 'Self-care has been identified as a life-long habit and culture ... the action individuals take for themselves and their families to stay healthy and manage minor and chronic conditions based on the knowledge and information available and working in collaboration with health care professionals where necessary.' Expert patient programmes are not simply about instructing patients about their condition and measuring success on the basis of patient compliance, they encourage patients to develop the confidence to use their own skills and knowledge to manage their own illness. They are patient-centred instead of disease-centred.

This all sounds rather utopian, but will it make a difference? Early indications look promising.[32] The Expert Patient Programme was implemented in 2002 and by 2004, it had reached over 11,000 people living with 300 different conditions across the UK.

Among the reported changes were included a reduction in depression, fatigue and the intensity of pain, an increase in self-confidence, fewer visits to the doctors, a reduction in days off work and a more effective dialogue with health professionals. These preliminary results indicate that when people are more involved in the management of their own long-term illness, there are not only improvements in patient well-being, but a less dependent and more effective system of health care. In time, people may learn to take control of their health in much the same way as they control their personal finances, family size and leisure time. By 2008, it is planned that the Expert Patient Programme should be available to patients with long-term medical conditions within every primary care trust in the country. It remains to be seen whether these early results would be maintained and whether it is suitable for everybody. Patients with specific illnesses, like irritable bowel syndrome, eating disorders or chronic fatigue syndrome may require a more specific programme. And since functional illnesses can last for years, self-management may require long-term support. So the UK government is seeking to fill these gaps by collaboration with the voluntary sector. Charities serving patients with specific illnesses are being encouraged to develop their own self-management programmes to dovetail with the Expert Patient Programme.

But would this make the doctor redundant? Not at all! It should instead lead to a more creative and productive therapeutic relationship. With more responsibility of health care invested in patients, consultations with doctors would be more a communication between experts. The doctor has extensive knowledge of how bodies work, what constitutes an unhealthy diet and lifestyle, how to treat illness with drugs and when to refer to a specialist. But patients are also experts. They have lived with the same body for all of their lives and they know how it is likely to react to certain situations. They also understand the stresses and strains in their family and workplace. So although doctors would offer interpretations, give advice and generally help their patients make informed choices about how best to manage his or her illness, the responsibility for whether they remain ill or recover would ultimately rest with the patient. This single shift in attitude can be liberating for both doctor and patient. I enjoyed medicine much more when I realised that I did not have to bear direct responsibility for curing my patients' illness but could allow myself the time and creative space to help them arrive at the solutions that would help them get better themselves. This attitude also freed my patients from a grudging dependence on me while allowing them to gain more confidence in looking after themselves. But while we should all welcome the opportunity for a more accountable health service based on a real partnership between doctor and patient, we must take care to avoid a return to the chaos and superstition that existed before the scientific revolution.

Such changes, although they are an important step in the right direction, are still missing the point. They still treat contemporary health care, whether it is delivered by doctors, therapists or patients themselves, as a kind of fire service, to be called upon when there is a crisis. A hundred years ago, improvements in public hygiene, sanitation, nutrition and living standards did more to reduce the enormous morbidity and mortality from infectious and nutritional diseases than any of the contemporary advances in medicine. Now we need another set of public health reforms in the way people live together in order to reduce the enormous burden of chronic functional illnesses on our modern Western societies.

In Chapter Five, I suggested that a combination of quite fundamental changes in social attitudes and an unprecedented degree of social isolation has undermined the ability of people to resolve the trials of modern life without becoming ill. But to expect doctors or any other combination of health workers to cure society is like asking generals to stop terrorism. The sickness is inherent in the social system and will only get better when the way in which people live changes. Victorian society responded to the cultural upheavals of the industrial revolution by putting in place the social structures that we all took for granted until recently – the churches, schools, police forces, hospitals, town councils, working men's clubs, women's institutes and so on. These gave people a sense of belonging, of identity and social cohesion. Now that the next enormous wave of social change is upon us and culture is once again fragmented by change, we will need to create new social structures. Emphasis will need to be placed on encouraging more social involvement, working in smaller groups, introducing incentives for community responsibility, creating new initiatives for the socialisation of our children.

Human beings are social animals. And social animals always get ill if they are cut off from their community. So the enormous advances in technology should be employed not so much to isolate individuals still further but to provide new opportunities for creative social interaction and a restoration of community and collective identity that transcends the morbid obsession with the self.

Notes

Introduction

1 Data on the decline of many common diseases in Britain were obtained from Karen Dunnell's article, 'Are We healthier?' for the Office of National Statistics report *The Health of Adult Britain 1841–1994* (Charlton & Murphy 1997; Dunnell 1997). Also read Dr R. Stallones's article 'The Rise and Fall of Ischaemic Heart Disease' (Stallones 1980).

2 The medical correspondent of the *Daily Telegraph*, Dr James LeFanu has documented the major milestones in medical discovery around the middle of the last century in the first part of his book, *The Rise and Fall of Modern Medicine* (LeFanu 1999).

3 By 2000, the expenditure of health in the UK was 7.3 per cent of GDP, exceeding the spending on defence and education, but still much lower than Switzerland (10.7 per cent), Germany (10.6 per cent), France (9.5 per cent) and the United States (13.0 per cent), according to OECD Health Data 2002 (www.oecd.org/document/22/0). The predictions for UK health expenditure to 2023 are outlined in 'NHS Funding and Reform: The Wanless Report', House of Commons Library, www.parliament.uk/commons/lib/research/rp2002/rp02-030.pdf

4 Consumer surveys on self-reported health integrate biological, psychological and social dimensions and therefore offer a more subjective and comprehensive assessment of the health of a nation. They also reflect the expectations people have about their health as well as the actual prevalence of sickness. Nevertheless, they have been shown to predict early mortality, psychological health and hospital utilisation. British figures are taken from the General Household Survey (Bridgewood *et al.* 1995; Office of National Statistics 2001). The European figures are derived from the European Community Household Panel (ECHP), coordinated by Eurostat, which showed that in 1998, 43.3 per cent of women and 36.1 per cent of men described their health as fair, bad or very bad, but there were large cultural differences in health perception. For example, over 75 per cent of people in Ireland, Denmark and Greece rated their health as good or very good compared to less than 50 per cent in Germany and Portugal (European Commission, Statistical Office of the European Communities 2002). More recent figures indicate that as many as 60 per cent of people in Europe thought their lives adversely affected by their health (Hungin *et al.* 2003). The Australian figures are taken from the Australian Institute of Health and Welfare,

www.aihw.gov.au/publications/aus/aho4. American data on self-perceived health was obtained from the Family Core Component of the 1997–2004 National Health Interview Surveys, the General Social Survey (1972–98) and from Robert Putnam's (pp. 331–2) presentation of consumer research/market intelligence data from Deaton and Parsons's article on 'Ageing and the Inequality of Health and Income' (Deaton & Parsons 1998; Putnam 2000). The discrepancies in the data from different countries and even within the same country reflect different assumptions as to what constitutes a long-standing illness or good health (Miilunpalo *et al.* 1997).

5 Trends in long-term illness in young people were obtained from the British General Household Survey (Office of National Statistics 2001) and from a paper entitled 'Long-term illness and psychosomatic complaints in children aged two to seventeen years in the five Nordic countries. Comparison between 1984 and 1996'. The largest increases were from Finland, and the prevalence for all countries was highest in low-income, low-educated, one-parent families (Berntsson & Kohler 2001). The European figures were obtained from the European Community Household Panel (European Commission, Statistical Office of the European Communities 2002). There is also a recent report of the asthma epidemic in children (Nowak, Suppli Ulrik & von Mutius 2004).

6 Dr Iain Sidford, a general practitioner tutor working in Redditch, Worcester-shire, reported a 75 per cent rise in consultations per patient between 1970 and 1995 (Sidford 1997). The General Household Survey reports that the proportion of people visiting their GP in the fourteen days prior to interview rose from 12 to 17 per cent between 1972 and 1993 and has remained reasonably static since that time, but these figures do not take into account the frequent attenders that occupy so much of the workload of the average GP. The data on prescriptions was obtained from the Mintel report on Ethical Medicines (Mintel 2000a) and the Prescription Pricing Authority (2004).

7 In 1989, Doctors Kurt Kroenke and David Mangelsdorff reviewed the records of 1,000 army personnel, their dependants and retired service members who attended the Brooke Army Medical Clinic for a range of common medical symptoms. A pathological diagnosis was established in just 14 per cent of cases. Some were given a psychological diagnosis, but this still left 74 per cent patients with no obvious pathological or psychological reason for their symptoms (Kroenke & Mangelsdorff 1989a). For surveys of the prevalence of medically unexplained symptoms, see Guo, Kuroki, & Koizumi 2001; Katon 1984; Katon, Sullivan, & Walker 2001; Khan *et al.* 2003; Kroenke & Mangelsdorff 1989b; Peveler, Kilkenny, & Kinmouth 1997; Thomas 1994; Wessley & Ismail 2002. The WHO has recently conducted a survey of medically unexplained somatic symptoms in five different cultures across the world (Isaac *et al.* 1995). The difference in numbers probably represents different doctors' beliefs of what constitutes an unexplained illness and to what extent the illness is the usual way of expressing psychosocial distress. The importance of recognition and appropriate management of medically unexplained symptoms to health care providers is emphasised in a 2005 paper in the *British Medical Journal* (Rosendal, Olesen, & Fink 2005).

8 Data from Japan was obtained from OECD publications and from a recent

paper on medically unexplained illness. See Guo, Kuroki, & Koizumi 2001; and Jeong & Hurst 2001.

9   In *Bowling Alone* Putnam used data on headaches, indigestion and insomnia from the DDB Needham Lifestyle Survey Archive 1975–99 to generate a score for 'malaise', which has increased in the last quarter of the twentieth century as social connectiveness has declined. The European figures were obtained from the European Community Household Panel (Statistical Office of the European Communities 2002) and relate to rates of illness from teenagers.

10 A recent postal survey showed that frequent medical attendance was more likely in people with medically unexplained symptoms and health anxiety (Little *et al.* 2000), while a systematic review of published papers revealed that particularly high attendance rates were associated with high rates of physical and psychiatric disease and social problems (Gill & Sharpe 1999).

11 In the UK, these include the ME Association, ReMEmber, Pain Concern, the Fibromyalgia Association, the National Back Pain Association, the Migraine Trust, Women's Health, Cyclical Vomiting Syndrome Association, Action Against Allergy, Hyperactive Children's Support Group, Allergy UK, Food Allergy Association, National Asthma Campaign, the IBS Network, the Eating Disorders Association, the Endometriosis Society, the National Association for Premenstrual Syndrome, the National Association for Crohn's and Colitis Sufferers, Mind, and many many more. Similar organisations exist in every country in the Western world.

12 £2.3 billion was spent on non-prescriptive medicines in the UK in 1999. By 2002, the total market for vitamins and minerals was estimated by Mintel at £350 million while the total market for complementary medicines was estimated at £130 million, an increase of 60 per cent since 1997. UK and European data on the purchase of 'over the counter' health remedies and nutritional supplements were obtained from the Target Group Index on the British Market Research Bureau (1998) and from the Euromonitor and Mintel reports (Euromonitor 1999; Mintel 2000b; Mintel 2003a; Mintel 2003b).

13 By 1993, more visits were made to providers of complementary and alternative medicine (425 million) in America than to primary care physicians (388 million) and more was spent on complementary therapies, tonics and vitamin and mineral supplements ($13.7 billion) than on all hospital admissions. Utilisation of complementary and alternative medicine has grown more rapidly in the United States than in other Western countries (Barnes *et al.* 2004; Eisenberg *et al.* 1993), but every indication suggests that other Western countries, including the UK, are catching up rapidly (Ernst 2000; Thomas, Nicholl, & Coleman 2001). Some countries, such as Germany, France and Japan, have more of a continuous tradition of complementary medicine and have integrated it into conventional health care.

Chapter 1: What kind of illness are we suffering from?

1   For an excellent account of the threats posed by virulent new plagues, infecting humans as a result of exposure to animal reservoirs, read *Virus X* (Ryan 2003).

2   *Candida albicans* is a fungus that is normally present on the skin, and in the

mouth, the vagina and the bowel. For most people, it is completely harmless, but under certain conditions when the resistance of a person is weakened, it may multiply and invade the skin and mucous membranes, causing itching and inflammation. It is most common in the vagina, where it may be recognised as adherent white plaques or patches. This is known as 'thrush'. Some practitioners, however, claim that many people have an allergy or hypersensitivity to *candida* and that this can cause a whole range of common, otherwise medically unexplained symptoms although there is no medical evidence for this. The leading exponents of '*candidiasis* hypersensitivity' have been C. Orian Truss MD of Birmingham, Alabama, and William G. Crook of Jackson, Tennessee. Crook became interested in yeast problems after reading one of Truss's papers and in 1983 published his popular book, *The Yeast Connection*. See also the paper on dubious yeast allergies by Stephen Barrett on www.quackwatch.org

3   For further information on these possibilities read *Human Colonic Bacteria: Role in Nutrition, Physiology and Pathology* (Gibson & MacFarlane 1995), *The Large Intestine in Health and Disease* (Cummings 1997) and 'A Gut Feeling' (Vines 1998).

4   To put things into perspective, plants contain a wide range of natural toxins to protect them from ingestion from animals. It is also possible that in years gone by, when large amounts of toxic arsenic, antimony and mercury salts were used to treat diseases, people were exposed to a much greater extent to toxic substances than today.

5   For example, further information on the effects of chronic fluoride intoxication is documented in a recent review in *Fluoride* (Waldcott 1998) and discussed in an open correspondence in *Gut Reaction* between me and Leonard Harley (spring 2004 issue www.ibsnetwork.co.uk). Mercury poisoning from dental amalgam is still a controversial issue. See the UK Amalgam Website (www.amalgam.ukgo.com).

6   For more information on the rise of allergies read 'Allergy, the Unmet Need, a Blueprint for Patient Care', a 2003 report from the UK Royal College of Physicians. The poor correlation between self-reported allergy and the results of allergy testing is documented in many publications (Bhat, Harper, & Gorard 2002; Krahnke *et al.* 2003) and may be in part related to local allergic reactions taking place in the lining of the gut and airways (Lin *et al.* 2002), which would not be detected by blood or skin tests.

7   Stress increases the permeability of the epithelial lining of the gut and the airways, allowing food substances and other substances access to the immunological defences (Groot *et al.* 2000). It releases the cytokines that induce inflammatory responses and excites immune responses, increasing mast cells, enteroendocrine cells and all the other components of allergic responses. So it stands to reason that things that cause alarm would excite allergic responses while anything that recruits the confidence and trust of a patient and induces a state of relaxation might well damp down allergic responses (Frieri 2003).

8   Recently the trend has been to talk about 'medically unexplained symptoms', implying they do not fulfil the criteria of any of the 5,000 or so medical diagnoses. But this might exclude conditions like anorexia nervosa, fibromyalgia and even irritable bowel syndrome, which many doctors regard as 'explained'.

9 It is called Stendhal's syndrome because the nineteenth-century French novelist is said to be the first to write about the head-spinning disorientation some tourists experience when they encounter Florentine masterpieces. For an entertaining account of the range of modern syndromes and illnesses, read *The Hypochrondriac's Handbook* (Naish 2004).

10 But this does not necessarily indicate some definite disease. Such changes could arise as a result of physical and emotional tension plus an increased sensitivity to some local change in blood flow, or exposure to particular environmental constituents such as particular foods.

11 Researchers and opinion leaders from both sides of the Atlantic continue to engage in this controversy. For a sample, read the MRC 2003 review of research into UK Gulf War veterans' illnesses at www.mrc.ac.uk

12 Evidence in support of the increase in prevalence of and health care seeking for functional illness can be obtained from the following sources. Headache: American Council for Headache Education, www.achenet.org (Cox, Blaxter, & Buckle 1987; Cypress 1981; Linet 1989). Functional Gastrointestinal Disorders: (Nguyen-Van-Tam & Logan 1997; McCormick, Fleming, & Charlton 1995). Backache: (Frymoyer & Cats-Baril 1991). Chronic Fatigue Syndrome: (Chen 1986; Cox, Blaxter, & Buckle 1987; Kellner 1994; Meltzer, Petticrew, & Hinds 1995; Wessley, Hotopf, & Sharpe 1998). Fibromyalgia: (Bakal 2000; Kellner 1994; Masi & Yunus 1986; Wessley, Nimnuan, & Sharpe 1999b; Wolfe & Cathey 1983). Non Cardiac Chest Pain: (Mayou *et al.* 2000). Obesity: (Lewis *et al.* 2000; Mokdad *et al.* 2001; National Audit Office 2001).

13 The indirect costs of IBS, such as absence from work and loss of productivity, the social cost of IBS has been estimated in excess of £200 million a year. For a breakdown of UK health care costs of irritable bowel syndrome, see Camilleri & Williams 2000; Donker, Foets, & Spreeuwneberg 1999; Wells, Hahn, & Whorwell 1997. For migraine, see Ferrari 1998; Hu 1999 and Bandolier/Sept 1999/band 67. For back pain see Maniakidis & Gray 2000. For obesity see the National Audit Office's 2001 report, 'Tackling Obesity', the 2003–4 report of the House of Commons Health Committee on Obesity, the US Surgeon General's call to action to prevent and decrease overweight and obesity (2001), and the WHO report, Global Strategy on Diet, Physical Activity and Health 2003.

14 Functional illness uses more health care resources than any other category. See Morris, Gask, & Ronals 1998; Robinson *et al.* 2003; Smith 1994.

15 There are several versions to this story. Three flies were sitting on a dung heap and along came an elephant. 'What on earth is that?' they said to each other. 'Let's take off and have a look.' After some minutes they landed back on their spot on the dung heap and, bursting with excitement, compared notes. 'Did you ever see anything like it, so white and smooth and shiny?' exclaimed the first fly, who had landed on one of the elephant's tusks. 'No, no, no. It isn't like that at all,' argued the second who had landed on the elephant's back. 'It is black, hard and dry and it goes on for ever.' 'You're both wrong,' said the third. 'It is pink and wet and there's always a strong wind blowing.' He had landed on the tip of the elephant's trunk. And so the arguments went on, each one convinced he had the right impression. But in fact, all of them were right, they were just seeing the

elephant from their own unique perspective (Wessley, Nimnuan, & Sharpe 1999b).

16 The prevalence of any illness always depends on the stringency of the diagnostic criteria. For example, within the spectrum of patients suffering from chronic fatigue syndrome, attempts have been made to establish a more specific diagnosis such as myalgic encephalomyelitis (ME) or chronic fatigue immune deficiency syndrome (CFIDS). CFIDS is a highly specific diagnosis that requires the following criteria: a substantial reduction of previous activity; a persistent or relapsing illness that lasts at least six months; a very definite onset; cannot be explained by mental or physical illness; four or more of the following symptoms – severely impaired memory or concentration, sore throat, tender lymph nodes, muscle pain, multi-joint pain without swelling or redness, headaches of new onset, unrefreshing sleep, post-exertion malaise. This does not mean that CFIDS necessarily exists as a separate diagnosis; it merely represents the attempts of international classification committees to ringfence a particularly severe form of fatigue to facilitate discovery of a definite cause. It is hardly surprising that the prevalence of CFIDS is less than a tenth of that of chronic fatigue syndrome. Similarly, of all the people who suffer with unexplained abdominal pain, only a fraction conform to the Rome diagnostic criteria for irritable bowel syndrome (Drossman *et al.* 2000).

17 Thus 60 per cent of patients with irritable bowel syndrome, for example, also have functional dyspepsia, 50 per cent have an erratic pattern of eating, 14 per cent have chronic fatigue syndrome, 30 per cent have fibromyalgia, 16 per cent have temporomandibular joint disorder, 38 per cent have chronic back pain and 18 per cent have premenstrual syndrome. Likewise patients with chronic fatigue syndrome frequently have features of fibromyalgia, irritable bowel syndrome, tension headache, premenstrual syndrome, food allergy and multiple chemical sensitivity. See Aaron & Buchwald 2001; Barskey & Borus 1999; Deary 2001; Katon, Sullivan, & Walker 2001; Wessley, Nimnuan, & Sharpe 1999b; Whitehead, Palsson, & Jones 2002. In a recent survey of 'medically unexplained' symptoms from different cultures, all of the patients included had a variety of somatic symptoms referable to different parts of the body. (See Isaac *et al.* 1995.)

18 Not only are women more likely to suffer from functional illness, but they are more likely to get them more severely, to seek help from their GPs and to be referred to hospital clinics (Cloninger *et al.* 1986; Kroenke & Price 1993; Melville 1987). Although the female-to-male ratio for irritable bowel syndrome in the community is about 3–2, consultant gastroenterologists regularly see about four times as many women with this condition than men.

19 The fact that women are more predisposed to these immunological diseases might either suggest that immunological factors underpin functional illnesses. On the other hand since emotional tension is known to enhance immune reactivity and instigate allergies (see Frieri 2003) and attacks of auto-immune disease and functional illness, it might suggest that women have a greater tendency to impaired emotional regulation (see Chapter 3).

20 There is extensive evidence to support the association between functional illness and psychological disorders (Bennett & Kellow 2002; Hamilton, Campos, &

Creed 1996; Katon, Sullivan, & Walker 2001; Kroenke & Price 1993; Pearson 1991; Russo *et al.* 1994; Simon & VonKorff 1991).

21 Mohammed Yunus, Professor of Rheumatology at Chicago University and an authority on fibromyalgia syndrome, has called this the 'third disease paradigm' (Yunus 2000).

22 Figures from the UK Department of Health Indicate 20 per cent of women and 13 per cent of men suffer from anxiety and depression but population surveys suggest a much higher prevalence (see Meltzer *et al.* 1995; Putnam 2000; Wolpert 1999; World Health Organisation 1999). More than 40 per cent of Americans suffer from serious anxiety and depression during their life span. Antidepressants are currently prescribed 20 million times a year in Britain, an increase of 700 per cent over the last ten years. It was recently reported that over 50 per cent of Britain's university students show signs of depression. This suggests an alarming increase since 1987, when figures for significant emotional disturbance among students were between 1 and 25 per cent. Suicide has become the commonest cause of death among young people, higher than road traffic accidents.

23 Then as now, functional illness was a complex mixture of somatic and emotional symptoms. For a wealth of references see *Hysteria: The History of an Illness* by Ilza Veith (Veith 1965), *Anatomy of Melancholy* by Robert Burton (Burton 2001), *Elizabethan Madness* by Videa Skultans (Skultans 1985), and *From Paralysis to Fatigue* by Edward Shorter (Shorter 1993).

24 Thomas Sydenham's contemporary, Georgio Baglivi (1668–1706), whom Pope Clement XI had appointed to the chair of medical theory in the Collegio della Sapienza in Rome, wrote that diseases of the mind tend to manifest themselves by gastrointestinal symptoms largely brought about by decreasing appetites and disinterest in food, thus making an early connection between psychological disturbance and functional gastrointestinal disorders and anorexia nervosa. He further considered that those of gentle breeding and more delicate emotional sensitivity were more susceptible to disease than the 'meaner' sort of person, stressing how some, through indignation and impatience, turned the slightest disorders into long and mortal diseases. He believed that almost all of the cure 'lay in the patient's own breast, that is in a mind well fortified with patience, fortitude, prudence, tranquillity and the other moral virtues without which all manner of remedies and all the efforts of physicians will be vain and useless'. See Veith 1965, pp. 146–51.

25 See *The English Malady* by Edward Cheyne (Cheyne 1734; Guerrini 2004).

26 George Beard's original observations were recorded in the *Boston Medical and Surgical Journal* (Beard, 1869). Eleven years later, Beard published his book entitled *A Practical Treatise on Nervous Exhaustion* (Neurasthenia), in which the diagnosis became expanded to accommodate every physical symptom imaginable and a number of mental ones as well. The development and extinction of neurasthenia as a medical paradigm is discussed by Edward Shorter, pp. 220–32. Nevertheless, the concept of neurasthenia was until recently alive and well in China and was also implicit in Dr Raymond Pujol's 1967 description of '*la nevrose des téléphonistes*' or receptionist's neurosis. There is even a suggestion that it could be revived (Sharpe & Carson 2001).

27   But hysteria did not disappear. The writer Elaine Showalter wrote of the
     epidemics of hysterical disorders, imaginary illnesses, rumour panics and
     hypnotically induced pseudo-memories that flooded the media in the 1980s and
     1990s and reached a crescendo at the time of the millennium: 'From chronic
     fatigue syndrome to tales of alien abduction, from Gulf War syndrome to tales
     of satanic ritual abuse, these epidemics of psychogenic disease and confabulated
     memory have much to tell us about the anxieties and fantasies of contemporary
     Western culture, and, in their erosion of reason and courage, pose as great a
     social threat as the plagues of the tropical rainforests' (Showalter 1997).

28   For a scholarly and readable development of this idea, read *Minding the Body*
     (Bakal 2000).

29   For a description of the concept of abnormal illness behaviour, see Dr Issy
     Pilowsky's original paper and his book of the same name (Pilowsky 1969). Also
     see Dr David Mechanic's paper 'Sex, illness, illness behaviour and the use of
     health services' (Mechanic 1978). And for a more amusing account of this
     phenomenon, read *The Hypochondriac's Handbook* by John Naish (Naish 2004).

30   For references on quality of life of functional gastrointestinal disorders
     compared with conditions that have a definitive pathological basis see Gralnek *et
     al.* 2000, and Pace *et al.* 2003.

31   See 'Neurohumoral Features of Myocardial Stunning Due to Sudden Emotional
     Stress'. (Wittstein *et al.* 2005). This would account for Cannon's Voodoo Death
     (Cannon 1957).

32   Health professional organisations are only now beginning to acknowledge the
     need to train doctors to understand and manage those illnesses that do not have
     a pathological basis but are probably caused by a person's psychological response
     to the events in his or her life (Rosendal, Olesen, & Fink 2005).

Chapter 2: What makes people ill?

1   It is a curious fact that people who have suffered a shattering traumatic
     experience earlier in their lives, tend, like a moth to a flame, to revisit the
     circumstances of the trauma. So people who have been abused in childhood can
     tend to find themselves in abusive relationships when they grow up. Freud
     thought that this 'compulsion to repetition' occurred in order to gain mastery
     over the experience by changing the story, but at times it seems almost like
     picking at a sore, a compulsion to relive the drama and the pain in order to
     validate the sense of who they are. This might explain why the repetitive re-
     enactment of the trauma as bodily illness is so difficult to cure. Some patients
     seem to cling on to the symptoms as part of themselves, the cross they have to
     bear.

2   Relationships between stressful life events and medically unexplained symptoms
     have been documented in numerous publications. Powerful anecdotal evidence
     from patient narrative has been confirmed by the more formal 'Life Events and
     Difficulties Schedule' devised by George Brown and Tirril Harris (Brown &
     Harris 1989). Ethelle Bennett and John Kellow from Sydney, Australia have
     written an excellent recent account of life events, functional gastrointestinal
     symptoms and other stress-related conditions (Bennett & Kellow 2002). For

more references, see 'Medical Symptoms Without Identified Pathology: Relationship to Psychiatric Disorders, Childhood and Adult Trauma and Personality Traits' (Katon, Sullivan, & Walker 2001).

3   Pierre Briquet's experience is quoted in books by Shorter (pp. 97–8) and Van der Kolk (p. 49) (Shorter 1993; Van der Kolk, McFarlane, & Weisaeth 1996).

4   *Life Events and Illness*, ed. by George Brown and Tirril Harris (Brown & Harris 1989) p. 3.

5   This study was nicely controlled since health interviews had been conducted a year previously as part of a wide-ranging epidemiological survey (Escobar *et al.* 1992). So it was possible to conclude that the symptoms had occurred since the disaster and only in those who had been involved in it. Similarly the Brisbane floods in 1974 were associated with increased number of visits to physicians (Abrahams 1976). More recent studies have demonstrated that symptoms are more marked if disaster victims have suffered the psychological symptoms of post-traumatic stress disorder (McFarlane *et al.* 1994).

6   Many papers have been written about the predisposition to ill health in veterans of many armed conflicts in the twentieth century. See Askevold 1976; Hyams, Wignall, & Roswell 1996; Kardiner 1941; Kolonoff, McDougall, & Clark 1976; Litz, Keane, & Fisher 1992; Shalev, Belich, & Ursano 1990; Solomon & Mukulineer 1987; Solomon, Mukulineer, & Kotler 1987; Stretch *et al.* 1995.

7   The following quote from a soldier who served in the Falklands conflict, published by Dr S. Hughes in the *British Medical Journal* (Hughes 1990), illustrates the sheer terror that soldiers experience.

> For no obvious reason, I had suddenly been overwhelmed by a crescendo of blind unreasoning fear, defying all logic and insight. Nothing that General Galtieri's men had generated compared with the terrors that my own mind invented that night. Having looked death full in the eye outside Goose Green and again, but two weeks later, on a barren hillside called Wireless Ridge, I think I can honestly say I no longer feared death or the things real and imagined that usually became the objects of phobias. I was afraid that night of the only thing that could frighten me still – myself. I was afraid of losing my control.

8   Ill health has been extensively documented in former prisoners of war (see Goulston, Dent, & Chapuis 1985). Survivors of the Nazi Holocaust have been investigated in more depth than any of group of prisoners. Physical symptoms can occur up to forty years later and include chronic tension, gastrointestinal conditions, cardiovascular ailments, headaches, joint pain and asthma. See also Bower 1994; Chodoff 1963; Eitinger 1964; Eitinger 1980.

9   Dr J.M. Da Costa documented the large number of previously healthy young men who suffered cardiac arrhythmias during the American Civil War. Although these cases might well have an infectious component – for example, typhus – the descriptions suggest that psychological factors played an important role. In the early Victorian era in Britain, trains were not as safe or comfortable as they are now and people suffered from crashes and joltings of the spine, which left them with chronic neck and back problems, similar to the long-term effects of whiplash injury nowadays (Erichsen 1866; Trimble 1981). In 1720, South

Sea stock had reached a height of £1,000 for a £100 investment, but it rapidly collapsed. Lots of people lost money, including Sir Isaac Newton, and many became ill. Dr John Midriff wrote up his 'Observations of the Spleen and Vapours, containing remarkable cases of persons of both sexes from the aspiring director to the humble bubbler, who have been miserably afflicted with those melancholy disorders, since the fall of The South Sea and other publick stocks' in *Applebee's Journal*, assuring his readers that 'the number of distempered heads is so strongly encreased for some months past by the sudden rising and falling of men's fortunes and families under the operation of the South Sea vomits' (Guerrini 2004).

10   The psychological symptoms of post traumatic stress disorder are described in a recent book, *Traumatic Stress; The Effect of Overwhelming Stress on Mind, Body and Society* (Van der Kolk, McFarlane, & Weisaeth 1996).

11   This was what Sigmund Freud and Joseph Breuer meant when they stated that 'hysterics suffer mainly from reminiscences (Freud & Breuer 1895). In a later paper, entitled 'Inhibitions, Symptoms and Anxiety', Freud wrote, 'The symptom may have originally had a function, but the original reason for it may have long gone, and it continues to function like an outlaw, a foreign body which was keeping up a constant succession of stimuli and reactions in the tissue in which it was embedded' (Freud 1925).

12   See *Emotional Factors in Pulmonary Tuberculosis* (Kissen 1958).

13   See Stallard, Velleman, & Baldwin 1998; and Shevlin *et al.* 1997.

14   While not wishing to deny the importance of severe physical or sexual abuse and its long term impact on the health of the victim, it would be grossly misleading to assume, as some do, that functional illness, especially that affecting the pelvis and its functions, is most probably the result of physical or sexual abuse, and that patients who fail to acknowledge it are in denial. However, abuse of some sort is common in our society. In a recent random survey of 1,245 American adolescents, 23 per cent had been victims of physical and sexual assault, but only a fifth of these developed emotional and physical illness (Kilpatrick & Saunders 1995). To some extent, everybody is at risk of what might be regarded as sexual abuse in the period of experiment and adventure between leaving home and the establishment of a new stable partnership. Research in this area does not necessarily elicit the context and rarely investigates the meaning to the individual. Finally, it is important to point out that sexual and physical abuse are not the only forms of abuse and may not necessarily be the most damaging. Considerable damage to a person's self-worth and to their health can be brought about by emotional forms of abuse, such as constant criticism and verbal attacks and even the persistent, undermining attitude of a dominant boss or partner.

15   There is an extensive bibliography of the relationship between physical and/or sexual abuse and a wide range of psychiatric and medical illnesses (Arnold, Rogers, & Cook 1990; Bryer *et al.* 1987; Drossman *et al.* 1990; Drossman *et al.* 1996; Felice *et al.* 1978; Fry 1993; Harrop-Griffiths *et al.* 1988; Leroi *et al.* 1993; Waller 1991). In one study, fourteen out of fifteen patients consulting at an outpatient clinic for constipation and abdominal pain had been victims of sexual abuse (Leroi *et al.* 1993).

16   Jean-Martin Charcot called this '*choc nerveux*' or traumatic neurosis. By 1886, he

concluded that paralyses elicited under hypnotism and paralyses following a psychic shock were identical. Symptoms were acquired as their mental representation rushed into a suppressed psyche (Shorter 1993, pp. 194–5).

17 Charles Hanley's book documents the massacre and a television documentary referred to the large number of soldiers who suffered ill health after this event (Hanley, Choe, & Mendoza 2001).

18 Primo Levi, who wrote about his experiences in Auschwitz in *Survival in Auschwitz* and *The Drowned and the Saved*, remarked that 'when all was over, the awareness emerged that we had not done anything or not enough against the system' (quoted in Hass 1990).

19 Knowing one's identity, name and biological parents, is considered essential to personality development and psychological well-being. Twenty-three Holocaust survivors who didn't know their true identity were compared with the same number who did. Those without an identity had higher somatisation, depression and anxiety scores fifty years later (Amir & Lev-Wiesel 2001). The same association is expressed in Margaret Humphrey's book, *Empty Cradles*, which describes the plight of 150,000 children, some just three or four years old, who were deported from British children's homes in the mid-twentieth century and shipped off to a life of abuse and slavery in Australia. Many did not know who they were and were told their parents were dead (Humphreys 1996).

20 See Engel & Schmale, 1967; and Schmale 1958. Similar observations were made for patients suffering from many different conditions, including acute leukaemia, ulcerative colitis and breast cancer. These are quoted in Taylor's account of 'Psychosomatic Medicine and Contemporary Psychoanalysis' (Taylor 1987, pp. 39–71).

21 The effects of bereavement on illness has been extensively documented 'Widows and Their Families' (Marris 1958) and 'The Psychosomatic Effects of Bereavement in Modern Transient Psychosomatic Medicine' (Parkes 1970). Widowers are more likely to suffer from illness than widows (see Parkes, Benjamin, & Fitzgerald 1969) but the effect is mitigated if they re-marry (see Helsing, Moyses, & Somstock 1981).

22 Freud has provided a useful distinction between death and divorce in his paper 'Mourning and Melancholia'. When the love object no longer exists, reality testing demands that all feeling is withdrawn from the object, and it is the gradual withdrawl of 'cathexis' that occurs during the process of mourning or grieving. Divorce is more like a prolonged state of melancholia or grievance, where the object cannot be released and so the ego is depleted and impoverished on a grand scale (Freud 1917).

23 For the first time in our history we have created a world in which marriage can be terminated at any time. Previously, society worked together to prevent separation. The effect on all participants can be devastating for men, women and children. This is documented in the shocking but important study of sixty families after divorce by Judith Wallerstein and Sandra Blakeslee (Wallerstein & Blakeslee 1989).

24 Increases in the rate of illness have been observed during the Bristol floods of 1968 (Bennett, 1970). Similar observations were made during the Brisbane floods in 1974 (Abrahams, Price, & Whitlock 1976) and have been described in a recent

report of the human health consequences of flooding (Defra Flood Management Division 2004; Erikson 1976, p. 236; Hajat *et al.* 2003; Tapsell 2000).

25   Refugees are likely to have experienced ill health not just because they have lost their home but because of the trauma they had experienced in their country of origin (see Alcock 2003; Frye & D'Avanzo 1994; Frye & McGill 1993; Van Ommeren *et al.* 2001).

26   From the Greek *nostos*, meaning 'a return home' and *algos*, meaning 'pain'. See *Nostalgia: A Swiss Disease* (Sanchez & Brown 1994; also Fried's classic study on the health impact of slum clearance (Fried 1963). The health effects of displacement and nostalgia are discussed in a recent paper in the *American Journal of Psychiatry* (Fullilove 1996).

27   Franz Alexander, founder of the Chicago Institute for Psychoanalysis and the foremost psychosomatic theorist of his generation, proposed that when the dependency needs of early childhood are interrupted, the overactivity of the parasympathetic nervous system can result in diseases such as peptic ulcer, ulcerative colitis and bronchial asthma (Alexander, French, & Pollock 1968). See also Chapter 3.

28   The investigation of the telephone company employees was known as the Cornell Medical Project (Hinkle & Wolff 1958). Several more recent studies have demonstrated that the presence of persistent threats causes people to develop functional illness (Bennett *et al.* 1998; Bennett & Kellow 2002; Katon, Sullivan, & Walker 2001). As an indication of the effect on the body of chronic threat, Battle of Britain pilots reported that they hated hanging around on the ground waiting for the bell to ring to signal a scramble. One always had to stop and be violently sick before clambering into his plane. And the world champion racing driver, Michael Schumacher has been recorded to have a much higher pulse just before a race while he is stationary on the grid than at any other time during the race.

29   See *The Stress of Life* (Selye 1956).

30   Recent neuroimaging studies have suggested that sadness has a particular brain map, which can be wiped out by thinking about something else, but then comes back again if one remembers the sad event (Damasio *et al.* 2000). Charles Darwin once wrote, 'It seems as soon as the stimulus of mental work stops, my whole strength gives way.' Not only did he suffer from exhaustion, he was also burdened with chronic intestinal disorders. Was it guilt? Darwin married twice and fathered several illegitimate children. He prescribed sexual intercourse as a cure for hypochondria. As the author and journalist John Naish commented in *The Hypochondriac's Handbook*, 'At least it took his mind off things.' (Naish 2004 p. 51).

31   Dr Wellington Machado from São Paulo, Brazil, interviewed 100 women in hospital on the day before they were due to undergo hysterectomy and administered standard psychological questionnaires. He also made systematic enquiries about their physical symptoms and noted the results of their laboratory tests. He then followed these women up for six months after the operation. Fourteen had developed abdominal pain and bowel disturbance that had started at the time of the operation. Looking back at the original

questionnaires, there was a significantly higher prevalence of depression in the women who developed chronic abdominal symptoms than those who did not.

32 As the self-psychologist Michael Shore put it, 'Hell hath no fury like a vulnerable person whose office is reduced in size or whose regular parking spot has been taken by someone else, or whose Volvo fails to start' (Shore 1980).

33 One of my colleagues calls this 'Bing's disease' after the singer and entertainer, Bing Crosby (the old groaner).

34 George Engel described this as the 'giving up, given up' complex. In clinical situations, this is often associated with such expressions as 'It's too much'; 'It's no use'; 'I can't take it any more'; 'I give up'. The patient feels less intact, less in control. He attributes his feelings of hopelessness to weakness, inadequacy and failures in himself (Engel 1968).

Chapter 3: Emotional regulation and the development of illness

1 Tom's narrative is reported in Wolf's books on the stomach and human gastric function (Wolf 1965; Wolf & Wolff 1943). Over a hundred years earlier, in 1825, the American army surgeon, Colonel William Beaumont, had documented the physiological effects of emotion in the exposed stomach of his patient, the French fur trapper, Alexis St Martin, who had been shot in the stomach in the retail store of the American fur company on Mackinac Island, Lake Michigan (Beaumont 1833). Since St Martin was destitute, Beaumont took him into his own home and St Martin survived for another sixty years after his accident. The observations of Beaumont and Wolf have been corroborated by recordings of motility and secretion made from the intact stomachs of human volunteers.

2 At around the same time as Stewart Wolf was working with Tom, another American physician, Dr Thomas Almy, showed that even the colon could express emotion (Almy & Tulin 1947). Almy conducted emotive interviews on patients while recording the contractile activity of the colon by inserting small balloons into the anus. These were connected via pressure transducers to a polygraph. As the discussion turned to 'unpleasant life situations productive of emotional conflict', Almy observed that the colon contracted vigorously, but when the discussion evoked sadness and the patient wept, the contractions ceased. It is for this reason that Almy coined the term 'the weeping gut' to describe the alterations in stomach and bowel function caused by emotional distress. In one notable experiment, Almy conducted an examination of the rectum of a student volunteer through an illuminated tube called a sigmoido-scope and pretended that he could see a cancer in the rectum. The lining of the bowel instantly turned a livid red and started contracting vigorously. These reactions ceased abruptly when Almy confessed that this was a hoax.

The Mexican word '*coraje*' refers to anger in women so powerful that it is associated with the vomiting of bile. But it is not only people who vomit when they are angry. Species as diverse as the Andean llama and the Fulmar petrel are said to protect themselves by vomiting in the face of their assailants.

3 See the recent paper entitled 'Subcortical and Cortical Brain Activity during Self-Generated Emotions' (Damasio *et al.* 2000).

4 The concept of the four humours (phlegm, blood, yellow bile and black bile) was

first coined by the philosopher Empendocles of Akragas in Sicily and grounded on the principle of the four supposed elements – earth, air, fire and water. All of the humours had to be in 'harmony' for health and happiness. As Roy Porter described it, 'this fourfold pattern offered a kind of universal hold-all, in which tastes, temperaments, and a surprising number of diseases could find loose accommodation'. Although Western doctors have long since abandoned humoural notions of medicine, the same words are used to describe a person's temperament – phlegmatic, choleric, melancholic and sanguine (Porter 1999, pp. 56–8).

5   The face is like our personal two-way video screen, a window on the soul, responding to events and advertising our feelings to others. It may be a worrying thought, but after a lifetime, as our skin dries and the creases in our skin become fixed by use, the emotional history of our lives is written in the lines of our face. It's all there, the joys in the lines at the sides of our eyes, the concerns and worries in the parallel lines of our foreheads, the tragedies in the drawing down of the sides of our mouths. Charles Darwin made the most comprehensive study of facial expression of emotions in his lesser known book *The Expression of Emotions in Man and Animals*, while more recently, Paul Ekman has made the comprehensive scientific study of human facial expression (Darwin 1872; Ekman 1984).

6   There are a range of brain structures associated with emotional response (MacLean, 1949). As well as the orbitofrontal cortex, they include: the cingulate gyrus, an evolutionarily ancient rim of cerebral cortex that is situated low down on the inner surface of each cerebral hemisphere and is responsible for coordinating emotional responses; the hypothalamus, which functions as a head ganglion for the autonomic nervous system and the endocrine (hormonal) systems; the hippocampus, which is responsible for contextual memory; and the amygdale, two almond-shaped structures situated deep in the temporal lobes of the brain which function as the emotional alarm bell. For a discussion of the role of the amygdala in emergency responses and in panic, see chapter 8 of Joseph LeDoux's *The Emotional Brain* (LeDoux 1998, pp. 225–66).

7   So new events are tagged and coded with a physiological signature according to past experience. In *Descartes Error*, Antonio Damasio calls these 'somatic markers' (Damasio 1994).

8   The release of cortisol is one component of the activation of the hypothalamo-pituitary adrenal (or HPA) axis, a cascade of responses to stress. Stress stimulates the production of corticotrophin releasing hormone (CRH) from the hypothalamus at the base of the brain. CRH enters the veins that drain the blood from the hypothalamus into the anterior pituitary gland, hanging like a cherry below it. There it stimulates the production and release of adreno-corticotrophic hormone (ACTH) and beta-endorphine, which has an analgesic and calming effect on the body, similar to morphine. ACTH in turn stimulates the adrenal gland, situated just above the kidney, to manufacture and secrete cortisol (Claes 2004; Mayer 2000; Selye 1936). Other hormones in the cascade, notably endorphins and ACTH and CRH itself, have additional effects such as the suppression of memory and pain, lightening of mood and the encouragement of rest.

Activation of the HPA axis supports the activation of the sympathetic nervous system by maintaining bodily functions and it augments the restorative and recuperative functions of the parasympathetic nervous system. As an example of this, marathon runners often report a period of severe exhaustion at about 20 miles, which they call 'hitting the wall', and many are embarrassed by a sudden urgency to defecate at around the same time. Scientists have recently shown that 'hitting the wall' is associated with a marked surge in the activity of the HPA axis.

9   The mechanisms that allow an animal to deal with external threat are the same as those that optimise its ability to survive injury or infection (Cannon 1929; Meyer 2000; Selye 1936). The two basic types of response are the 'high-energy reactions', what the American physiologist Walter Cannon described as fight or flight responses, and the 'low-energy, adaptive responses', which the pioneer of behavioural medicine, George Engel, characterised as conservation and withdrawal (Cannon 1929; Engel & Schmale 1972). Acute threat and painful stimuli to the skin activate the sympathetic circuit, causing us to respond by aggression or flight, but a chronically distressing situation activates the parasympathetic circuit in the same way as when we have a headache or an infection; we experience an overwhelming desire to lie down and rest. In many stressful situations, sympathetic and parasympathetic strategies are reciprocally coupled; when the high-energy sympathetic responses are active, the low-energy parasympathetic responses are damped down and vice versa. This is advantageous, because it allows for consistent shifts that are more likely to lead to rapid resolution. For example, an acute threat stimulates a rapid sympathetic response to protect the individual followed by a slower parasympathetic response to promote recovery. But it would be a mistake to think that one system is activated at the expense of the other. In many chronically stressful situations, both types of response may be activated to a variable extent alongside elevations in cortisol. This state of chronic overdrive often leads to illness.

10   Hans Selye (1907–82) became world famous for proving that stress was a major factor in the causing of disease. Educated in Prague, he moved to America and eventually became Professor and Director of the Institute of Experimental Medicine at McGill University, Montreal. An endocrinologist by training, Selye was one of the first to recognise that stressors of various sorts – infection, starvation, injury and psychological threat – all induced a stereotyped physiological response that seemed to be mediated through the hypothalamo-pituitary-adrenal axis and the secretion of cortisol. Selye called this combination of responses the 'general adaptation syndrome'. Although he recognised that such changes help the body to respond to injury and resolve threats, if the stress is prolonged and resolution is impeded, then the exaggerated activity of this HPA axis could predispose to a range of 'diseases of adaptation'. Thus he and others saw many of the common illnesses of civilisation as a failure to adapt to stressful life events. More than anyone else, Seyle demonstrated the importance of emotional responses in causing much of the wear and tear experienced by human beings throughout their lives and suggested a possible mechanism (Selye 1936; Selye 1956; Selye 1982). People who gave up developed elevated levels of

corticosteroids and tended to become ill (Engel 1968) while those who retained a
positive attitude and engaged with the situation would remain healthy.

11   In the years before modern standards of hygiene, public health and antibiotics,
the numerous stresses of contemporary life would have suppressed the immune
system and made people seriously ill with infections. Nowadays, the exaggerated
HPA responses and high cortisol levels induced by insoluble life situations and
tragic life events are more likely to contribute to the epidemic of obesity by
encouraging eating and redistributing body fat to abdominal regions. High levels
of cortisol increase the fat and sugar levels in the blood, predisposing to diabetes,
elevate the blood pressure, enhance the tendency of the blood to clot and raise
cholesterol levels, and increase the risk of strokes and heart attacks (Bjorntorp &
Rosmond 2000; Chrousos 1995; McEwen 1998; Repetti, Taylor, & Seeman 2002;
Sternberg 2000). They also stimulate acid secretion in the stomach and impair
healing of inflammation and erosions, increasing the risk of ulcers. Prolonged
stimulation of the HPA axis is also associated with depression (Checkley 1996),
and many functional illnesses (Chrousos 1995; Demitrack *et al.* 1991; McEwen
1998; Sharpe & Carson 2001; Whitehead, Palsson, & Jones 2002). Recent
experimental observations suggest that coping strategies involving the parasympathetic nervous system and the HPA axis increase the permeability of the gut,
predisposing to infections and allergies (Groot *et al.* 2000).

12   The philosopher Ludwig Wittgenstein once commented: 'The best insights of
the human soul are through the body.' And Freud considered that 'the Ego is
first and foremost a bodily ego'. In 1884, the American physiologist William
James wrote a paper for the philosophical journal *Mind* entitled 'What Are
Emotions?' in which he posed the question: 'Do we run from a bear because we
are afraid or are we afraid because we run?' Professor James suggested that the
sensation of fear was generated by the changes in heart rate, blood pressure,
respiration and gut motility that occurred as a result of the perception of the
dangerous situation. He said that he found it impossible to imagine an
emotional experience occurring in the absence of the body responses that
accompany it (James 1884). The physiologist Walter Cannon argued against this
interpretation on the grounds that emotions form very quickly and a feedback
loop through the body would take too long to account for that (Cannon 1927).
This is certainly true when we think of the sort of non-specific shock or alarm
reactions we might experience if somebody shouts at us, but we now know that
our alarm response is short-circuited through the amygdala before we have a
chance to feel anything. But surely the emotional content of a frightening
experience comes a little time later when our heart accelerates and we begin to
shake and think of the danger we were in. And much of what we would
recognise as emotion, such as anxiety, sadness, guilt, love and joy, seems to form
quite slowly and would be well able to incorporate feedback. Antonio Damasio
has also argued that once that link between certain experiences and bodily
feelings has been consolidated by experience, the brain is able to generate the
same feeling instantly, even if the connections between the brain and viscera had
been damaged. He called this an 'as-if' loop (Damasio 1999). Joseph LeDoux
developed the argument in *The Emotional Brain* (LeDoux 1998).

If emotion comes from bodily experience, then people who have suffered neurological injuries in which they have been disconnected from their bodies should experience no emotion. The answers are ambiguous. An early study claimed that patients with the most severe spinal injury had a dulling of intensity of emotional feelings (Hohmann 1966), but this was subsequently challenged (Bermond *et al.* 1995). However, spinal injury spares the vagus nerve, which transmits information about visceral feeling to the brain and it also allows feedback from facial movements. More convincing is the data from those unfortunate people who have neurological lesions just in front of the midbrain and lose all control of their body with the exception of the movement of their eyes. See *The Feeling of What Happens* (Damasio 1999, pp. 292–3). Although such patients are confined to a state of nearly complete imprisonment, they mercifully do not experience the anguish and turmoil that would be expected from their terrible plight, but are said to experience a new sense of tranquillity (Bauby 1997; Mozerkey 1996).

13 These experiments were stimulated by the serendipitous observation that when lipid solutions were infused into rats they groomed and went to sleep. As subjects had no idea what was going into their intestines and the same feelings were not generated when the solutions were infused into the blood stream, the feelings had to be coming from the gut and conveyed to the brain by visceral nerves. See 'Influence of Fat and Carbohydrate on Postprandial Sleep, Mood and Humour' (Wells *et al.* 1997). These observations may explain, at least in part, why people take milky drinks to help them go to sleep, why athletes take glucose tablets to help them run faster, and why the banquet with plenty of rich fatty food and alcohol forms such an important part of any international conference.

14 So perhaps that should be seen as a strategy to induce the necessary rest, immobility and seclusion for healing to take place. Sickness, like fear, or reproduction, is a state that causes the organism to organise its priorities. See *Depression, Stress and Immunological Activation* (Connor & Leonard 1998).

15 For example, a sense of peace and deep relaxation can also be experienced during light stroking of the skin and gentle massage of the large muscles of the back and limbs. By contrast, a sharp slap, a scratch, a burn can have quite the opposite effect, triggering an alarm response. Although gentle stroking or rubbing of the forehead, the scalp, the shoulders, and the back can be deeply relaxing, the same stimuli applied to the genital areas can have quite different effects, transforming relaxation into excitement and desire. Experiments have demonstrated that light touch and muscular massage stimulates delta fibres that provide input to the limbic system and can lower plasma cortisol levels and raise oxytocin (Uvnas-Moberg 2003). Therapies such as acupuncture, shiatsu, therapeutic massage and reflexology use the remarkable emotional sensitivity of the skin to help to calm tension and heal disease (see Chapter 9).

16 This is similar to Paul MacLean's proposal that emotions involved the integration of impressions arising from the external environment with visceral sensations from the body (MacLean, 1949). The orbitofrontal cortex is able to integrate and make sense of information about other people – facial expression, the sound of the voice, smell, touch, the social context, data on the physical environment, knowledge of the culture and information about our internal environment (how I feel) – in order to generate an emotion and execute the

most appropriate response to change. See *The Feeling of What Happens* (Damasio 1999, pp. 280–1). In his latest book, *Searching for Spinoza*, Damasio has argued that emotional responses are played out in the theatre of the body and are evolutionary in origin, like hunger, sadness and fear, whereas feelings are played out in the theatre of the mind, but he chooses the broader definition of feeling as some variant of pain and pleasure, as it occurs in emotions. I find it less confusing to regard feelings as bodily sensations – irrespective of whether they are induced by a physical stimulus or a life situation – and emotion as the condensation of feeling and context.

17   The word 'emotion' is derived from the latin '*e-motio, e-movere*' to move away. According to Freud, we are driven to seek pleasure and minimise displeasure (Freud 1920). We could say that the psyche abhors tension and seeks to relieve it through thought and action. Emotions instigate adaptive behaviour to specific situations and they help prepare the body for such changes. *The Feeling of What Happens* (Damasio 1999, pp. 53–4). The importance of being in touch with our bodily feelings and emotions is the subject of *Minding the Body: Clinical Uses of Somatic Awareness* (Bakal 2000).

18   This principle was brought home to me recently while on holiday in the Cotswolds. My partner Joan and I decided to have dinner about 3 miles from the farm where we were staying. When we had finished it was dark and we could not see landmarks and signs. So we retraced our footsteps using the landmarks in our head, the memory traces generated by the events that had occurred on the way down, the people we met, the dog that barked, where we had the conversation about the parlous state of our finances, where we saw the owl. We didn't make a single mistake.

My son, Alex, knows the scores of all the matches that Sheffield Wednesday have played since 1989 when we first started supporting them. I have only got to say to him, 'Queens Park Rangers at home, 1995,' and quick as a flash, he will say, 'Three–nil; Pearson, Hyde and Hirst.' How does he manage this amazing feat of recall? He identifies so strongly with his team that the results serve to consolidate his identity as a Wednesdayite. People revising for exams or preparing reports would do well to realise that the more invested and excited they can become about what they are reading, the easier it is to recall it and write about it.

19   Thus, events and situations are coloured or tagged with visceral (or somatic) markers so that we can recognise their specific emotional qualities and respond in a manner that is compatible with our life experience of other events that have the same qualities (Damasio 1994). As the psychoanalyst Susie Orbach recently commented in a lecture 'The body is the physical sense of memory; it holds the trauma.' Some species do actually change colour with emotion. Every morning as the sun rises, Australian sea horses (*Hippocampus whitei*) greet each other with an elaborate dance, during which they change colour to a bright orange – a kind of seahorse blushing.

20   Recent studies in vision have shown that most of what we see is constructed from a brain image of what we expect to see, prompted by cues in the real world. The same applies to what we hear or smell or feel. Susan Greenfield provides a clear account of this in chapter 4 of her highly accessible book *The Brain Story*

(Greenfield 2000). Of course, after the best part of a lifetime, we all become more fixed in our views. We become skilled at interpreting events to fit in with our experience and we tend to accumulate the companions and the interests that consolidate our world view. Children tend to criticise their parents for having rigid, old-fashioned ideas, and to a large extent they are right. But that is no bad thing since it provides children with points of anchorage as they are growing up and a focus of resistance during their struggles to become separate and individual.

21 We can all feel near the edge at times. Many women find that their ability to cope is attenuated just before a monthly period. Alcohol and most other recreational drugs remove our cognitive containment over our emotions. So while emotions oil the wheels of social intercourse, making life feel more friendly or fun, they also release Plato's wild horses (see p. 60). Intoxicated people no longer respond in a thoughtful way to novel situations and are more likely to act on impulse; they may hit out at somebody who bumps into them and spills their drink; they may drive their car too fast without thinking; they may allow a stranger who looks nice to be intimate with them. Most crimes of violence are carried out by people who have had too much to drink; most car accidents occur when drivers are under the influence of alcohol; and 50 per cent of young people say that their first sexual experience occurred when they were drunk.

22 Recent studies using brain imaging have challenged the notion of lateralisation of function that was derived from observations of patients with brain tumours, strokes or injuries involving one side of the brain. It now appears that while intuitive, analytic and linguistic capabilities are mainly lateralised, they are by no means entirely so (Canli *et al.* 1998; Davidson 1992; Rotenberg 2004; Wager *et al.* 2003).

23 This process is known by psychoanalysts as projective identification.

24 Evidence for the differential action of the branches of the autonomic nervous system on gastrointestinal function is provided in the review by Emeran Mayer (2000).

25 Franz Alexander proposed that when the dependency needs of early childhood are interrupted, the over-activity of the parasympathetic nervous system can result in diseases such as peptic ulcer, ulcerative colitis and bronchial asthma. On the other hand, when effort and aggressiveness are blocked, over-activity of the sympathetic nervous system may lead to diseases such as rheumatoid arthritis, essential hypertension and hyperthyroidism (Alexander, French, & Pollock 1968).

26 See *Dietary fibre and personality factors in determinants of stool output* (Tucker, Sandstead, & Logan 1981). These emotional connotations probably explain why relaxation and laxative have the same etymological derivation.

27 Graeme Taylor developed the proposal that people with psychosomatic illness suffer a disturbance of psychobiological regulation in *Psychosomatic Medicine and Contemporary Psychoanalysis* (Taylor 1987).

28 Activation of the hypothalamo-pituitary axis with release of cortisol appears to be associated with emotional tension. This is apparent in the observation that people with irritable bowel syndrome who oscillate between diarrhoea and constipation exhibit high levels of cortisol (Read 2000; Whitehead, Palsson, &

Jones 2002). Cortisol levels are also elevated in anorexia nervosa as well as those with binge eating (Boyar *et al.* 1977). In contrast, people who are not in touch with their emotions have very low levels of cortisol (Henry 1997; McEwen 1998).

29 People going to the gas chambers, facing firing squads or being involved in disasters are often said to be unnaturally calm, as if detached from what is happening. The same applies to people suffering from post-traumatic stress disorder (Van der Kolk 2003). Mason and his colleagues described how, during the prolonged stress of the fatal illness, some parents of leukaemic children behaved as if nothing was wrong (Mason *et al.* 1990). They were shown to have very low levels of cortisol, and the death of a child on the same ward reduced levels still further; they could not acknowledge it. I wonder whether the same phenomenon can occur when any of us are suffering from severe pain or nausea, when all that seems to matter is to remove all sensory input by lying perfectly still in a darkened room with eyes closed and ears covered.

30 Some people exhibit a periodicity in which detachment oscillates with times of emotional connectivity. Psychiatrist J.P. Henry described a forty-year-old woman with a traumatic childhood and unhappy marriage who developed regular manic depressive cycles. When she was manic, she worked but was cold and rude if anybody interrupted her. Then, between midnight and 3 a.m., the mood would change and she would become depressed and express regret for her abrasive acts of the previous day. There was a strong correlation between her mood and cortisol excretion. When she was manic and out of touch with her emotion, then cortisol levels were suppressed; when she was depressed and exhibited regret and contrition, then cortisol levels were elevated. See *Psychological and Physiological Responses to Stress* (Henry 1997).

31 Graeme Taylor (Taylor 1987, p. 75) describes how it was two French psychoanalysts, Marty and de M'Uzan, who were in fact the first to describe such an emotional dissociation after studying a wide variety of physically ill patients. They reported that many of their patients seemed to have a very stunted imagination with little ability to fantasise and think emotionally. The way they communicated was mundane, unimaginative and tied to reality. Marty and de M'Uzan coined the term '*pensée opératoire*' or 'operational thinking' (Marty & de M'Uzan 1963). The significance of this finding was not really appreciated. John Nemiah and Peter Sifneos studied twenty patients with psychosomatic illness and found that sixteen of them showed 'a marked difficulty in expressing or describing their feelings and an absence or striking diminution of fantasy' (Nemiah & Sifneos 1970a; Nemiah & Sifneos 1970b; Sifneos 1973).

32 Wickramasekere interviewed his patients about emotionally sensitive issues while recording physiological data on skin temperature, blood flow or muscular activity (Wickramasekere *et al.* 1998; Wickramasekere 1998; Wickramasekere, Davies, & Davies 1996). I recently interviewed a young woman called Cheryl, whose early life was a horror story of rejection and abuse. She was sent to me because her food would not go down and she had persistent vomiting. Communication was difficult to begin with. She was withdrawn, seemed suspicious of me and complained that her lunch was just sitting on her chest like a heavy weight. As we talked, she relaxed and began to open up in an emotional sense, expressing her sense of frustration at doctors and the restrictions in her

life. I listened to her and fed back my understanding of what she was saying. Half an hour into our session, she announced that her food was going down. It was her suspicion and fear that seemed to produce the long periods of inertia in the gullet. Relaxation of that tension released the spasm, allowing the food to be taken in and digested.

33 There is a strain of rat called the Lewis rat that has a genetic reduction in HPA activity with suppression of cortisol. This animal is very susceptible to rheumatoid arthritis and other autoimmune inflammatory diseases.

34 See *Specific Brain Processing of Facial Expressions in Alexithymia* (Kano *et al.* 2003). The same pattern of reduced activity in the right frontal lobe has also been observed in people suffering with autism, schizophrenia, depression and several inflammatory and functional illnesses (Rotenberg 2004).

35 See Damasio 1994; Harlow 1868.

36 As Elliott commented, 'I know this is horrible but I don't feel the horror.' A life without emotion, without the highs of joy or love or the lows of sadness or anger, is no life at all, but at least you would think that such a person would have an enhanced ability to make rational decisions in a crisis. Not a bit of it. Elliott found it hard to make the simplest decision or to complete any project. At work he would waste a whole day on some unimportant detail while urgent tasks went unheeded. The root of Elliott's problem was that, without emotion, he was unable to evaluate one thing over another. Faced with a situation that called for decisive action, he could generate a full range of appropriate responses but none of them felt any more right than another. In *Mapping the Mind*, Rita Carter described how a very senior American judge caused huge embarrassment after a severe right brain stroke because he insisted on continuing at the bench despite having lost his ability to weigh evidence. He maintained an exceptionally jolly courtroom, happily allowing serious criminals to go free while occasionally dispatching minor offenders to long prison sentences (Carter 2001).

37 See *Men are from Mars, Women are from Venus* for an entertaining account of gender differences in personality and behaviour (Gray 1993). Numerous studies support the idea that women are more in touch with their feelings (Grossman & Wood 1993). When visceral sensitivity is recorded by distending balloons in the gut, filling the bladder with water, infusing nutrients into the small intestine, women feel sensations at lower thresholds than men (Sun, Donnelly, & Read 1989). Women also have sharper hearing, a broader field of vision and are more sensitive to touch. See chapter 1 of *Brain Sex* (Moir & Jessel 1989). But it is not just physical feelings; the poet Lord Byron summed it up when he wrote: 'Man's love is of man's life a thing apart, Tis woman's whole existence'. For recent studies on gender differences in brain imaging of emotion, see Canli *et al.* 1998; Davidson 1992; Kring & Gordon 1998; Wager *et al.* 2003. When exposed to pain or threat of pain, men tended to activate the more analytical prefrontal cortex while women activate the more emotional parts of their brains (Nabiloff *et al.* 2003). Observations in animals show that behaviour and cortisol responses to separation and stress are greater in female chicks and rats than they are in males. Alexithymia is more often a feature of men than women, particularly men that have a particularly logical and rational way of dealing with experience, such as

scientists and mathematicians. In fact, it is said that 50 per cent of scientists have features of alexithymia.

Chapter 4: Why some people get ill and others don't

1   As St Ignatius of Loyola, founder of the Society of Jesus, said, 'Give me the child for the first seven years and I shall show you the man.' But although our personality is moulded during childhood, life's trauma still has the capacity to break the mould.

2   See 'Relationship of Child Abuse and Household Dysfunction to many of the leading Causes of Death in Adults', the Adverse Childhood Experiences Study (Felitti *et al.* 1998b).

3   Use of the term 'mother' here is not meant to be gender specific nor does it necessarily imply a biological relationship. It is used in a generic sense to apply to any person, male or female, who fulfils a maternal role in early infancy.

4   For studies of illness seen in orphans kept in institutions (hospitalism) see Spitz 1945; Spitz & Wolf 1946; Hoksbergen *et al.* 2003; MacLean 2003; O'Connor & Rutter 2000.

5   Chaotic and unpredictable early environments, trauma, neglect and separation from parents can impair the ability of the growing child to regulate his physiology and behaviour and predict a tendency to life-long illness. Repetti, Taylor and Seeman reviewed the evidence for this in their recent review, 'Risky Families: Family Social Environments and the Mental and Physical Health of Offspring (Repetti, Taylor, & Seeman 2002). The accruing evidence linking adverse early-life events and lasting neurobiological changes predisposing to illness was also the topic of a recent major conference, 'Effects of Early-Life Events on Mind Brain Body Interactions' (Mayer & Nemeroff 2003). Maternal deprivation can even cause illness in animals. Kittens parted from their mothers have a tendency to develop asthma, whereas rat pups separated early can go on to develop gastric ulcers, infections and cancer (Taylor 1987, p. 67).

6   When the epidemiologist David Barker examined the birth and post-natal records of people in their fifties, he was able to demonstrate that those suffering from obesity, hypertension, diabetes, angina, heart attacks, strokes and bronchitis – the so-called diseases of civilisation – had low birth weights and also weighed less at the age of one (Barker 1992). It is well known that maternal stress can lead to miscarriage, premature birth, low birth-weight infants as well as failure to thrive in early life. For example, mothers exposed to the earthquake in Irvin, California during the first trimester of pregnancy, gave birth to infants of low birth weight. Maternal stress can also reset cortisol metabolism in the foetus which may be partly responsible for an increased tendency to obesity, diabetes, high blood pressure and cardiovascular illness in later life (Seckl 2001; Weinstock 1997). This begs the question as to whether the recent epidemic of childhood obesity might represent impaired psychobiological regulation caused by experience of emotional deprivation in early life.

7   Studies have shown that rat pups exposed to unpredictable stress in the first few days of life and even *in utero* developed an exaggerated cortisol response to

stress, which was lessened if the pups were subjected to regular handling. The same pattern occurred if pups were given endotoxin (Shanks, Larocque, & Meaney 1995). Similar changes can occur with severe disruptions in maternal care. Michael Meaney from McGill University in Montreal, Canada showed that rat dams which failed to care sufficiently for their pups by licking and grooming them not only had exaggerated cortisol responses themselves, they induced exaggerated cortisol responses in their pups, who seemed more vigilant and fearful. These changes could last throughout the life cycle and predisposed to a variety of illnesses. If these same pups were taken and fostered by high lickers and groomers, then their cortisol responses and behaviour was normalised (Meaney *et al.* 1985; Plotsky & Meaney 1993). Further studies have shown that maternal separation induces alternations in hippocampal development in later life indicative of memory loss (Andersen & Teicher 2004), changes in drug sensitivity suggestive of a vulnerability to compulsive drug taking (Brake *et al.* 1919), changes in fear responses (Daniels *et al.* 1919), and a predisposition to colitis (Milde, Enger, & Murison 2004).

8 The process of attunement and imprinting are described in detail in chapters 6–9 of *Affect Regulation and the Origin of the Self* (Schore 1994).

9 Initially, the infant can only focus on objects that are about ten inches away (Haynes, White, & Held 1965), the same distance separating the infant from a parent's face when held.

10 Faces seem more attractive when the pupils are dilated. It is the gleam in the eye, probably a corneal reflection against the darkness of the retina, that makes the connection (Stern 1977, p. 19). In experiments with painted balloons, infants responded positively when they could see the glistening darkness of the eyes. (Spitz 1965). Experiments carried out on human infants have shown how brief flashes of light against a dark background produce quite large electrical discharges over the right hemisphere and may serve to 'print' the moment of emotional communication in the working memory. Studies on the electrical activity of the human brain have revealed that brief flashes of light produce larger than average evoked potentials over infants' visuospatial right hemisphere (Hahn 1987). When I am taking photographs of birds or mammals I try to capture this reflection, this gleam in the eye, because this is what makes the photograph seem 'alive'. For the same reason, the large, glistening black orbs of a baby elephant seal are more endearing to me than the heavily pigmented lozenges of a sheep or even the vertical slits of a cat.

11 The facial skin has a higher density of touch, stretch, pressure and temperature sensors than any other area of the body. These not only respond to the mechanical deformations that result from changes in facial expression, they also pick up the temperature changes that accompany emotionally induced changes in blood flow associated with anger, embarrassment and fear. More neural space in the brain is devoted to the face than any other part of the body. When Paul Ekman, Professor of Psychology at the University of California in San Francisco and a world expert on emotional expression, had subjects move certain facial muscles their mood was strongly influenced by the expression they were wearing. This has been demonstrated by experiments in which expressions are

induced on one side of the face by electrical stimulation without the subject being aware of the expression that is produced (Adelman & Zajonc 1989; Ekman 1984; Ekman 1993). So putting on a happy face may not be such a bad idea when you are feeling blue. We are also strongly influenced by the expression on somebody else's face. Professor David Thompson from Manchester University told me recently that when people look at a fearful face compared with a neutral face, the part of the brain that subserves emotional responses lights up, and if the oesophagus is being distended at the same time, they are more likely to complain of pain and nausea (Phillips *et al.* 2003).

12 Thus our earliest memory traces are encoded by a prototype of our mother's (or father's) emotionally expressive face, which Margaret Mahler has compared to a beacon, to which the growing child refers back to guide his growing capacity for self-regulation (Mahler 1972).

13 See 'Read my Mind' by Alison Motluk in the *New Scientist* (27 January 2001).

14 Excellent accounts on attunement are to be found in books on child development by Daniel Stern (1977), Margaret Mahler (1972) and Daniel Siegel (2000).

15 Jason hated all the paraphernalia of hospital and investigations. He felt it an intrusion, and it undoubtedly made his illness more difficult to treat. It was important therefore that I found a way of communicating with Jason that encouraged collaboration instead of resistance. The improvement in his illness came about through a shared interest in military history.

16 Jaak Panksepp has shown that separation distress is alleviated by opiates, suggesting not only that opiates are good antidepressants, but opiate addiction is a substitute for socialisation. It reduces tail-wagging and face-licking in dogs and leads to detachment resembling autism in humans. Autism is a high endorphine state of self-sufficiency and can be 'treated' with the opiate antagonist *naloxone.* Opiate withdrawal, on the other hand, gives rise to a clinical picture that is the same as separation distress (Panksepp 1998).

17 It is important to understand that the parasympathetic and sympathetic nerves exist to regulate the physiological systems of the body from before birth, but the relationship with a parent allows the infant to develop autonomy over his visceral and emotional responses. For a description of the neurohumoral hypothesis for the development of the sympathetic limbic loop, see Schore 1994, chapter 10.

18 Freud regarded shame as a psychic dam to the child's instinctual life, curbing dangerous arousal, restricting mobility and opposing activity (Freud 1905). Jean-Paul Sartre described it more dramatically 'as a crack in my universe' and 'leakage through a drain hole in the centre of one's being' (Sartre 1957). See also Schore 1994, chapter 25.

19 Schore also describes the evidence supporting the notion that shame sets in train the hormonal changes that deactivate development of the sympathetic loop and activates the development of the parasympathetic limbic loop (Schore 1994).

20 See Baker & Merskey 1982; Craig *et al.* 1993; and Patterson *et al.* 1992. John Bowlby used the term 'environmental failure' to describe the impact of disturbances in early parenting on development. He quoted evidence from

prospective studies in infants to show how insecure attachments in infancy were likely to predispose children to react adversely to stressful life events, resulting in the development of illness (Bowlby 1973; Bowlby 1980).

21 The paediatrician and psychoanalyst Donald Winnicott pointed out how important it was for a mother to be neither neglectful nor over-solicitous of their charges. For development of the concept of the 'good-enough mother', read *Home is Where We Start From* (Winnicott 1986) and *The Family, the Child and the Outside World* (Winnicott 1964).

22 When developmental psychologist Katherine Tennes rated the distress of one-year-old human infants to an hour-long separation from their mothers, she found that they showed quite marked differences in behaviour which were related to their hormone responses (Tennes 1982). Mary Ainsworth (1913–99) also documented distinct patterns of behaviour during separation and reunion (Ainsworth 1985), and suggested these might predict the way the child would develop. Parker has described three types of dysfunctional attachment between parent and infant: avoidant; overindulgent; or ambivalent (Parker 1979). Hypochondriasis has been associated with more maternal over-protection (Baker & Merskey 1982).

23 Recent scientific evidence supports the notion that chaotic and unpredictable early environments, trauma, neglect and separation from biological caregivers all exert lasting influences on the neurobiology of the developing child and that these influences may represent a common pathway in the development of illness and poor outcomes, irrespective of social influences (Kaufman & Charney 2001; Mayer & Nemeroff 2003; Meaney *et al.* 1985; Plotsky & Meaney 1993; McEwen 1998.

24 Recent observations indicate that patients with binge eating disorder (Ghiz & Chrisler 1995) and those with diarrhoea (Read 2000) appear both viscerally and emotionally uncontained and have suffered from deficiencies of nurturing experience early in life, while those with anorexia and constipation (Read 2000) have often been subjected to a more controlling environment. For example, see Arthur Crisp's *Let Me Be* (Crisp 1980) and Hilde Bruch's *The Golden Cage* (Bruch 1977).

25 See Eric Brenman's recent paper on hysteria (Brenman 1985).

26 See Winnicott 1951; Kohut 1971.

27 The presence of father, siblings, grandparents and other relatives and family friends all have an important social influence on the growing child. They give him the space and the different viewpoints to develop an independent sense of identity. Many people with eating disorders, chronic fatigue syndrome, irritable bowel syndrome and other functional illnesses report that their father was either physically or emotionally absent when they were growing up and they could not achieve the necessary separation from their mothers.

28 This involves the development of a region to the front and sides of the frontal lobes – associated with the creation of abstract mental representations – the growth of the left frontal lobe, and increasing neural connections between the two sides of the brain. So if the orbitofrontal cortex is linked to the dilated pupils, the smile of excitement and the rumbling guts of shame, the dorsolateral

frontal cortex in connection with the 'stiff upper lip'. See Schore 1994, chapter 17, pp. 231–40.

29   Wilfred Bion described it in terms more familiar to a nuclear physicist. He called a child's raw emotions 'alpha particles' and the mother's processed feelings, which are returned to the infant, 'beta particles' (Bion 1962).

30   In her insightful book *The Theatres of the Body*, the psychoanalyst Joyce McDougall, who until recently still practised in Paris, wrote how the growing ability of the infant to cope with separation through the creation of mental representations or symbols would seem to lead to the progressive 'desomatisation' of mental distress as the infant grows up.

31   For the role of bodily feelings and their regulation in the development of a sense of identity, read *The Feeling of What Happens* (Damasio 1999). The idea that emotional regulation predominantly takes place in the right frontal cortex has not been fully supported by recent studies of brain imaging (Wager *et al.* 2003).

32   When somebody feels that their identity is intruded upon by another, they will find some way of frustrating the person or organisation that is controlling them. This is why an adolescent with over-invested parents might refuse to eat, work or find a job, but if their rebellion results in illness it solves the conflict over dependency by keeping them at home as somebody who needs very special attention. Sometimes a person feels the need to go way out to find themselves. As long as this isn't harmful, it is often best to let them find their own way. There is nothing worse you can do to an artist struggling in a garret than to re-house him. It strips him of his special identity.

33   The illness and depression associated with environmental failure in early life are often caused by self-attack. Unable to blame others for the way they feel, fragile, insecure people can attack their own neediness, further inhibiting thought and self-expression and impairing self-regulation (see Glasser 1992; Guntrip 1964).

34   Famous people cannot seem to find the more mundane middle ground of more stable people, but when asked, they would probably not want it anyway. According to the legend, Achilles lost his mother when very young and was fostered by Chiron, King of the Centaurs, who brought him up tough on a diet of marrow-bone and honeycomb. As he grew up, he was offered the choice between a long, happy and inglorious life, or great renown as a warrior but death in battle while still young. He of course chose the latter since at least it would provide him with a strong but brief sense of identity and purpose. People like Achilles have to work very hard to create a sense of identity and importance that would provide them with admiration and respect on a vast scale. Indeed, we could logically argue that the only reason that man is so successful is because he cannot face the pain of his own loneliness.

35   From *Shadows on the Wasteland* (Stroud 1994).

36   We are all narcissistic to some extent. Indeed some degree of narcissism is necessary and desirable. It is important to be special to our partner, children, parents and friends. It is important to have a role in society; we all like to feel that we have areas of expertise and that we do a good job. So narcissism is healthy up to a point. It is when people feel so vulnerable and precious that they avoid interaction with others and have to withdraw behind a defensive wall of their own self-importance that narcissism can become unhealthy.

Chapter 5: Why modern life is making us ill

1 Alvin Toffler described the current revolution as the third wave of change, a technological revolution that is likely to sweep across the planet in little more than a few decades, changing our whole concept of life. In this bewildering context, Toffler describes how businesses swim against erratic economic currents, politicians see their ratings bob wildly up and down, universities, hospitals and other institutions battle desperately against inflation. Value systems splinter and crash, while the lifeboats of family, Church and State are hurled about (Toffler 1981, p. 15).

2 In what might be regarded as one of the last ripples of the agricultural revolution, the Australian government settled tens of thousand of Australian Aborigines in reservations between 1890 and 1950. Enormous numbers became ill and died. And to this day, the health of Aborigines is much worse than that of other Australians by virtually every health status measure. Aboriginal mortality is 2.5 to three times that of the total Australian population, and Aborigines can expect to live about eighteen years less than other Australians. The rates of hospitalisation of Aborigines are also 2.5 to three times those of other Australians. The causes of the poor health of Aborigines are complex, reflecting a combination of historical, cultural, social and economic factors. Australia-wide, the social and economic disadvantages of Aborigines have been seen as of central importance in determining current health status. These disadvantages, related to Aboriginal dispossession and characterised by poverty and powerlessness, are reflected in measures of education, employment, income and housing. Source: Overview of Aboriginal Health Status in Western Australia. Australian Institute of Health: Reconciliation and Social Justice Library (http://www.austhi.edn.au/au/special/rsproject/rslibrary/aih/wa/index.html).

3 In *Somatic Fictions: Imagining Illness in Victorian culture* (Vrettos 1995).

4 See *Chance Witness* (Parris 2002, pp. 125–6).

5 But this is not the only age in which man has faced apocalyptic scenarios. And the plagues, famines, floods and wars of times past were arguably much worse than they are today because societies lacked the predictions and protection of modern technology. But the only people affected were those in the immediate disaster area; the rest of the world was blissfully ignorant. And expectations were different then. In the past, people just placed their faith in their Gods and prayed for deliverance. Now we have science. But contemporary science depends on the methodological principle of doubt, the creation of plausible possibilities that one then tries to disprove, often quite successfully (Popper 1934). We may have 'specialists' to guide us, but they only know the codes of their own particular subject; their expertise is measured by their capacity to define issues with ever-increasing clarity and precision. The danger is that we all come to know more and more about less and less, and expert knowledge does not necessarily create stable solutions. Consider, for example, atomic fission or human cloning.

6 In his book, *The Body and Society*, Turner develops the notion of the 'somatic society', where major political features are expressed through the body. This applies as much to what we eat and how we play as to how we become ill (Turner 1996a). The same notion is implicit in the psychological concept of embodiment.

7 In the 1950s, women accounted for about a third of total employment in the UK.

Since then the figure has gradually increased to reach 50 per cent and in the thirty-five-to-forty-five age group (key child-rearing years) more than 70 per cent of women are in paid employment, though about half of these work part-time in the unskilled and casual sector of the market. The hourly rate of pay for women is about 80 per cent that for men. More than three-quarters of female part-time employment is taken by married women with employed husbands. The limited maternity leave for working mothers, and the fact that few fathers take time off to support their wives, means that many infants are entrusted to the care of a stranger at a very vulnerable stage in their development. This inevitably generates conflicts and creates an additional burden of guilt for the struggling mother. The number of unmarried working mothers in the UK tripled between 1972 and 1994, and by 2003, 56 per cent of lone mothers were working compared with 72 per cent of those who were married or co-habiting (Abrams 1995; Central Statistical Office 1996; Flanders 1994; Office of National Statistics 2004a; Turner 1996b).

8   As early as the sixth century AD, Siddhartha Gautama, the Buddha or Awakened One, observed that sorrow is experienced because of the impermanence of things, but he could have had no idea of the rate at which life was to change in the decades leading up to the third millennium.

9   'For the yuppies of the 1980s, success took on a different meaning. As members of the baby boom generation they were forced by virtue of sheer numbers to work harder and do better than previous generations to obtain jobs and to advance quickly to keep pace with spiralling inflation. Employers capitalised on the economics and demographics of the time by creating a climate in which long hours, multiple responsibilities and fast-paced productivity were the norm. Do it all and do it now became the watchword of the corporate and professional worlds. These changes in the definition of success gave rise to the development and legitimation of ways of living characterised by long working days, competing demands and frantic pace. They are cultural underpinnings of the exhausting lifestyles described by sufferers of chronic fatigue syndrome. In this sense, the fatigue these individuals experience is emblematic of their social experience, a metaphor for the over-committed life.' *Modernity and Self-Identity* (Giddens 1991).

10   Randolph Nesse and George Williams pointed out in their book, *Evolutionary Medicine*, that many of the biological diseases we suffer from might be regarded as evolutionary in origin, diseases of adaptation (Nesse & Williams 1994).

11   When I was appointed a university professor after publishing many papers on the physiology of the pelvic floor that none but the anally retentive really cared about, my friend, Dr David Rumsey, gave a speech commenting on my shiny new 'chair' and how whenever I sat down they would all get the reflected glory. His amusing comment had the desired effect of bringing me gently down to earth.

12   *Bowling Alone* took its title from the decline in major-league bowling in American towns and suburbs, which Putnam argues is representative of the gradual erosion of a sense of 'community' that has taken place in America over the last half of the twentieth century. Drawing on data from the Roper Social and Political Trends and the DDB Needham Life Style Survey, this book

documents the extent to which Americans have become disconnected from family, friends, neighbours and social structures (Putnam 2000). They have lost 'social capital' and this is associated with an erosion in trust, health and happiness (Lindstrom 2004). Also in his book, *Politics and Progress*, the British MP (previously Home Secretary) David Blunkett argued that genuine freedom consists of self-government, by which he meant that people are truly free when they act together as members of a community to govern their own lives (Blunkett 2001). See also *The Psychology of Happiness* (Argyle 1992).

13 See Egolf *et al.* 1979. The Roseto studies are also quoted in *Bowling Alone*, p. 329.

14 In the General Social Survey of America, the proportion of all Americans currently married fell from 74 per cent in 1982 to 56 per cent in 1998. Single-parent families more than doubled since 1950. The proportion of families with both parents and children living at home fell from 40 to 26 per cent from 1970 to 1997. In Britain, the proportion of families headed by a lone parent increased from nearly 8 per cent in 1971 to 27 per cent in 2002 (Office of National Statistics 2004b). In the UK, there were seven times the number of divorces occurring in 2001 compared with 1961. By 2002, less than half the women between 18 and 49 were married (Office of National Statistics 2004b). Fewer and fewer couples are choosing to make the commitment of marriage, knowing that the chances of them still being married by the time the children leave home are slim. Another indicator of our lonely and disconnected society is the proliferation of dating agencies and singles clubs.

15 See George Ritzer's book, *The McDonaldisation of Society* (Ritzer 2000 Wager *et al.* 2003). McDonald's has been held up as the model for corporate control. In 1937, Mac and Dick McDonald applied assembly-line procedures, familiar to the Ford motor car industry, to the preparation of food in their restaurant in Pasadena, California. The brothers broke down food preparation to simple repetitive tasks that could be learned quickly by novice cooks and developed regulations dictating what workers should do and even what they should say. The watchwords of the McDonald's hamburger chain were efficiency, calculability, predictability and control. Since the quality of the product was not allowed to vary by more than a little, the effort focused on how quickly and economically it could be produced. There was little room for individuality in the McDonald's service; the interaction between the staff and their customers was as prescribed as the meal that they help to produce. The product tasted much the same whether it was purchased in Chicago, Rome or Bangkok. The aim was not to create a nourishing and relaxing experience for tired and hungry people, but to provide a brief refuelling stop for busy workers.

16 'Capital could profit from the accumulation of men and the enlargement of markets only when the health and docility of the population had been made possible by a network of regulations and controls. The human factor is placed in an iron cage of rationalism' (Weber 1965).

17 See *An Evil Cradling*, Bryan Keenan's account of his incarceration in Lebanon (Keenan 1992). Dame Ellen MacArthur, who sailed around the world single-handedly in the Vendée Globe challenge (and more famously in her record-breaking voyage in 2004–5), described how she developed a bond with her boat that was so great she could not bear to be parted from her when she reached home.

18   In a comprehensive review of the health consequences of loneliness, one scholar
      concluded: 'Loneliness is linked with more reported feelings of ill health and
      visits to physicians as well as to physical disease' (West 1986). The notion is also
      implicit in Putnam's links between health and 'social capital' (Putnam 2000)
      and a recent comprehensive medical review on the effect of loneliness on
      neuroendocrine, cardiovascular and inflammatory responses to stress in middle-
      aged people (Steptoe *et al.* 2004). For more references see Taylor's book on
      psychosomatic medicine (Taylor 1987, pp. 287–92) and the review 'Social
      Modulation of Stress Responses' (DeVries, Glasper, & Detillion 2003). Lisa
      Berkman, one of the leading researchers in the field, has even suggested that
      social isolation is a chronically stressful condition, to which the organism
      responds by ageing faster (Berkman 2003).

19   The screening of violence on television has increased since the 1950s to such an
      extent that in 1992, it was reported that by the time the average American child
      leaves elementary school, he or she will have seen 8,000 murders and more than
      100,000 rapes and assaults on network television. At the same time, violent crime
      rates had increased by nearly eight times. Scientific studies point overwhelmingly
      to a causal relationship between media violence and aggressive behaviour in
      some children (Bushman & Anderson 2001; Huesmann *et al.* 2003; Huston
      2003). See also a joint statement on the impact of entertainment violence on
      children: Congressional Public Health Summit, 26 July 2000, www.senate.gov/
      ~brownback/violence.pdf

20   Sugar has been said to constitute empty calories as it can only be used to supply
      energy and does not provide any of the essential nutrients for growth and repair.

21   Fourteen thousand readers applied for a factsheet on ME offered by the *Observer*
      magazine in 1986. And a 'chronic fatigue story' transmitted by TV Ontario
      prompted more than 51,000 viewers to try to phone the station during the 45-
      minute segment. See *The Media and Loss of Medical Authority* (Shorter 1993,
      pp. 314–19).

22   A controlled study conducted in Fiji suggested that the introduction of television
      resulted in great body image concerns among adolescent girls and disordered
      eating (Becker *et al.* 2002). Also the recent explosion of television from the West
      showing idealised images of women has made Georgian women more self-
      conscious and judgemental about their own weight, and may have led to an
      increase in problems such as bulimia (press release from the Institute of
      Psychiatry's Eating Disorders Unit: Eastern Europe, 2003). Robert Putnam
      reported a strong correlation between dependence on television for entertain-
      ment and self-reported symptoms of malaise – headaches, tiredness and
      indigestion (Putnam 2000 figure 68, pp. 240–1). Irritable bowel syndrome is rare
      in rural African communities but becomes much more common when they
      move to the cities and have more access to television (Olubuyide, Olawuyi, &
      Fasanmade 1995; Segan & Walker 1984).

23   In his book, *Affect Regulation and the Origin of the Self* (pp. 540–1), Allan Schore
      concluded that in the first eighteen months of life, infants' socio-emotional
      environment indelibly influences the evolution of brain structures responsible
      for their emotional functioning for the rest of their lives. These conclusions raise
      worrying concerns if day care, as typically provided in American society and

increasingly in British society, begins in the first year of life. A recent British report showed that when mothers and fathers work full-time and childcare is conducted by unpaid family members, there are insecure attachment patterns and negative effects on the child's behaviour and cognitive function, but when arrangements for childcare are organised and paid for on a formal basis, there is little evidence that the child's welfare is impaired (Gregg & Washbrook 2003).

24   Surveys in the 1940s and 1950s found that younger people were happier and suffered less 'malaise' than older people. By the mid-1970s, the frequency of these symptoms did not differ significantly by age. On average, people in their sixties were neither more nor less likely than their children or grandchildren to suffer from upset stomachs, migraines and sleepless nights. Over the next two decades, malaise among the elderly declined while more middle-aged and younger people became ill. By 1999, 45 per cent of adults younger than thirty suffered frequent malaise compared with 30 per cent of adults over sixty. See Putnam 2000, chapter 14. These figures parallel the rates of depression, which has increased to affect over 50 per cent of university students, compared with 25 per cent of total population. Between 1950 and 1995, the rate of suicide among the young quadrupled while in the older age groups it declined (Rutter & Smith 2004).

25   Over the same time children have become less sociable. By 1990, between 13 and 22 per cent of American children were said to be maladjusted. Depression and illness among the young are highest in states where people are less likely to socialise with one another. Putnam ascribes the increase in illness and depression among the young to lack of social connectivity. Young people in 1972–5 were twice as likely to read a daily newspaper, one and half times as likely to go to church, three times as likely to be a union member, two and half times as likely to attend a public meeting, twice as likely to write to their congressman, and twice as likely to trust their neighbours. See Putnam 2000, chapter 14. Psychiatrist Martin Seligman commented that the growth of depression among younger Americans is caused by 'rampant individualism coupled with a lack of commitment to the traditional institutions of society'. He added that without social support, 'helplessness and failure can all so easily become hopelessness and despair' (Seligman 1988).

26   The recent British National Survey of Sexual Attitudes (2001) indicates that young people are doing it more frequently with more people, at a younger age and in more varied ways than ever before. There are rises in the numbers of heterosexual and homosexual partnerships, in concurrent sexual partnerships, in underage sex, anal sex, orogenital sex and I am sure that sex on national monuments is up, too. One in twelve men and one in twenty-eight women admitted sleeping with more than ten different people in the previous five years and one in seven men and one in eleven women said that they had overlapping sexual relationships in the last year. If we can believe the statistics, a significant proportion of young people have sex with partners they only met a few hours previously (*Times*, 10 February 2001). So if sex is not about love, let alone procreation, might it represent a restless, almost desperate quest for some meaning in life? When the Swedish physician Dr Axel Munthe went to Naples in 1888 to help with the cholera epidemic, he observed that people were engaged in

an orgy of sex, as if in the presence of death there was a desperate urge for life (Munthe 1929).

27   The psychologist Michael Shore commented, 'We all live in a rich and nutrient broth of self-objects. They support our identity, express our aspirations, locate us in society and maintain our sense of self-confidence and esteem (Shore 1980).

28   A recent UK survey concluded that women who undergo breast reconstruction tend not to consult their partners beforehand. It is something they need to do to feel better about themselves, a narcissistic enterprise that rarely gives long-lasting satisfaction.

29   This idea is explored in *Status Anxiety* (De Botton 2004), in which the author writes that every adult life could be said to be defined by two great love stories. The first – the story of our quest for sexual love – is well known and well charted. The second – the story of our quest for love from the world – is a more secret and shameful tale. And yet this second love story is no less intense than the first. People without status remain unseen, they are treated brusquely, their complexities are trampled upon and their identities ignored. De Botton claims that the reason for the strange melancholy that haunts us in the midst of abundance is the anxiety we have over our own status and the envy of those to whom we consider ourselves equal.

30   It is not just our envy that diminishes us. The envy of others can create conflict between ambition and the need to be loved with the result that some people may sabotage their own success to remain popular. Freud wrote that he would probably not have discovered psychoanalysis if his father had not died. He felt held back by his father's envy. People are more likely to have a breakdown after a success than a failure probably because a success leads to destructive envy and perhaps social isolation.

Chapter 6: The meaning of illness and the purpose

1   In the spring of 1980 in the town of Chowchilla, California, three youths held up a bus of twenty-six children at gunpoint, kidnapped the children and drove them for eleven hours in two blackened vans without food or toilet stops and then buried them alive for sixteen hours in a truck trailer. Two of the kidnapped boys dug the group out and they all survived, albeit severely traumatised. When the children were interviewed four years after the event, several of them continued to suffer from symptoms which directly reflected their individual experience of that severely traumatic episode. These included difficulty in breathing, stomach aches whenever they were anxious, urinary incontinence, claustrophobia and inability to go to public toilets. These symptoms were more likely if they were upset about something else. They also included weight gain, since several of the victims had reacted to the trauma by eating and putting on weight (Terr 1983).

2   *Studies on Hysteria* (Freud & Breuer 1895, pp. 56–8).

3   *The Psychosomatic Concept in Psychoanalysis* (Deutsch 1953).

4   The concept of 'the unthought known' is discussed in detail in *The Shadow of the Object* (Bollas 1987).

5   Post-infectious diarrhoea has been documented after attacks of gastroenteritis

experienced during the Second World War but it is only recently that prospective studies have been conducted to document the factors that predict the development of long-standing symptoms. (Gwee 1996; Gwee 1999; Rodriguez & Rugiomez 1999). Infections such as glandular fever and acute viral illnesses such as meningitis and 'flu' have been implicated in the development of myalgic encephalomyelitis and chronic fatigue syndrome ever since they were first described. Prospective studies have shown that psychological distress before and during the acute viral illness is predictive of post-infectious fatigue (Buchwald 2000: Cope 1994; Hotopf 1996; Wessley, Hotopf, & Sharpe 1998). A prospective study conducted on patients admitted to an infectious diseases ward showed that emotional upset at the time of the acute illness predicted chronic symptoms, which for up to six months were similar to the acute illness (Lewis 2002).

6 Dr Wellington Machado from São Paulo, Brazil interviewed 100 women in hospital on the day before they were due to undergo hysterectomy and administered standard psychological questionnaires. He also made systematic enquiries about their physical symptoms and noted the results of their laboratory tests. He then followed these women up for six months after the operation. Fourteen of them had developed abdominal pain and bowel disturbance that had started at the time of the operation. Looking back at the original questionnaires, there was a significantly higher prevalence of depression in the women who developed chronic abdominal symptoms than those who did not.

7 For evidence supporting the notion that emotional and psychological factors may condition the persistence of pain following injury or surgical trauma, see Benedikt & Kolb 1986; Costa & McCrae 1985: Duckro, Chibnall, & Tomazic 1995; Melzack 1973; Pearce 2001; Solomon 2001; Venable, Carlson, & Wilson 2001). Edwin Shorter speculates that perhaps it was due to the increase in visits to the dentist after the First World War that many patients began complaining of unendurable facial pain following minor dental procedures (Gayford 1969; Lesse 1956).

8 Conditioned responses also occur for aversive stimuli. For example, a team of Canadian scientists has demonstrated how food intolerances could be conditioned. First they made rats allergic to a specific protein, so that every time they received food with that protein in it, they got diarrhoea. They then coupled the administration of that food to a flashing light and a buzzer. After a few trials, the rats would get diarrhoea every time the lights flashed and buzzer sounded, even when no food was given (MacQueen *et al.* 1989).

9 Dr Joire's description was reported in chapter 10 of *From Paralysis to Fatigue* (Shorter 1993, p. 286). This remarkable phenomenon is supported by recent observations using brain mapping, which have shown that when a person empathises with the pain of a loved one, they show the same pattern of activation of the emotional areas of the brain as if they had pain themselves (Singer *et al.* 2004).

10 For a fascinating account of the power of suggestion read *Voodoo Death* (Cannon 1957). Nowadays, hypnosis is more often employed to heal illness,

rectifying the movements of the bowel, lowering blood pressure and suppressing pain (Whorwell, Prior, & Faraghar 1984).

11   Dreaming provides us with some insight into how experience is organised for storage in long-term memory. It seems to replay the thoughts and events of the day, arranging them into a narrative, an allegory, that expresses a particular emotional theme that may be troubling us. No wonder Freud called dreams the 'royal road to the unconscious'. Dream thoughts are not organised in a logical temporal sequence, neither do they obey normal spatial configurations; events of the previous day can be joined to events that happened years ago. The story can flit effortlessly from one scene to another with no sense of disjunction. The dreamer can play the different characters in the dream. All that seems to matter is how the narrative contributes to the emotional meaning. Thus in dreams our ideas and experience seem to be organised according to the predominant emotion – sadness, fear, shame, guilt, desire – and choreographed with physiological change. People who are under threat can be awakened with heart thumping, or wake others up by screaming; those who are lonely and preoccupied with sexual desire may find with some surprise that they have an erection when they wake up or that they have expelled semen (wet dreams). Recurrent dreams can seem to depict in terrifying detail the fears that preoccupy them, their constant sense of guilt or unworthiness, the theme of victimisation.

People who don't dream, insomniacs who can't sleep or people who are too busy to find time to relax can find it very difficult to see their experience in perspective. Such individuals are often depressed, and can be bothered by paranoid and psychotic delusions, unprocessed emotion and renegade ideas which have not been properly organised and packed away. Volunteers who are prevented from sleeping for more than two nights can be seriously disturbed by quite florid delusions.

12   Wilhelm Stekel was a member of Freud's circle and coined the term somatisation. This case history is described in Shorter, 1993, p. 260.

13   'My word, you do look queer', by Bob Weston and Bert Lee, as narrated by Stanley Holloway.

14   Sacks discussed how illness can become an expression of the individual in his book *Migraine* (Sacks 1981, p. 224). Migraine similarly gathers identity from stage to stage, for it starts as a reflex, but can become a creation.

15   Groddeck wrote extensively about the symbolism of our lives. Everything we do, he asserted, has meaning. According to Groddeck, when a person has bad breath, his unconscious does not want to be kissed, and when he coughs, he wants something not to happen; when he vomits, he wants to get rid of something harmful, and when he loses his sight, he does not want to notice things. Freud apparently had many reservations regarding Groddeck's fanciful theories, but the two men established a friendship, which continued until Groddeck's death in 1934.

16   As Bob Trowbridge expressed it, 'When the body is ill, life is experienced almost exclusively through the lens of that illness. When you hurt your toe, the whole world becomes a sore toe.' See *The Hidden Meaning of Illness* (Trowbridge 1996, pp. vii–xv).

17   See *Inhibitions, Symptoms and Anxiety* (Freud 1925).

18 *The Diary of Alice James* quoted in *Somatic Fictions* (Vrettos 1995, p. 48).

19 'This was a terrible time. Families were split and people did not know where their children or parents were or even whether they were dead or alive. Professionals who had been deprived of their occupation and moved to the countryside remained angry and resentful and longed to return to city life. Young adults searched for ways to recoup lost years of education, and former elites continued to hope for rehabilitation.' *Culture and Somatic Experience* (Ware & Kleinman 1992, p. 551).

Chapter 7: Cultural ailments

1 Simon Read, 'Seamarks', 1991. Southampton Art Gallery, Plymouth Art Centre, and James Hockney Gallery, Farnham.

2 The culture creates templates for how we greet each other, how we express affection, work together, deal with aggression, bring up our children, mourn the loss of our loved ones. It instils attitudes about issues such as race, religion, single parents, homosexuality, sport, nuclear power, and the environment. And it determines our bodily functions; how and what we eat, how we cough, spit, expel our urine and faeces, expose our bodies, and how and with whom we can engage sexually. For example, spitting is no longer considered polite behaviour in the streets of Northern Europe or America, but it is quite natural for Japanese to spit in public and it seems to be *de rigueur* for professional footballers. In contrast it is not considered respectable for Japanese to blow their noses, though this is considered polite behaviour in England, providing one uses a handkerchief or paper tissue. Snorting the mucus back or expelling it through one nostril while blocking the other, as seen in some southern European and Arabic nations is, however, considered quite offensive by the English. Touching young women on the bottom may well be tolerated on the streets of Rome but might elicit a slap in the face if attempted in Tunbridge Wells. Norbert Elias's *The Civilising Process* is a classic study of how society is incorporated into diet and eating practices, tracing the development of table manners from a communal activity with minimal regulation to a highly regulated hierarchical behaviour determined by social etiquette (Elias 1978).

3 Turner develops the notion of the 'somatic society' where major political features are expressed through the body. This applies as much to what we eat and how we play as to how we become ill (Turner 1996a).

4 *Somatic Fictions* provides fascinating insights into what illness meant in Victorian culture (Vrettos 1995).

5 From *Hysteria: The History of a Disease* (Veith 1965).

6 The term for this, which is still in current medical usage, is '*globus hystericus*'.

7 Veith gives an extensive account of the diseases that arose from witchcraft (Veith 1965, pp. 55–73). A detailed discussion of St Augustine's philosophy is to be found in Gerald Walsh and Daniel Honan's translation (Walsh & Honan 1954), although some have concluded that the theory of bewitchment was invented by doctors to account for epidemics of unexplained illnesses (Estes 1984). In his notes to his play *The Crucible*, Arthur Miller explored the psychology and politics that created the Salem witch hunt. Salem, Miller wrote, 'was a perverse

manifestation of the panic which set in among all classes when the balance began
to turn towards individual freedoms. The witch hunts served as a catalyst and
focus for repressed emotions, a long overdue opportunity for everybody to
express his guilt and sins under cover of accusations of the victims' (Burr 1959;
Miller 1953).

The belief that possession by spirits could cause illness was not just a product
of Western religion. In China it was thought the spirits of one's ancestors could
enter the body and cause illness. Especially vulnerable to ancestral mischief were
young girls whose marriageable age had passed without the appearance of a
suitable husband. Isolated, deprived of a proper place in society and unbalanced
by shame, they believed themselves haunted. In Japan, spirits were believed to
exist as foxes, who would disguise themselves as beautiful young girls (foxy
ladies) in order to seduce men. In her monograph on hysteria, Veith describes
how a young woman, showing unmistakable signs of fox possession, was cured
after revealing that her mother, a widow, regularly had illicit intercourse with a
silk merchant. The widow was sent back to her native village and the girl was
completely restored to health. Her contextual illness was caused by the onerous
feelings of shame at having to keep her mother's immoral secret. To this day, ill
health among low-income Afro-Americans is often ascribed to voodoo, hoodoo,
crossing up, fixing or hexing. Outbreaks of upridosh, possession by evil spirits or
Jinns, were recently reported by people of Bangladeshi origin living in London.
The symptoms were not unlike those of medieval bewitchment. And people
possessed of evil spirits in Malaysia are said to go crazy. So throughout history,
illness attributed to sorcery and witchcraft has been manifested by a theatrical
combination of emotional and bodily symptoms. Fear of cultural prohibition
was particularly strong in such societies and symptoms probably represented
feelings of guilt and shame. But it was not so much the external demons that
made people ill, but the internal demons conjured up by cultural strictures.
References for examples of illnesses that are believed to be caused by spirits in
our current age are to be found in chapter 5 of Culture, Health and Illness
(Helman 2001).

8   Diseases in Young Women (Johnson 1849 quoted in Shorter 1993, pp. 30–1). But it
    was probably the foreign travel that cured them rather than the water. For a
    description of the adventures of Isabella Bird, see a report of the exhibition Three
    Centuries of Women Travellers, held at the National Portrait Gallery in 2004
    (Foster 2004).

    Robert Edes, while working at the Adams Nervine Asylum, wrote a long paper
    entitled 'The New England Invalid' in which he described a typical patient in
    this way: 'This is the invalid with nothing to do and who requires a household to
    help her do it. She has no hardships, she has studied moderately at school, and
    perhaps has had a fall or an acute sickness, but she does not convalesce beyond a
    certain point, and is, or thinks she is, as helpless as any other. She is apt to think
    that all she wants is rest, when she has never done anything that ought to tire her
    and has had nothing but rest for years.' (Edes 1895, quoted in Shorter 1993, p.
    282.)

9   So in Elizabeth Gaskell's Cousin Phillis, we read how Phillis developed 'brain
    fever' and nearly died when she heard that Holdsworth had married in Canada.
    And in Charlotte Brontë's Shirley, Caroline Helstone responds to her lover's

indifference through a process of self-starvation. In so doing, she chooses to become the embodiment of her lover's rejection; she literally wastes away and becomes nothing in his eyes. Although many nineteenth-century doctors (all male) felt a sense of confusion when confronted by such mystery illnesses, women were able to read this language of feeling as 'disappointment'. The quote and the subsequent examples are all taken from *Somatic Fictions* by Athena Vrettos.

10   Henri Schaeffer was a specialist in psychotherapy, who had trained at Salpêtrière (Schaeffer 1929, quoted in Shorter 1993, p. 293).

11   Reference to this interpretation of Elizabethan melancholy can be found in 'Seventeenth-Century Melancholy', Appendix B, in *Drama and Society in the Age of Jonson* (Knights 1937, pp. 315–52).

12   Leopold Lowenfeld, a nerve doctor from Munich, made the following comment on urban life in 1894:

> The ceaseless hurry and disruption of business life, the feverish pace one has to adopt to get anywhere, the clamour of the wagons in the business streets, the endless variety that strikes the eye everywhere, all the entertainments that exhaust body and soul and continue until late at night: all these circumstances entrain indisputably an excessive use of nervous energy and do not permit the proper restoration of the exhausted system.

13   At the age of just twenty-eight, Dr William Griesenger coined the term 'irritable weakness' in the textbook on psychiatry he wrote following his two-year experience as assistant physician at the Winnenthal Asylum in Germany (Griesenger 1861). As William Osler wrote in his classic book, *The Principles and Practice of Medicine* (Osler 1892): 'The individual loses the distinction between essentials and non-essentials, trifles cause annoyance and the entire organism reacts with unnecessary readiness to slight stimuli and is in a state which older writers call irritable weakness.' George Beard's book was entitled *Neurasthenia or Nervous Exhaustion* (Beard 1869). In 1893, Freud, who considered himself neurasthenic, wrote to Wilhelm Fleiss that he was seeing so many neurasthenics that, 'I may be able to confine myself to this type of patient in the course of the next two or three years.'

14   C.G. Helman discusses the concept of psychosomatic illness among non-Western cultures in chapters 5 and 10 of *Culture, Health and Illness*, and refers to descriptions of cultural illnesses, such as heart distress (Good 1977), the sinking heart (Krause 1989) and the angry liver (Ots 1990).

15   See chapter 10 of *English Madness* (Skultans 1985).

16   Food safety and fears of contamination were important factors in Joan Ransley's thesis, entitled 'The Meaning of Food to Patients with Irritable Bowel Syndrome' (Ransley 1997).

17   Shopping has become one of the most popular out-of-home leisure activities in Western countries. In 2004, 84 per cent of the adult population in the UK enjoyed browsing for goods in person, while 33 per cent enjoyed browsing on line. People in the UK spend at least one hour a week shopping for pleasure. Groups with above-average inclination to leisure shop include 15–34-year-olds, working managers, working women and better-off families (Mintel 2004).

18 The Adverse Child Experiences study noted that people with exposure to adverse experiences during childhood had increased rates of alcoholism, drug abuse, smoking, promiscuity and severe obesity (Felitti *et al* 1998a). Other studies have shown a strongly positive relationship between binge eating and both compulsive buying and impulsive behaviours. (Favaro *et al.* 2003; Lee, Lennon, & Rudd 2000; Sansone, Levitt, & Sansone 2005).

19 See *Fetal and Infant Origins of Adult Disease* (Barker 1992). For evidence that nutritional deprivation in the foetus resets biochemical regulation leading to a more conservative metabolism and a tendency to overconsume in adult life see: Seckl 2001; Weinstock 1997.

20 For example, mothers exposed to earthquakes early in pregnancy had a much greater tendency to give birth to premature infants of low birth-weight. This was particularly likely if their spouse was injured or killed (Chang *et al.* 2002; Glynn *et al.* 2001).

21 For psychological studies on emotional deprivation see: Lissau & Sorensen 1994; Riva 1996.

22 For a recent review on the 'thrifty genotype' and evolutionary theories cause of obesity read: Lev-Ran 2001.

23 Different psychosocial perspectives are expressed in *The Gilded Cage* (Bruch 1977), *Let Me Be* (Crisp 1980) and *Hunger Strike* (Orbach 2003).

24 For a discussion on Victorian perceptions of women with tuberculosis and the effects of corsets, see *Somatic Fictions* (Vrettos 1995, p. 193).

25 This is similar to what Friedrich Nietzsche described as the struggle between Apollo representing rationalism and Dionysius representing sensual satisfaction, arguing that it was only through the reconciliation of these two dimensions that human beings could achieve any balance in their lives.

26 From *The Social Course of Illness in Neurasthenia and Chronic Fatigue Syndrome* (Ware & Kleinman 1992).

27 One famous example was Florence Nightingale. In 1857, the year after she returned from the Crimea, Nightingale took to her bed, convinced her life was in imminent danger. But she lived until she was ninety, dying in 1910. Lytton Strachey wrote that she remained an invalid, but an invalid of curious character. She was too weak to walk downstairs but worked harder than most cabinet ministers, (Naish 2004, p. 53).

28 See *Modern Disorders of Vitality* (Henningsen & Priebe 1999).

Chapter 8: The medicalisation of illness

1 I am sure that the role of the clinician's white coat is more to shield his mind from the patient's emotions than to protect his clothes from the patient's bodily fluids. This was reinforced when I was training to be a gastroenterologist. My chief was given a clean white coat before every ward round and wore it buttoned up to the neck as he progressed from bed to bed. At the end of the ward round, there were always a few patients who required a rectal examination to be conducted in the treatment room. Although this was invariably a messy procedure, what happened to the white coat? It was removed and hung on the back of the door.

2   *Observations on the Nature, Causes and Cure of those Disorders which have been commonly called Nervous, Hypochondria or Hysteric to which are prefixed some remarks on the Sympathy of the Nerves* (Whytt 1765). For comment, see *From Paralysis to Fatigue* (Shorter 1993, pp. 22–3).

3   The whole thing may appear quite bizarre when viewed from the lofty plane of twenty-first-century medicine, but a similar pattern of illness can be evoked by modern medical science. I recently offered a young woman, an accountant, seven sessions of psychotherapy. She clearly found the whole experience very difficult. By the third session, she developed pains in her flank accompanied by tiredness and headaches and tingling in her fingers. Alarmed, and unimpressed by my reassurances, my patient made an urgent appointment with a neurologist, who advised that she have an MRI scan to rule out the slight chance that she might have multiple sclerosis. Although he had indicated that he really did not think she had any neurological disease, the damage was done. By the next week, her symptoms had expanded. The pains were worse and she had developed some weakness of the legs. She felt too ill to attend any more sessions. She later wrote to tell me that the scan was normal and her symptoms had in any case begun to abate after our last appointment. I suspect my colleague had provided the patient with what she had wanted, an excuse to abort the therapy she was finding so disturbing.

4   Frederick Skey of St Bartholomew's Hospital wrote in 1855 about past decades of spinal illness, commenting on the ease with which patients could reproduce the symptoms of true neurological afflictions (Skey 1855, quoted in Shorter 1993, p. 32).

5   Women were considered more susceptible to illness because 'their pelvic organs were in a condition of permanent irritation'. Battey published his findings in 1876 but not all surgeons were so impressed (Frederick 1895).

6   Charcot even developed a special instrument called an ovarian compressor to diagnose them. See Shoiter 1993, pp. 166–200. The movements of hysterical fits were much more purposeful than the tonic spasms and clonic jerking of the limbs, tongue biting and involuntary micturition of classic epileptic seizures.

7   Poirry was Professor of Medicine in Paris in the mid-nineteenth century and 'collected' numerous cases of motor hysteria (Poirry 1850). This is also quoted in Shorter 1993, p. 97.

8   Munthe worked at the Salpêtrière with Charcot and documented his experiences in his beautiful book, *The Story of San Michele* (Munthe 1929, pp. 302–3).

9   The coup de grâce for hysterical fits was delivered by another of Charcot's disciples, Joseph Babinski, who provided the basis for the modern clinical diagnosis of neurological disorders. He described how, if the lateral side of the foot is stroked firmly with a thumbnail or other pointed object, the big toe usually turns down, but if the patient has disease of the brain or the spinal cord, it will turn upwards. This is still known as the Babinski reflex. For the first time, neurologists had a means of diagnosing organic disease of the central nervous system, thus doing away with vague talk about weakened nerves. But if hysteria was not a neurological disease, what was it? Babinski was in no doubt. Hysteria

was 'any symptom that could be induced by suggestion and abolished by persuasion', thus making a link with Sigmund Freud and Joseph Breuer's contemporary notion of hysteria as 'a disease at the level of the idea' (Babinski 1901, quoted in Shorter 1993 pp. 197–8).

10 Reference to the changing pattern of illness at the Cery Hospital in Lausanne is to be found in a 1984 article by J. Frei, and discussed in Shorter 1993, pp. 268–9.

11 I once visited the ward of a particularly eminent London ophthalmologist, who specialised in treating people with exophthalmos or protruding eyes. To walk down the length of the ward in the gathering dusk created the unnerving impression of walking a gallery of portraits; twenty-four pairs of eyes seemed to follow me. And browsing through my bookshelves the other day, I came across a comparatively recent book on constipation. It was 400 pages long, contained forty-seven chapters and over a thousand references. It contained everything a superspecialist would wish to know about constipation – and a lot the rest of us wouldn't (Kamm & Lennard-Jones 1994).

There are now thousands of different medical journals that report the latest research findings on a myriad of different specialities. Every speciality has its own annual meeting. The American meetings tend to be the largest. The annual meeting of the American Gastroenterology Association regularly has more than 10,000 delegates, but meetings of cardiologists and anaethesiologists are even larger. Cynical observers might note how rarely the many thousands of abstracts contain any new conceptual advance and wonder therefore whether the real function of these meetings is to encourage the members to keep faith with a system that is under threat.

12 *Functional Somatic Syndromes, One or Many* (Wessley, Nimnuan, & Sharpe 1999a).

13 I have for a long time been critical of the need of some medical opinion leaders to classify medical illness that has no basis in pathology (American Psychiatric Association 1994; Drossman *et al.* 2000), regarding this as an exercise in control rather than an attempt to understand the illness or improve the lot of the patient. In one paper I wrote: 'The categorisation of functional gastrointestinal disorders might be compared to the "Grab for Africa" in the nineteenth century. The straight borders and right angles that separate different countries may have satisfied the tidy minds of colonial administrators sitting in their neat offices in London, Paris or Brussels, but they reflected a singular lack of concern or understanding for tribal boundaries and allegiances, and just sowed the seeds for future turmoil and confusion' (Read 1998).

14 *The Diseases of the Stomach* (Brinton 1859).

15 *The Logic of Scientific Discovery* (Popper 1934).

16 The latest version of *The Oxford Textbook of Medicine* consists of three bulky catalogues, each weighing 6 kg and containing about 1,500 pages with 1,000 words packed in two columns on each page. These mighty tomes classify every known illness, all 5,342 of them, each with its own set of symptoms, signs, pathology, aetiology (causes), differential diagnosis (what else it might be) and treatment. They remind me of similarly weighty volumes, which depict in loving detail the distinctive features of all 9,305 of the world's different bird species,

though I must admit I was always more intrigued by the promiscuous behaviour of the hedge sparrows that I saw in the garden, of which nothing was mentioned, than I ever was by the finer distinguishing features of the large family of leaf warblers (*Phylloscopus*).

17 Topical and controversial, *The Tyranny of Health* exposes the dangers of the explosion of health awareness for both patients and doctors. Fitzpatrick suggests that health propaganda is having a very unhealthy effect on the nation. Patients are made unnecessarily anxious as a result of health scares which have greatly exaggerated the risks of everyday activities such as eating beef, sunbathing and having sex. This is not a new idea. In *The Remembrance of Things Past*, Marcel Proust wrote, 'For each illness that doctors cure with medicine they provoke it in ten healthy people by inoculating them with the virus that is a thousand times more powerful than any microbe, the idea that one is ill.'

18 As Shakespeare wrote, 'There's nothing either good or bad, but thinking makes it so' *Hamlet*, Act II, Sc ii. See *The Amplification of Somatic Symptoms* (Barskey *et al.* 1988).

19 In *The Political Anatomy of the Body* (Armstrong 1983).

20 In *The Body and Society: Explorations in Social Theory* (Turner 1996a, p. 201).

21 See *The Illness Narratives: Suffering, Healing and the Human Condition* (Kleinman 1988).

22 See chapter 6 of *The Tyranny of Health* (Fitzpatrick 2001).

23 As early as 1964, psychiatrist R.D. Laing wrote: 'The experience and behaviour that gets labelled as schizophrenic is a special strategy that a person invents in order to live in an untenable situation.' See chapter 5 of *The Politics of Experience* (Laing 1967).

24 From 'Mind Beyond the Brain: Some Implications of Cognitive Neuroscience for Cultural Psychiatry' (Henningsen 2001).

25 Prescription volume has risen to over 667 million items in 2004 and the net ingredient cost has increased to £7,786 million, with the main increases being for drugs used in cardiovascular, endocrine and central nervous disease (Prescribing Pricing Authority 2004).

26 Other examples include the marketing of the new psychiatric condition 'social phobia' alongside a new antidepressant drug and the heightening of public perception of ADD (attention deficit disorder) together with a specific drug to treat it.

27 For more information on the ways in which the pharmaceutical corporations frame public and medical opinion, read *Selling Sickness: The Pharmaceutical Industry and Disease Mongering* (Moynihan, Heath, & Henry 2002) and *Disease Mongers* (Payer 1992).

28 The list of side effects on even quite straightforward medication is rather frightening if we stop to think about it. Most of us don't. For a stimulating and provocative account of this topic, read Ivan Illich's classic diatribe, *Limits to Medicine, Expropriation of Health* (Illich 1977).

29 By calling his syndrome 'the English malady', Cheyne was in fact flattering his readers. He saw the syndrome as arising from English wealth, civilisation and refinement. Just as today's celebrities talk of food intolerances, burn-out and

exhaustion, and check into health spas, clinics and retreats, so the eighteenth-century elite also believed themselves particularly susceptible to nervous disorders and dietary complaints. The rich tended to eat too much rich food and exercise too little. Their breeding and education made them naturally refined and more sensitive, both physically and mentally, and more vulnerable to nervous disorders. *The English Malady* includes case studies and Cheyne's own autobiography. The patients described in the case notes are not all suffering from problems of digestion and obesity, although diet forms a significant part of the treatment for all. Rather they suffer from a combination of nervous and physical symptoms. To Cheyne, mind, body and spirit were intimately linked, and a better diet and more healthy regime were necessary parts of treatment for a wide range of mental and physical illness.

30 *Quacks: Fakers and Charlatans in English Medicine* (Porter 2000, p. 193). During the seventeenth century, the most commonly used medical therapies were self-treatment and treatment rendered by lay people (Beier 1987).

31 For reference on Edward Ewel's Panaseton, see Porter 2000, p. 126. Self-help was the norm in Georgian England. People from all walks of life were deeply involved in health care. Wet-nurses, maids, stable hands and cooks all fancied their skills in mixing a poultice, lancing a vein or drawing teeth. Self-instruction manuals, such as *Every Man His Own Doctor* (republished by Pryor Publications, Whitstable in 1998) existed in every affluent household. Every kitchen contained a shelf full of herbal ingredients. The garden and hedgerow provided raw materials for hundreds of herbal remedies, while grocers sold medicinal spices, such as cumin, nutmeg and cinnamon, from the Far East. As Roy Porter commented, 'Today's bathroom cabinet with its pain killers, cough medicines and antiseptics hardly bears comparison to the medicine chests, one for gentlemen, one for ladies and one for horses, advertised in *The Domestic Guide* at the beginning of the nineteenth century' (Porter 2000, p. 45).

32 Since the time of Hippocrates, doctors have believed that regular bowel movement is very important for a person's health. In 1932, the New Health movement advocated the use of roughage in the diet to reduce the incidence of intestinal disease. Thirty years later, Dennis Burkitt, working as a doctor in Africa, observed a much lower incidence of colonic cancer among Africans living in a rural environment and consuming relatively large quantities of dietary fibre. Burkitt subsequently expanded his theory to encompass many other diseases of civilisation (Burkitt, Walker & Painter 1972). This caught the attention of the media and for a while high-fibre diets were all the rage. Then slowly data began to emerge to indicate that there was not such a direct link with dietary fibre, and that other differences of lifestyle may also be implicated, as well as possible genetic differences. For example, the Mormons of Utah also have a low incidence of colonic cancer but they eat a very low fibre diet.

33 The full context of the quotation from Dr John Moore (1729–1802) is to be found in Hunter and MacAlpine's account of the birth of psychiatry (Hunter & MacAlpine 1963, p. 498) and the same passage is quoted in *Quacks* (Porter 2000, p. 26).

34 Cited in *Complementary Therapies in Context* (Graham 1999, p. 280).

Chapter 9: Breaking the mould

1   A new guide for patients launched in 2004 by the *British Medical Journal*, entitled *BMJ Best Treatments* declares that for many conditions there is no good evidence that any specific treatment works. As the editor, Luisa Dillner, says: 'The big myth about medicine is that the professionals know what works . . . There is a tendency for doctors to exaggerate the benefits of what they do because they want to help.' *Best Treatments* is based on another BMJ publication, *Clinical Evidence*, in which 500 of the world's leading doctors sort through the results of thousands of research studies to decide what really works and what doesn't (see www.besttreatments.co.uk).

2   Carl Binger (1889–1976) is quoted in *The Greatest Benefit to Mankind* (Porter 1999, pp. 669–70).

3   The importance of hearing, understanding and changing the patient's narrative was emphasised by Michael Balint in his classic book, *The Doctor, the Patient and the Illness* (Balint 1957). In recent years there has been a resurgence of interest in narrative-based medicine (Elwyn 1996; Greenaugh 1999; Kleinman 1988).

4   For an account of the use and evidence for CBT and psychoanalytical therapies in irritable bowel syndrome, read my article 'Harnessing the Patient's Powers of Recovery: The role of the Psychotherapies in the Irritable Bowel Syndrome' (Read 1999).

5   For recent reviews, read *Body Psychotherapy* (Stanton 2002).

6   For a beautiful allegory of the process, progress and indeed the feeling of psychotherapy, read *Journey to Ixtlan* (Castaneda 1972).

7   Recent studies into the science of memory have revealed that memory is not fixed. Karim Nader from McGill University in Canada recently demonstrated in animal experiments that memories fixed biochemically can become unfixed again when the brain is confronted with a similar situation, allowing memories to be modified. This might explain why our autobiographical memories constantly reshape as we go through life (Nader 2003).

8   *Letters from England* (Southey 1951).

9   This negative connotation is implicit in the origin of the word. In Latin, *placebo* means 'I shall please'. It is the first word of the vespers for the dead, which, according to Christian liturgy, contain verse nine of Psalm 114, beginning, '*Placebo domino in regione vivorum*' (I shall please the Lord in the land of the living). In the twelfth century, these vespers were commonly referred to as placebos, a popular term of derision applied to their incomprehensible nature (Simini 1994). By the fourteenth century, the term had become secular and pejorative, suggesting a flatterer or sycophant – a meaning probably derived from the deprecation of professional mourners, who were paid to sing placeboes. So even in the Middle Ages, the placebo was applied to help the aggrieved cope with their loss and feel better. When the word entered medical terminology, the negative connotation stuck.

10   For such trials the cohort of patients are divided randomly into two equal groups of similar age and sex distribution. One group of patients is prescribed the active drug. The other group is prescribed an inactive substance or blank, packaged in a tablet or capsule that looks identical to the 'active' treatment. The

blank is called the placebo. It attempts to control for the non-specific effects of confidence and belief conferred by such factors as the relationship with the doctor, the attention the patient receives for taking part in the trial and what he or she may have heard about the active treatment. The trial is termed 'double-blind' as neither the patient nor the doctor knows which patients have received the active treatment. This information is coded and kept locked away in a sealed envelope, often in the offices of the pharmaceutical company. The patient is followed up for a prescribed period of time, usually between one and three months and disease indicators are examined. After the trial has been completed, the randomisation code is broken, and the efficacy of the active and placebo treatment are compared by statistical analysis.

11   Placebos can be remarkably effective. Placeboes have effects on the brain activity that are almost identical to antidepressants (Mayberg *et al.* 2002). When prescribed with conviction by an enthusiastic practitioner to a suggestible patient, the response rate is near 100 per cent and the effect can last for years. For example, good or excellent cures of cold sores were reported in 85 per cent patients taking the immunomodulating drug Levimasole, even though its efficacy was not supported by double-blind control trials (Roberts *et al.* 1993). Even in double-blind trials, it is often necessary to study hundreds of patients to demonstrate statistical significance. The powerful effects of expectation or belief in such trials is explicit in the observation that the placebo demonstrates the same range of unwanted side effects and the same increase in efficacy on increasing the dose as the active drug (Rosensweig, Brohier, & Zipfield 1993). Even if the trial is successful, the result may be spurious since, despite concealing the identity of the tablets, patients often know when they have received the active drug. In one crossover study, in which this was measured, 70 per cent of the patients knew whether they had received the active drug (Greenberg & Fisher 1989). It may, for example, have a bitter, drug-like aftertaste, or it may cause some detectable physiological change such as drowsiness, dryness of the mouth or a rumbling sensation in the gut. So, aware of the identity of the new treatment, dependent and suggestible patients duly comply with the expecta-tions. This fact has quite enormous implications. If so much of a drug's action is caused by belief and expectation, then what is the value of the cocktail of quite toxic drugs that are consumed in such a haphazard fashion by so many elderly people as well as younger people with chronic functional illness? At least placeboes and complementary therapies are not poisonous.

12   See *BMJ News Round-Up*, 6 March 2004. Pfizer will not apply for a licence for Sildenafil for women. (Mayor 2004).

13   In another example, Dr Stewart Wolf (see also p. 49) gave a woman who was suffering from continuous vomiting the emetic syrup of Ipecac, but told her this was a medicine that would abolish her nausea. Within twenty minutes the vomiting stopped and the stomach showed normal contractile activity. Again, the patient was responding to the idea (Wolf 1949). Faith has always been an essential aspect of healing. As Robert Burton commented as early as 1628, in his *Anatomy of Melancholy*: 'An empiric oftentimes and a silly chirurgeon doth more strange cures than a rational physician.'

14   For references on the importance of belief and expectation see: Kirsch 1996;

Wickramaseker 1980. For many people, the fear of illness induces an attitude of learned helplessness, in which they feel lost and dependent on others. Harold Benson has suggested that if they can have something that allows them to gain control of their illness, then they can replace their learned helplessness by 'remembered wellness' (Benson & Friedman 1996).

15   Voudouris enhanced the credibility of an analgesic cream with a simple act of deception. He was using the cream to treat the pain induced by applying an electrical current for the forearm (Voudouris, Peck, & Coleman 1990). In half of the subjects, the current was reduced, giving the impression of greater analgesia. The subjects in whom the current was reduced continued to experience greater analgesic effects of the cream for some time afterwards.

16   Understanding and caring make people feel better. It was always the case. Little children have always responded better to medicine when it is given with a cuddle, and very often the cuddle is enough by itself. I am not necessarily suggesting that doctors go around cuddling their patients, though they could do worse. I worked for over twenty years with somebody who possessed that capacity for making people feel better. Her name is Carmel Donnelly. She was able to relieve patients who had been severely constipated for years by simply talking to them, offering some homespun Celtic nostrums and massaging the abdomen with aromatic oils.

17   This personal communication by Dr Jean Worrall is to be found in *The Placebo Concept in Medicine and Psychiatry* (Grunbaum 1986). Many traditional forms of healing used dance and theatre to create an atmosphere of authority and awe. The healing temples of Ancient Greece, the chanting and dances of the African witch doctors, the Red Indian medicine men and the aboriginal healers all conveyed the impression of a special communion with a powerful spirit world. And in the Middle Ages, when all illness was thought to be related to possession by the devil, only the grave monks in their black robes had the God-given authority and power to exorcise demons. An anecdote attributed to Denis, Dean of Durham, 1684–91, described a French doctor whose patient was convinced he was possessed by the devil. The doctor called in a priest and a surgeon, meanwhile equipping himself with a bag containing a live bat. The patient was told it would take a small operation to cure him. The priest offered up a prayer and the surgeon made a slight incision in the man's side. Just as the cut was given, the doctor let the bat fly, crying, 'Behold, the devil is gone.' The man believed it and was cured. (Quoted in *Trust Me, I'm a Doctor*, bbc.co.uk 2000.)

18   Ward rounds are pure theatre, and as in all dramatic productions, props are important. So the consultant's suit, his shiny black shoes and waistcoat, the old-fashioned stethoscope poking out of his pocket evoke an attitude of authority. By contrast, the sloppy-jo jumpers, open-neck shirts and 'hush puppies' that so many GPs wear these days may create the notion of a friendly neighbour you can talk to over the garden fence but may not inspire confidence in everybody. After all, who wants to talk about their piles to their neighbour!

19   It is not just what you prescribe, it is the way you prescribe it (Chaput de Saintonge & Herxheimer 1994). And injections are more powerful than tablets (Blackwell, Bloomfield, & Buncher 1972; Evans 1974). Patients in the Villa Maria Roman Catholic mission hospital in Masaka, Uganda, where I worked in 1967,

would insist on having a Murphy, the injection of coloured saline named after the Irish doctor who had popularised it.

20 In the 1950s there was a fashionable belief that ligation of the internal mammary artery, which runs down the inside of the chest wall alongside the sternum, could abolish the pain of angina. Thousands of people submitted themselves to this operation and many showed a complete recovery. The scepticism of the medical profession caused Edmund Dimond to carry out a controlled trial in which ligation of the artery was compared with a sham operation in which an incision was made in the chest wall but nothing else was done and the chest was closed up again. The sham operation was more effective than the real one (Dimond, Kittle, & Crocket 1960).

21 As Lawrence Kirmayer put it, healing provides 'imaginative possibilities and rhetorical supplies' (Kirmayer 1993).

22 Dr Ian Wickramasekere called this the Missouri effect because Missouri car bumper plates used to proclaim it as the 'show me' state (Wickramasekere 1998; Wickramasekere 1999).

23 The effects of hypnotherapy on rectifying physiological responses has been demonstrated in several studies. For example, see Kopi 1988; Whorwell, Prior, & Faraghar 1984.

24 Ludwig Wittgenstein once said, 'The best insights of the human soul are through the body.' Since our emotions and our concept of self come from the body (see Chapter 3), body therapies can be used to modulate emotion and re-establish a sense of harmony and personal integration. For further information, look on the European Association of Body Psychotherapy website – www.eabp.org

25 The large body of evidence supporting the effectiveness of different complementary therapies in reducing stress hormones, rectifying physiological functions and treating functional illnesses is described in chapters 6–13 of Helen Graham's excellent book, Complementary Therapies in Context (Graham 1999). These effects are often dismissed by conventional medicine as being due to the placebo effect. The importance of integrating the placebo or healing effect in any evaluation of effectiveness of treatment is argued by Kaputchuk, Edwards and Eisenberg in Complementary Medicine: Beyond the Placebo Effect (1996).

26 The essential difference between these two therapeutic philosophies is the contrast between the reductionist, bottom-up approach of orthodox medicine, where disease is seen to be a defect at the level of the cell, the receptor or the gene, and the holistic, top-down approach of psychotherapies and complementary therapies in which illness is seen as a disturbance in the relationship between the whole person and his environment (Sperry 1987).

27 On 29 June 1983, HRH the Prince of Wales wrote a letter to the British Medical Association, of which he was president, in which he urged the medical profession to pay more attention to complementary therapies. 'Western medicine without the patient focus and holistic emphasis of the complementary approach loses its essential humanity. Complementary medicine without Western scientific discipline risks a return to chaos and superstition ... Sophistication is only skin-deep and when it comes to healing people, it seems to me that account has to be taken of sometimes long-neglected complementary methods of healing, which, in the right hands, can bring considerable relief, if not hope to an increasing

number of people.' Twenty years later, or so it seems, his plea has been answered. In 2000, a select committee was set up by the House of Lords to examine Complementary and Alternative Medicine. Unfortunately, the report concluded that more research on complementary therapies should be carried out so that some of them may come to fulfil the criteria that could lead to their inclusion within orthodox medicine. This, in my opinion, would seem to miss the point. Complementary therapies represent a different therapeutic philosophy that depends less on evidence and more on trust, time and confidence.

28 The mission statement of the Prince of Wales Foundation for Integrated Health Care is to promote the development and integrated delivery of safe, effective, and efficient forms of health care to patients and their families by encouraging greater collaboration between all forms of health care. (http://www.princeofwales.gov.uk/trusts/integrated-medicine.html)

29 But what personal qualities and skills would a practitioner in integrated health care need? Above all, such a person would need to be sensitive, trustworthy and empathic. He or she should have good enough communication skills to be able to facilitate insight into the meaning of the illness by exploring links between symptoms and life situations. She should have sufficient insight to make appropriate suggestions that could lead to a reduction in symptoms. An approved training programme in integrated health care would have to impart sufficient medical knowledge to appreciate when the patient's pattern of symptoms indicate organic disease. It would also need to include a holistic understanding of functional illness, a vocational training in communication and counselling skills, and an understanding of the philosophy and science of healing. Perhaps it is possible to envisage a future where such integrated health practitioners would do most of the work of advising and helping the patients get better, while the doctors and practice nurses focus on the relatively small percentage of patients who require medical investigation and treatment.

30 This message is implicit in the recent UK government report, *Building on the Best* (Wanless 2003).

31 The Expert Patient: a new approach to chronic disease management for the twenty-first century. http://www.doh.gov.uk/cmo/ep-report.pdf

32 Emerging trends from pilot studies indicate that visits to GPs and outpatients are down by 9 per cent, while 30 per cent of people showed a significant reduction in depression and 30 per cent felt better prepared for consultations with professionals.

Bibliography

Aaron, L. A. & Buchwald, D. 2001. A review of the evidence for overlap among unexplained clinical conditions. *Annals of Internal Medicine*, vol. 134, no. 9, pp. 868–81

Abrahams, N. J., Price, J., & Whitlock, F. A. 1976. The Brisbane floods, January 1974, their impact on health. *Medical Journal of Australia*, vol. 2, pp. 936–9

Abrams, R. 1995. All work and low pay. *Guardian*, 10.8.1995

Adelman, P. K. & Zajonc, R. 1989. Facial expression and the experience of emotion. *Annual Review of Psychology*, vol. 40, pp. 249–80

Ainsworth, M. D. S. 1985. Patterns of infant–mother attachments: antecedents and effects on development. *Bulletin of the New York Academy of Medicine*, vol. 61, pp. 771–91

Alcock, M. 2003. Refugee Trauma – the Assault on Meaning. *Psychodynamic Practice: Individuals, Groups and Organisations*, vol. 9, pp. 291–336

Alexander, F., French, T. M., & Pollock, G. H. 1968. *Psychosomatic Specificity.* University of Chicago Press, Chicago

Almy, T. P. & Tulin, M. 1947. Alterations in colonic function in man under stress. *Gastroenterology*, vol. 8, pp. 616–26

American Psychiatric Association 1994. *Diagnostic and Statistical Manual of Mental Disorders: DSM IV*, 4th edn, American Psychiatric Association, Washington DC

Amir, M. & Lev-Wiesel, R. 2001. Does everyone have a name? Psychological distress and quality of life among child holocaust survivors with lost identity. *Journal of Traumatic Stress*, vol. 14, pp. 859–69

Andersen, S. L. & Teicher, M. H. 2004. Delayed effects of early stress on hippocampal development. *Neuropsychopharmacology*, vol. 29(11), pp. 1988–93

Argyle, M. 1992. *The Psychology of Happiness.* Methuen, London

Armstrong, D. 1983. *The Political Anatomy of the Body: Medical Knowledge in Britain in the Twentieth Century.* Cambridge University Press, Cambridge

Arnold, R. P., Rogers, D., & Cook, D. A. 1990. Medical problems of adults who were abused in childhood. *BMJ*, vol. 300, pp. 705–8

Askevold, F. 1976. War Sailor Syndrome. *Danish Medical Bulletin*, vol. 27, pp. 220–3

Babinski, J. 1901. Definition de l'hystérie. *Revue Neurologique*, vol. 9, pp. 1074–80

Baglivi, G. 1723. *The Practise of Physick, reduced to the ancient way of observations, containing a just parallel between the wisdom of the ancients and the hypotheses of modern physicians.*, 2nd edn, Midwinter, London

Bakal, D. 2000. Self medication versus self soothing. In *Minding the Body: Clinical uses of Somatic Awareness.* Guilford Press, London, pp. 82–129

Baker, B. & Merskey, H. 1982, 'Parental representations of hypochondriacal patients from a psychiatric hospital', *British Journal of Psychiatry*, vol. 141, pp. 233–8

Balint, M. 1957. *The Doctor, the Patient and the Illness.* Pitman, London

Barker, D. J. P. 1992. *Fetal and Infant Origins of Adult Disease.* BMJ Books, London

Barnes, P. M., Powell-Griner, E., McFann, K., & Nahin, R. L. 2004. *Complementary and Alternative Medicine Use Among Adults: United States, 2002.* US Dept of Health and Human Sciences National Center for Health Statistics, Washington, 343

Barskey, A. J. & Borus, J. F. 1999. Functional Somatic Syndromes. *Annals of Internal Medicine*, vol. 130, no. 11, pp. 911–21

Barskey, A. J., Goodson, J. D., Lane, R. S., & Cleary, P. D. 1988. The Amplification of Somatic Symptoms. *Psychosomatic Medicine*, vol. 50, pp. 510–19

Battey, R. 1876. Extirpation of functionally active ovaries for the remedy of otherwise incurable diseases. *American Gynaecological Society Transactions*, vol. 1, pp. 101–20

Bauby, J.-B. 1997. *Le Scaphandre et le Papillon.* Editions Robert Laffont, Paris

Beard, G. 1869. Neurasthenia or Nervous Exhaustion. *Boston Medical and Surgical Journal*, vol. 80, pp. 217–21

Beaumont, W. 1833. *Experiments and Observations on the Gastric Juice and Physiology of Digestion.* F. P. Allen, Plattsberg

Becker, A. E., Burwell, R. A., Gilman, S. E., Herzog, D. B., & Hamburg, P. 2002. Eating behaviours and attitudes following prolonged exposure to television among ethnic Fijian adolescent girls. *British Journal of Psychiatry*, vol. 180, pp. 509–14

Beier, L. 1987. *Sufferers and Healers.* Routledge, London

Benedikt, R. A. & Kolb, L. C. 1986. Preliminary findings on chronic pain and post-traumatic stress disorder. *American Journal of Psychiatry*, vol. 143, pp. 908–10

Bennett, E. & Kellow, J. E. 2002. Relations between chronic stress and bowel symptoms. In *Irritable Bowel Syndrome: Diagnosis and Management*, M. Camilleri & R. Spiller, eds., W. B. Saunders, Edinburgh, pp. 27–36

Bennett, E., Tennant, C. C., Piesse, C., Badcock, C. A., & Kellow, J. E. 1998. Level of chronic stress predicts clinical outcome in IBS. *Gut*, pp. 256–61

Bennett, G. 1970. Bristol Floods 1968. Controlled survey of effects on health of a local community disaster. *BMJ*, no. 3, pp. 454–58

Benson, H. & Friedman, R. 1996. Harnessing the power of the placebo response and calling it remembered wellness. *Annals Rev Medicine*, vol. 47, pp. 193–9

Berkman, L. 2003. The changing and heterogenous view of ageing and longevity: a social and biomedical perspective. *Annual Review of Gerontology and Geriatrics*, vol. 8, pp. 37–68

Bermond, B., Nieuwnhuyse, B., Fasiotti, L., & Sheurman, J. 1995. Spinal cord lesions, peripheral feedback and intensities of emotional feelings: *Cognition and Emotion*, vol. 5, pp. 201–10

Berntsson, L. T. & Kohler, L. 2001. Long-term illness and psychosomatic complaints in children, aged 2 to 17 years in the five Nordic countries. *European Journal of Public Health*, vol. 11, pp. 35–42

Bhat, K., Harper, A., & Gorard, D. A. 2002. Perceived food and drug allergies in functional and organic gastrointestinal disorders. *Alimentary Pharmacology and Therapeutics*, vol. 16, pp. 969–73

Bion, W. R. 1962. *Learning from Experience.* Heinemann, London

Bjorntorp, R. & Rosmond, R. 2000. The metabolic syndrome – a neuroendocrine disorder. *British Journal of Nutrition,* vol. 83, no. 1, pp. S49–S57

Blackwell, B., Bloomfield, S. S., & Buncher, C. R. 1972. Demonstrations to medical students of placebo responses and non drug factors. *Lancet* XX, pp. 1279–82

Blunkett, D. 2001. *Politics and Progress: Renewing Democracy and Civil Society.* Politico's Press, London

Bollas, C. 1987. The Psychoanalyst and the Hysteric. In *The Shadow of the Object,* Free Association Books, London, pp. 189–99

Bottiger, A. 1987. Über Neuasthenie und Hysterie und die Beziehungen beider Krankheiten zu einander. *MMW,* vol. 44, pp. 554–8

Bower, H. 1994. The Concentration Camp Syndrome. *Australian and New Zealand Journal of Psychiatry,* vol. 28, pp. 391–7

Bowlby, J. 1973. *Attachment and Loss: Separation, Anxiety and Anger.* Penguin, London

Bowlby, J. 1980, *Attachment and Loss: Sadness and Depression.* Basic Books, New York

Boyar, R. M., Hellman, L. D., Raffwerg, H., Katz, J., Zumoff, B., O'Connor, J., Bradlow, H. L., & Fukishiama, D. K. 1977. Cortisol secretion and metabolism in anorexia nervosa. *New England Journal of Medicine,* vol. 296, pp. 190–3

Braid, J. 1853. *Neurypnology: The Rationale of Nervous Sleep Considered in Relation with Animal Magnetism.* J. Churchill, London

Brake, W. G., Zhang, T. Y., Diorio, J., Meaney, M. J., & Gratton, A. 1919. Influence of early postnatal rearing conditions on mesocorticolimbic dopamine and behavioural responses to psychostimulants and stressors in adult rats. *European Journal of Neuroscience,* no. 7, pp. 1863–74

Brenman, E., 1985. Hysteria. *International Journal of Psychoanalysis,* vol. 66, pp. 423–32

Bridgewood, A., Malbon, G., Lader, D., & Matheson, J. 1995. *Health In England 1995.* Office for National Statistics, London

Brinton, W. 1859. *The Diseases of the Stomach: with an introduction on its anatomy and physiology; being lectures delivered at St Thomas Hospital.* J. Churchill, London

Briquet, P. 1881. De la prédisposition a l'hystérie. *Bulletin de l'Académie de Médicine de Paris,* vol. 10, pp. 1135–53

Brown, G. W. & Harris, T. 1989. *Life Events and Illness.* The Guilford Press, London

Bruch, H. 1977. *The Golden Cage.* Aronson, New York

Bryer, J. B., Nelson, B. A., Miller, J. B., & Krol, P. A. 1987. Childhood sexual and physical abuse as factors in adult psychiatric illness. *American Journal of Psychiatry,* vol. 144, pp. 1426–30

Buchwald, D. 2000. Acute infectious mononucleosis; characteristics of patients who report failure to recover. *American Journal of Medicine,* vol. 109, pp. 531–7

Burkitt, D. P., Walker, A. R., & Painter, N. S. 1972. Effect of dietary fibre on stools and the transit-times, and its role in the causation of disease. *Lancet,* vol. 30, no. 2 (7792), pp. 1408–12

Burr, G. L. 1959. *Narrative of the Witchcraft Cases.* Barnes and Noble, New York

Burton, R. 2001. *Anatomy of Melancholy.* New York Review Books, New York

Bushman, B. & Anderson, C. A. 2001. Media violence and the American Public: Scientific facts versus Media Misinformation. *American Psychologist,* vol. 56, pp. 477–89

Camilleri, M. & Williams, D. E. 2000. Economic Burden of Irritable Bowel Syndrome. *Pharmaco-economics*, vol. 17, pp. 331–8

Canli, T., Desmond, J. E., Zhao, Z., Glover, G., & Gabrieli, J. D. 1998. Hemispheric asymmetry for emotional stimuli detected with f-MRI. *Neuroreport*, vol. 9, pp. 3233–9

Cannon, W. B. 1927. The James Lange theory of emotion: a critical examination and an alternative theory. *American Journal of Psychology*, vol. 39, pp. 106–24

Cannon, W. B. 1929. *Bodily Changes in Pain, Hunger, Fear and Rage*. Appleton, New York

Cannon, W. B. 1957. Voodoo Death. *Psychosomatic Medicine*, vol. 19, pp. 182–90

Carter, R. 2001. *Mapping the Mind*. Weidenfeld and Nicolson, London

Castaneda, C. 1972. *Journey to Ixtlan*. Washington Square Press, Washington

Castin, P. & Sisteron, M. 1912. Travailles nerveux functionelles; leur re-éducation. *Dauphine Médicale*, vol. 36, pp. 124–9

Central Statistical Office 1996. *Social Trends 26*, HMSO, London

Chang, H. L., Chang, T. C., Lin, T. Y., & Kuo, S. S. 2002. Psychiatric morbidity and pregnancy outcome in a disaster area of Taiwan 921 earthquake. *Psychiatry & Clinical Neurosciences* vol. 56(2), pp. 139–44

Chaput de Saintonge, D. M. & Herxheimer, A. 1994. Harnessing placebo effects in health care. *Lancet*, vol. 344, pp. 995–8

Charlton, J. & Murphy, M. 1997. *The Health of Adult Britain 1841–1994*. The Stationery Office, London

Checkley, S. 1996. The neuroendocrinology of depression and chronic stress. *British Medical Bulletin*, vol. 52, pp. 597–617

Chen, M. K. 1986. The epidemiology of self-perceived fatigue among adults. *Preventive Medicine*, vol. 15, pp. 74–81

Cheyne, G. 1734. *The English malady, or a treatise of nervous diseases of all kinds, as spleen, vapours, lowness of spirits, hypochrondriacal and hysterical distempers*. Strahan and Leake, London

Chodoff, P. 1963. Late effects of concentration camp syndrome. *Archives of General Psychiatry*, vol. 8, pp. 323–7

Chrousos, G. P. 1995. The hypothalamo-pituitary-adrenal axis and immune mediated inflammation. *New England Journal of Medicine*, vol. 332, pp. 1351–62

Claes, S. J. 2004. Corticotropin-releasing hormone (CRH) in psychiatry: from stress to psychopathology. *Annals of Medicine*, vol. 36, no. 1, pp. 50–61

Cloninger, C., Martin, R., Guze, S., & Clayton, P. 1986. A prospective follow-up and family study of somatisation in men and women. *American Journal of Psychiatry*, vol. 143, pp. 873–8

Coker, W. J., Bhatt, B. M., Blatchley, N. F., & Graham, T. 1999. Clinical findings for the first 1000 Gulf War veterans in the Ministry of Defence's medical assessment programme. *BMJ*, vol. 318, pp. 290–4

Connor, T. J. & Leonard, B. E. 1998. Depression, Stress and Immunological Activation. *Life Sciences*, vol. 62, pp. 583–606

Cope, H. 1994. Predictors of chronic post viral fatigue. *Lancet*, vol. 344, pp. 864–8

Costa, P. T. & McCrae, R. R. 1985. Hypochrondriasis, neuroticism and ageing. *American Journal of Psychology*, vol. 40, pp. 19–28

Cox, B., Blaxter, M., & Buckle, A. 1987. *The Health and Lifestyle Survey*. Health Promotion Research Trust, London

Craig, T. K. J., Boardman, A. P., Mills, K., Daly-Jones, O., & Drake, H. 1993. The south London somatisation study I: longitudinal course and the influence of early life experiences. *British Journal of Psychiatry*, vol. 163, pp. 579–88

Crisp, H. 1980. *Let Me Be*. Lawrence Earlbaum, Hove

Cummings, J. 1997. *The Large Intestine in Nutrition and Disease*. Institute Danone, Belgium

Cypress, B. K. 1981. *Headache as a Reason for Office Visits. National Ambulatory Case Survey: US 1977–1978*. National Center for Health Statistics, Washington, 67

Da Costa, J. M. 1871. On irritable heart: a clinical study of a form of function cardiac disorder and its consequences. *American Journal of the Medical Sciences*, vol. 61, pp. 17–52

Damasio, A. 1994. *Descartes Error, Emotion, Reason and the Human Brain*. Grossert, New York

Damasio, A. 1999. *The Feeling of What Happens: Body, Emotion and the Making of Consciousness*. Heinemann, London

Damasio, A. 2003. *Looking for Spinoza. Joy, Sorrow and the Feeling Brain*. Heinemann, London

Damasio, A. R., Grabowski, T. J., Bechara, A., Damasio, H., Ponto, L. L., Parvizi, J., & Hichwa, R. D. 2000b. Subcortical and cortical brain activity during the feeling of self-generated emotions. *Nature Neuroscience*, vol. 3, no. 10, pp. 1049–56

Daniels, W. M., Pietersen, C. Y., Carstens, M. E., & Stein, D. J. 1919. Maternal separation in rats leads to anxiety-like behaviour and a blunted ACTH response and altered neurotransmitter levels in response to a subsequent stressor. *Metabolic Brain Disease*, no. 1–2, pp. 3–14

Darwin, C. 1872. *The Expression of Emotions in Man and Animals*, 1965 edn. University of Chicago Press, Chicago

David, A., Ferry, S., & Wessley, S. 1997. Gulf War illness. *BMJ*, vol. 314, p. 239

Davidson, R. J. 1992. Anterior brain asymmetry and the nature of emotion. *Brain and Cognition*, vol. 20, pp. 125–51

De Botton, A. 2004. *Status Anxiety*. Hamish Hamilton, London

Deary, I. J. 2001. 'A taxonomy of medically unexplained symptoms', *Journal of Psychosomatic Research*, vol. 47, no. 1, pp. 51–9

Deaton, A. & Parsons, C. H. 1998. Ageing and the inequality of health and income. *American Economic Review*, vol. 88

Defra Flood Management Division 2004. *The Appraisal of Human Related Intangible Impacts of Flooding*. Defra, London

Demitrack, M., Dale, J. K., Straus, S. E., Laue, L., Listwak, S. J., Kreusi, M. J., Chrousos, G. P., & Gold, P. W. 1991. Evidence for impaired activation of the hypothalamo-pituitary adrenal axis on patients with chronic fatigue syndrome. *Journal of Clinical Endocrinology and Metabolism*, vol. 73, pp. 1224–34

Deutsch, F. 1953. *The Psychosomatic Concept in Psychoanalysis*. International Universities Press, New York

DeVries, A. C., Glasper, E. R., & Detillion, C. E. 2003. Social modulation of stress responses. *Physiology & Behavior*, vol. 79, no. 3, pp. 399–407

Dimond, E. C., Kittle, C. F., & Crocket, J. E. 1960. Comparison of internal mammary ligation and sham operation for anginal pectoris. *American Journal of Cardiology*, vol. 5, pp. 483–6

Donaghy, M. 2004. Symptoms and the perception of disease. *Clinical Medicine*, vol. 4, pp. 541–4

Donker, A., Foets, M., & Spreeuwneberg, P. 1999. Patients with irritable bowel syndrome, health status and the use of health care services. *British Journal of General Practice*, vol. 49, pp. 787–92

Drossman, D., Corazziari, E., Talley, N., Thompson, G., & Whitehead, W. 2000. *Rome II: The Functional Gastrointestinal Disorders*. Degnon Associates, McLean, VA

Drossman, D., Li, Z., Gluch, H., & Toomey, T. C. 1990. Sexual and physical abuse in women with functional or organic gastrointestinal disorder. *Ann. Int. Med.*, vol. 113, pp. 828–33

Drossman, D., Zhiming, L. I., Leserman, J., Toomey, T. C., Yuming, J. B., & Hu, H. 1996. Health status by gastrointestinal diagnosis and abuse history. *Gastroenterology*, vol. 110, pp. 997–1007

Duckro, P. N., Chibnall, J. R., & Tomazic, T. J. 1995. Anger, depression and disability – a path analysis of relationships in a sample of chronic posttraumatic headache patients. *Headache*, vol. 35, pp. 7–9

Dunnell, K. 1997. Are we healthier?. In *The Health of Adult Britain 1841–1994*, J. Charlton & M. Murphy, eds. Stationery Office, London, pp. 173–81

Edes, R. T. 1895. The New England Invalid. *Boston Medical and Surgical Journal*, vol. 133

Egolf, B., Lasker, J., Wolf, S., & Potvin, L. 1979. The Roseto Effect, a fifty-year comparison of mortality rates. *American Journal of Epidemiology*, vol. 109, pp. 186–204

Eisenberg, D. M., Kessler, R. C., Foster, C., Narlock, F. E., Calkins, D. R., & Delblanco, T. L. 1993 Unconventional medicine in the United States: prevalence costs and patterns of use. *New England Journal of Medicine* vol. 328, pp. 246–52

Eitinger, L. 1964. *Concentration camp survivors in Norway and Israel*. Universitetsforlaget, Oslo

Eitinger, L. 1980. *The concentration camp Syndrome and its Last Sequelae in Survivors, Victims and Perpetrators*. Hemisphere, Washington DC

Ekman, P. 1984. Expressions and Nature of Emotion. In *Approaches to Emotion*, K. Scherexu & P. Ekman, eds. Lawrence Earlbaum, Hillsdale, N.J., pp. 319–43

Ekman, P. 1993. Facial Expression and Emotion. *American Physiologist*, vol. 48

Elias, N. 1978. *The Civilising Process*. OUP, Oxford

Elwyn, G. J. 1996. So many precious stories: a reflection narrative of patient-based medicine in general practice. *BMJ*, vol. 315, pp. 1659–63

Engel, C. C., Liu, X., McCarthy, B. D., Miller, R. F., & Ursano, R. J. 2000. Relationship of physical symptoms to post-traumatic stress disorder among veterans seeking care for Gulf War related health concerns. *Psychosomatic Medicine*, vol. 62, pp. 739–45

Engel, G. L. 1968. A life setting conducive to illness: The giving up, given up complex. *Ann. Int. Med.*, vol. 69, pp. 293–300

Engel, G. L., Reichsman, F., & Segal, H. L. 1956. A study of an infant with a gastric fistula. I. Behaviour and the rate of gastric secretion. *Psychosomatic Medicine*, vol. 18, pp. 374–98

Engel, G. L. & Schmale, A. H. 1967. Psychoanalytic theory of somatic disorder. Conversion, specificity and the disease onset situation. *Journal of the American Psychoanalytical Association*, vol. 15, pp. 344–65

Engel, G. L. & Schmale, A. H. 1972. Conservation withdrawal: A primary regulatory process for organismic homeostais. In *Physiology, Emotion and Psychosomatic Illness*, Ciba Foundation Symposium edn. Elsevier, Amsterdam

Erichsen, J. E. 1866. *On Railway and Other Injuries of the Nervous System*. Walton and Moberley, London

Erikson, K. 1976. *Everything in its Path; Destruction of Community in the Buffalo Creek Flood*. Simon and Schuster, New York

Ernst, E. 2000. Prevalence of use of complementary/alternative medicine: a systematic review. *Bulletin of the World Health Organisation*, vol. 78, pp. 252–6

Escobar, J. I., Canino, G., Rubio-Stipec, M., & Bravo, M. 1992. Somatic symptoms after a natural disaster. *American Journal of Psychiatry*, vol. 149, pp. 965–7

Estes, L. L. 1984. The Medical Origins of the European Witch Craze. *Journal of Social History*, vol. 17, pp. 270–84

Euromonitor 1999. Vitamins and dietary supplements. London, Euromonitor plc

Evans, F. J. 1974. The placebo response in pain reduction. *Advances in Neurology* 4, pp. 289–96

Favaro, A., Zanetti, T., Tenconi, E., Degortes, D., Ronzan, A., Veronese, A., & Santonastaso, P. The relationship between temperament and impulsive behaviors in eating disordered subjects. *Eating Disorders: the Journal of Treatment and Prevention* vol. no., 1, pp. 61–70

Felice, M., Grant, J., Reynolds, B., Bold, S., Wyatt, M., & Heald, F. P. 1978. 'Follow-up observations of adolescent rape victims. Rape may be one of the more serious afflictions of adolescence with respect to long-term psychological effects. *Clinica Paediatrica*, vol. 17, pp. 311–15

Felitti, V. J., Anda, R. F., Nordenberg, D., Williamson, D. F., Spitz, A. M., Edwards, V., Koss, M. P., & Marks, J. S. 1998a. Relationship of childhood abuse and household dysfunction to many of the leading causes of death in adults. The Adverse Childhood Experiences (ACE) Study. *American Journal of Preventive Medicine*, vol. 14(4), pp. 245–58

Ferrari, M. D. 1998. The economic burden of migraine to society. *Pharmacoeconomics*, vol. 13, no. 6, pp. 667–76

Fitzpatrick, M. 2001. *The Tyranny of Health*. Routledge, London

Flanders, S. 1994. The markets: sex and the labour market. *Financial Times*, 5.9.1994

Foster, S. 2004. *Off the Beaten Track: Three Centuries of Women Travellers*. National Portrait Gallery Publications, London

Frederick, C. C. 1895. Neurasthenia accompanying and simulating pelvic disease. *American Journal of Obstetrics*, vol. 32, pp. 829–34

Frei, J. 1984. Contribution a l'étude de l'hystérie. Problémes de définition et évolution de la symptomatologie. *Archives Suisse de Neurologie, Neurochirurgerie et Psychiatrie*, vol. 134, pp. 93–129

Freud, S. 1905. *Three Essays on the Theory of Sexuality*. 1953 edn. Hogarth, London

Freud, S. 1920. Beyond The Pleasure Principle. In *On Metapsychology*, vol. 11. Penguin, London

Freud, S. 1925. Inhibitions, Symptoms and Anxiety. In *On Psychopathology*, A. Richards, ed., Penguin, London, pp. 227–315

Freud, S. & Breuer, J. 1895. *Studies on Hysteria*. Penguin, London

Freud, S. F. 1917. Mourning and Melancholia. In *On Metapsychology*. A. Richards, ed. Penguin, London, pp. 245–68

Fried, M. 1963. Grieving for a Lost Home. In *The Urban Condition: People and Policy in the Metropolis*, L. J. Dohl, ed. Basic Books, New York, pp. 151–71

Frieri, M. 2003. Neuroimmunology and inflammation: implications for therapy of allergic and autoimmune diseases. *Annals of Allergy, Asthma and Immunology*, vol. 90, pp. 34–40

Fry, R. 1993. Adult physical illness and childhood sexual abuse. *Journal of Psychosomatic Research*, vol. 37, pp. 89–103

Frye, B. A. D'Avanzo, C. 1994. Themes in managing culturally defined illness in the Cambodian refugee family. *Journal of Community Health Nursing*, vol. 11, pp. 89–98

Frye, B. A & McGill, D. 1993. Cambodian refugee adolescents: cultural factors and mental health nursing. *Journal of Child and Adolescent Psychiatric and Mental Health Nursing*, vol. 6, pp. 24–31

Frymoyer & Cats-Baril. 1991. Musculoskeletal Disorders. In *The Health of Adult Britain: 1841–1994*, J. Charlton & M. Murphy, eds. HMSO, London, p. 254

Fullilove, M. T. 1996. Psychiatric Implications of Displacement: contributions from the psychology of place. *American Journal of Psychiatry*, vol. 153, pp. 1516–23

Gayford, J. J. 1969. Atypical Facial Pain. *Practitioner*, vol. 202, pp. 657–60

Gibson, G. R. & MacFarlane, G. T. 1995. *Human Colonic Bacteria: Role in Nutrition, Physiology and Pathology*, Boca Raton, CRC Press

Giddens, A. 1991. *Modernity and Self-Identity: Self and Society in the Late Modern Age*. Polity Press, Cambridge

Gill, D. & Sharpe, M. 1999. Frequent consulters in general practice: a systematic review of studies of prevalence, associations and outcome. *Journal of Psychosomatic Research*, vol. 47, no. 2, pp. 115–30

Glasser, M. 1991. Core conflict: problems in the psychoanalysis of certain narcissistic disorders. *International Journal of Psychoanalysis*, vol. 73, pp. 493–503

Glynn, L. M., Wadhwa, P. D., Dunkel-Schetter, C., Chicz-Demet, A., & Sandman, C. A. 2001. When stress happens matters: effects of earthquake timing on stress responsivity in pregnancy. *American Journal of Obstetrics & Gynecoloty*, vol. 184(4), pp. 637–42

Good, B. 1977. The heart of what's the matter: the semantics of illness in Iran. *Culture, Medicine and Psychiatry*, vol. 1, pp. 25–58

Goulston, K. J., Dent, O., & Chapuis, P. 1985. Gastrointestinal morbidity among World War II prisoners of war: 40 years on. *Medical Journal of Australia*, vol. 143, pp. 6–10

Graham, H. 1999. *Complementary Therapies in Context: The Psychology of Healing*, 2nd edn. Jessica Kingsley Publishers, London

Gralnek, I. M., Hays, R. D., Kilbourne, A., Nabiloff, B., & Mayer, E. A. 2000. The impact of irritable bowel syndrome on health-related quality of life. *Gastroenterology*, vol. 119, pp. 654–60

Gray, J. 1993. *Men are from Mars, Women are from Venus*. HarperCollins, New York

Greenaugh, T. 1999. Narrative-based medicine in an evidence-based world. *BMJ*, vol. 318, pp. 323–5

Greenberg, R. P. & Fisher, S. 1989. Examining antidepressant effectiveness. Findings, ambiguities and some vexing puzzles. In *The Limits of Biological Treatments for Psychological Distress*, R. P. Greenberg & S. Fisher, eds. Earlbaum, Hillsdale, NJ

Greenfield, S. 2000. The Mind's Eye. In *Brain Story*. BBC Worldwide, London, pp. 65–80

Gregg, P. & Washbrook, E. 2003. *The Effects of Early Maternal Employment on Child Development in the UK*. University of Bristol, Bristol, CMPO Working Paper Series No. 03/070

Griesenger, W. 1861. *Die Pathologie und Therapie der Psychischen Krankheiten*. Krabbe, Stuttgart

Groddeck, G. 1923. *The Book of the It*, 1949 edn. Vintage, New York

Groddeck, G. 1925. *The Meaning of Illness. Selected Psychoanalytical Writings*. Hogarth Press, London

Groot, J., Bjilsma, P., Van Kalkeren, A., Kiliaan, A., Saunders, R., & Perdue, M. 2000a. Stress-induced decrease of the intestinal barrier function: the role of muscarinic receptor activation. *Annals of the New York Academy of Sciences*, vol. 915, no. 1, pp. 237–46

Grossman, M. & Wood, W. 1993. Sexual differences of the intensity of emotional experience: a social role interpretation. *Journal of Personality, Sociology and Psychology*, vol. 65, pp. 1010–22

Grunbaum, A. 1986. The placebo concept in medicine and psychiatry. *Psychological Medicine*, vol. 16, pp. 19–38

Guerrini, A. 2004. *Obesity and Depression in the Enlightenment: The Life and Times of George Cheyne*. Weinstein, London

Guntrip, H. 1964. Ego weakness and the problem of psychotherapy. *International Journal of Psychoanalysis*, vol. 33, pp. 163–84

Guo, Y., Kuroki, T., & Koizumi, S. 2001. Abnormal illness behaviour of patients with functional somatic symptoms: relation to psychiatric disorders. *General Hospital Psychiatry*, vol. 23, pp. 223–9

Gwee, K. A. Graham, J. C., McKendrick, M. W., Collins, S. M., Marshall, J. S., Walters, S. J., Read N. W. 1996. Psychometric scores and persistence of irritable bowel after infectious diarrhoea. *Lancet*, vol. 347, pp. 150–3

Gwee, K. A. Leong, Y. L., Graham, C., McKendrick, M. W., Collins, S. M., Walters, S. J., Underwood, J. E., Read, N. W. 1999. The role of psychological and biological factors in post-infective gut dysfunction. *Gut*, vol. 44, pp. 400–6

Hahn, W. K. 1987. Cerebral Lateralisation of Function: From Infancy through childhood. *Psychological Bulletin*, vol. 101, pp. 376–92

Hajat, S., Ebi, K. L., Kovats, S., Menne, B., Edwards S., & Haines, A. 2003. The human health consequences of flooding in Europe and the implications for public health: a review of the evidence. *Applied Environmental Science and Public Health*, vol. 1, no. 1, pp. 13–21

Hamilton, J., Campos, R., & Creed, F. 1996. Anxiety, depression and management of medically unexplained symptoms in medical clinics. *Journal of the Royal College of Physicians*, vol. 30, pp. 18–21

Hanley, C. J., Choe, S. H., & Mendoza, M. 2001. *The Bridge at No Gun Ri*. Henry Holt, New York

Harlow, J. M. 1868. Recovery from the passage of an iron bar through the head. *Publications of the Massachusetts Medical Society*, vol. 2, pp. 327–47

Harrop-Griffiths, J., Katon, W., Walker, E., Holm, L., Russo, J., & Hickok, L. 1988. The association between chronic pelvic pain, psychiatric diagnoses and childhood sexual abuse. *Obstetrics and Gynaecology*, vol. 71, pp. 589–94

Hass, A. 1990. *In the Shadow of the Holocaust*. Cornell University Press, Ithica: New York

Haynes, H., White, B. L., & Held, R. 1965. Visual accommodation in human infants. *Science*, vol. 148, pp. 528–30

Helman, C. G. 2001. *Culture, Health and Illness*, 5th edn. Arnold, London

Helsing, K. J., Moyses, S., & Somstock, G. W. 1981. Factors associated with mortality after widowhood. *American Journal of Public Health*, vol. 71, pp. 802–9

Henningsen, P. 2000. Mind beyond the net: some implications of cognitive neuroscience for cultural psychiatry. *Transcultural Psychiatry*, vol. 34, pp. 467–94

Henningsen, P. & Priebe, S. 1999. Modern disorders of vitality: the struggle for legitimate incapacity. *Journal of Psychosomatic Research*, vol. 46, pp. 209–14

Henry, J. P. 1997. Psychological and physiological responses to stress: the right hemisphere and the hypothalamo-pituitary-adrenal axis, an enquiry into problems of human bonding. *Acta Psychiatrica Scandinavica*, vol. 640, pp. 10–25

Hinkle, L. E. & Wolff, H. G. 1958. Ecologic Investigations of the relationship between illness, life experiences and the social environment. *Ann. Int. Med.*, vol. 49, pp. 1373–88

Hohmann, G. W. 1966. Some effects of spinal cord lesions on experienced emotional feelings. *Psychophysiology*, vol. 3, pp. 143–6

Hoksbergen, R. A. C., ter Laak, J., van Dijkum, C., Rijk, S., Rijk, K., & Stoutjesdijk, F. 2003. Post-traumatic stress disorder in adopted children from Romania. *American Journal of Orthopsychiatry*, vol. 73, pp. 255–65

Hotopf, M. 1996. Chronic fatigue and minor psychiatric morbidity after viral meningitis: a controlled study. *Journal of Neurology, Neurosurgery and Psychiatry*, vol. 60, pp. 504–9

House of Lords Select Committee, 2000, *Complementary and Alternative Medicine. The sixth report from the House of Lords Select Committee on Science and Technology* HMSO, London HL Paper 123

Hu, X. H. 1999. Burden of Migraine in the United States. *Archives of Internal Medicine*, vol. 159, pp. 813–18

Huesmann, L. R., Moise-Titus, J., Podolski, C.-L., & Eron, L. D. 2003. Longitudinal relations between children's exposure to TV violence and their aggressive and violent behaviour in young adulthood: 1977–1991. *Development Psychology*, vol. 39, pp. 201–21

Hughes, M. D. 1990. Inside Madness. *BMJ*, vol. 301, pp. 1476–8

Humphreys, M. 1996. *Empty Cradles*. Corgi, London

Hungin, A. P., Whorwell, P. J., Tack, J., Mearin, F. 2003. The prevalence, patterns and impact of irritable bowel syndrome: an international survey of 40,000 subjects. *Ailment Pharmacol Ther.* vol. 17. pp. 643–50

Hunter, R. & MacAlpine, I. 1963. *Three Hundred Years of Psychiatry 1535–1860*. OUP, Oxford

Huston, A. C. 2003. *Big World, Small Screen. The Role of Television in American Society*. University of Nebraska Press, Lincoln

Hyams, K., Wignall, S., & Roswell, R. 1996. War syndromes and their evaluation: from the US Civil War to the Persian Gulf War. *Ann. Int. Med.*, vol. 125, pp. 398–405

Illich, I. 1977. *Limits to Medicine: The Expropriation of Health*. Penguin, London

Isaac, M., Janca, A., Costa e Silva, J. A., Acuda, S. W., Altamura, A. C., Burke, J. D., Chandrasekar, C. R., Miranda, C. T., Tacchini, G., 1995. Medically unexplained somatic symptoms in different cultures: a preliminary report from phase I of the WHO International Study of Somatoform Disorders. *Psychother Psychosom*, vol. 64, pp. 88–93

James, A. 1982. *The Diary of Alice James*. Penguin, London

James, W. 1884. What is an Emotion?. *Mind*, vol. 9, pp. 188–205

Jeong, H. S. & Hurst, J. 2001. *An Assessment of the Performance of the Japanese Health Care System*, OECD Directorate for Education, Employment, Labour and Social Affairs, Paris, 56

Johnson, W. 1849. *An Essay on the Diseases of Young Women* London

Joire, P. 1892. Contribution a l'étude de la contagion hystérique ou des crises par imitation. *Bulletin médical du Nord*, vol. 31, pp. 505–17

Kamm, M. A. & Lennard-Jones, J. E. 1994. *Constipation*. Wrightson, Petersfield

Kano, M., Fukudo, S., Gyoba, J., Kamachi, M., Tagawa, M., Mochizuki, H., Itoh, M., Hongo, M., & Yanai, K. 2003. Specific brain processing of facial expressions in people with alexithymia: an H2150-PET study. *Brain*, vol. 126, no. 6, pp. 1474–84

Kaputchuk, T. J., Edwards, R. A., & Eisenberg, D. M. 1996. Complementary medicine: efficacy beyond the placebo effect. In *Complementary Medicine: An Objective Appraisal*. E. Ernst, ed. Butterworth-Heinemann, Oxford, pp. 42–70

Kardiner, A. 1941. *The Traumatic Neuroses of War*. Hoeber, New York

Katon, W. 1984. The prevalence of somatisation in primary care. *Comprehens. Psychiatry*, vol. 25, no. 208, p. 215

Katon, W., Sullivan, M., & Walker, E. 2001. Medical Symptoms without identified pathology: relationship to psychiatric disorders, childhood and adult trauma and personality traits. *Annals of Internal Medicine*, vol. 134, no. 9, pp. 917–25

Kaufman, J. & Charney, D. 2001. Effects of early stress on brain structure and function: implications for understanding the relationship between child maltreatment and depression. *Development and Psychopathology*, vol. 13, no. 3, pp. 451–71

Keenan, B. 1992. *An Evil Cradling*. Vintage, London

Kellner, R. 1994. Psychosomatic syndromes, somatisation and somatiform disorders. *Psychother Psychosom*, vol. 61, pp. 4–24

Khan, A. A., Khan, A., Harezlak, J., Wanzhu, T., & Kroenke, K. 2003. Somatic symptoms in primary care: etiology and outcome. *Psychosomatics*, vol. 44, pp. 471–8

Kilpatrick, D. G. & Saunders, B. E. 1995. *The National Survey of Adolescents*. Medical Faculty of South Carolina, Charleston, SC

Kirmayer, L. J. 1993. Healing and the invention of metaphor: the effectiveness of symbols revisited. *Culture, Medicine and Psychiatry*, vol. 17, pp. 161–5

Kirsch, I. 1996. Hypnosis as an adjunct to cognitive behavioral psychotherapy: a meta-analysis. *Journal of Consulting and Clinical Psychology*, vol. 64, pp. 517–19

Kissen, D. M. 1958. *Emotional Factors in Pulmonary Tuberculosis*. Tavistock, London

Kleinman, A. 1988. *The Illness Narratives: Suffering, Healing and the Human Condition*. Basic Books, New York

Knights, L. 1937. *Drama and Society in the Age of Jonson*. Chatto and Windus, London

Kohut, H. 1971. *The Analysis of the Self*. International Universities Press, New York

Kolonoff, H., McDougall, G., & Clark, C. 1976. The Neuropsychological, psychiatric and physical effects of prolonged and severe stress: 30 years later. *Journal of Nervous and Mental Disorders*, vol. 163, pp. 247–52

Kopi, I. 1988. The mechanism of the psychophysiological effects of placebo. *Medical Hypotheses*, vol. 27, pp. 261–4

Krahnke, J. S., Gentile, D. A., Cordoro, K. M., Angemini, B. L., Cohen, S. A., Doyle, W. J., & Skoner, D. P. 2003. Comparison of subject-reported allergy versus skin test results in a common cold trial. *American Journal of Rhinology*, vol. 17, pp. 159–62

Krause, I. B. 1989. Sinking heart: a Punjabi communication of distress. *Social Sciences and Medicine*, vol. 29, pp. 563–75

Kring, A. M. & Gordon, A. H. 1998. Sex differences in emotion, expression, experience, and physiology. *Journal of Personality, Sociology and Psychology*, vol. 74, pp. 686–703

Kroenke, K. & Mangelsdorff, D. 1989. Common symptoms in ambulatory care: incidence, evaluation, therapy and outcome. *American Journal of Medicine*, vol. 86, pp. 262–6

Kroenke, K. & Price, R. 1993. Symptoms in the community; prevalence, classification and psychiatric co-morbidity. *Archives of Internal Medicine*, vol. 153, pp. 2474–80

Krystal, H. 1978. Trauma and Affects. *Psychoanalytic Study of the Child*, vol. 33, pp. 81–116

Laing, R. D. 1967. *The Politics of Experience*. Routledge and Kegan Paul, London

Latham, R. C. 1848. *The Words of Thomas Sydenham MD*. C. and J. Adland, London

LeDoux, J. 1998. *The Emotional Brain*. Weidenfeld and Nicolson, London

Lee, S. H., Lennon, S. J., & Rudd, N. A. Compulsive consumption tendencies among television shoppers. *Family & Consumer Sciences Research Journal*, vol. 28, no. 4, pp. 436–88

LeFanu, J. 1999. *Rise and Fall of Modern Medicine*. Little, Brown, London

Leroi, A. M., Bernier, C., Watier, A., Hemond, M., Goupil, G., Black, R., Denis, P., & Devroede, G. 1993. Prevalence of sexual abuse among patients with functional disorders of the lower gastrointestinal tract. *International Journal of Colorectal Disease*, vol. 10, pp. 200–6

Lesse, S. 1956. Typical Facial Pains of Psychogenic Origin. Complications of their Misdiagnosis. *JNMD*, vol. 24, pp. 346–51

Lev-Ran, A. 2001. Human obesity: an evolutionary approach to understanding our bulging waistline. *Diabetes/Metabolism Research Reviews*, vol. 17, no. 5, pp. 347–62

Lewis, C. E., Jacobs, D. R., McCreath, H., Kiefe, C. I., Schreiner, P. J., Smith, D. E., & Williams, O. D. 2000. Weight gain continues in the 1990s: 10-year trends in weight and overweight from the CARDIA study. *American Journal of Epidemiology*, vol. 151, pp. 1172–81

Lewis, I. 2002. Prospective study of factors influencing the persistence of symptoms in hospitalised patients with acute infection. *Journal of Psychosomatic Research*, vol. 54, no. 4, pp. 307–11

Lin, X. P., Magnusson, J. Ahlstedt, S., Dahlman-Hoglund, A., Hanson, L. A., Magnusson, O., Bengtsson, U., & Telemo, E. 2002. Local allergic reaction in food-hypersensitive adults despite a lack of systemtic food-specific IgE. *Journal of Allergy and Clinical Immunology*, vol. 109, pp. 879–87

Lindstrom, M. 2004. Social capital, the miniaturisation of community and self-reported global and psychological health. *Social Science and Medicine*, vol. 59, pp. 595–607

Linet, M. S. 1989. An Epidemiological Study of Headache among Adolescents and Young Adults. *Journal of the American Medical Association*, vol. 261, pp. 2211–16

Lissau, I. & Sorensen, T. I. A. 1994. Parental neglect during childhood and increased risk of obesity in young adulthood. *Lancet*, vol. 343, pp. 322–7

Little, P., Somerville, J., Williamson, I., Warner, G., Moore, M., Wiles, R., George, S., Smith, A., & Peveler, R. 2000. Psychosocial, lifestyle, and health status variables in predicting high attendance among adults. *British Journal of General Practice*, vol. 51, no. 12, pp. 987–94

Litz, B. T., Keane, T. M., & Fisher, L. 1992. Physical health complaints in combat related post traumatic stress disorder. *Journal of Traumatic Stress*, vol. 5, no. 1, pp. 131–41

Lowenfeld, L. 1894. *Pathologie und Therapie der Neurasthenie und Hysterie*. Bergmann, Wiesbaden

MacLean, K. 2003. The impact of institutionalisation on child development. *Development and Psychiatry*, vol. 15, pp. 853–84

MacLean, P. 1949. Psychosomatic disease and the visceral brain: recent developments bearing on the Papaz theory of emotion. *Psychosomatic Medicine*, vol. 11, pp. 338–53

MacQueen, C., Marshall, J., Purdue, M., Siegel, S., & Bienenstock, J. 1989. Pavlovian conditioning of rat muscosal mast cells to secrete mast cell protease. *Science*, vol. 243, pp. 83–5

Mahler, M. 1972. On the first three subphases of the separation individuation process. *International Journal of Psychoanalysis*, vol. 53, pp. 333–8

Maniakidis, N. & Gray, A. 2000. The Economic Burden of Back Pain in the UK. *Pain*, vol. 84, pp. 95–103

Marris, P. 1958. *Widows and their Families*. Routledge and Kegan, London

Marty, P. & de M'Uzan, M. 1963. La 'pensée operatoire'. *Revue Française Psychoanalytique*, vol. 27, pp. 1345–56

Masi, A. T. & Yunus, M. B. 1986. Concepts of illness in populations as applied to fibromyalgia syndromes. *American Journal of Medicine*, vol. 81, pp. 19–25

Mason, J. W., Giller, E. L., Kosten, T. R., & Yehuda, R. 1990. Psychoendocrine approaches to the diagnosis and management of PTSD. In *Biological Assessment and Treatment of Post-traumatic Stress Disorder*, E. L. Giller, ed. American Psychiatric Press, Washington

Mayberg, H. S., Silva J. A., Brannan, S. K., Tekell, J. L., Mahurin, R. K., McGinnis, S., & Jarabek, P. A. 2002. The functional neuroanatomy of the placebo effect. *American Journal of Psychiatry*, vol. 159, no. 5, pp. 728–37

Mayer, E. & Nemeroff, C. 2003. Effects of early life events on mind brain body interactions. Unpublished

Mayor, S. 2004. Pfizer will not apply for a licence for sildenafil for women. *BMJ*, vol. 328, no. 7439, p. 542

Mayou, R., Bass, C., Hart, G., Tyndal, S., & Bryant, B. 2000. Can clinical assessment of chest pain be made more therapeutic? *Quarterly Journal of Medicine*, vol. 93, pp. 805–11

McCormick, A., Fleming, D., & Charlton, J. 1995. *Morbidity Studies from General Practice: Fourth National Study 1991–2*. HMSO, London

McEwen, B. S. 1998. Protective and damaging effects of stress mediators. *New England Journal of Medicine*, vol. 338, pp. 171–9

McFarlane, A. C., Atchison, M., Rafalowicz, E., & Papay, P. 1994. Physical symptoms in post-traumatic stress disorder. *Journal of Psychosomatic Research*, vol. 38, pp. 715–26

Meaney, M. J., Aitken, D. H., Bodnoff, S. R., Iny, L. J., Tatarewicz, J. E., & Sapolsky, R. M. 1985. Early postnatal handling alters glucocorticoid receptor concentrations in selected brain regions. *Behavioural Neuroscience*, vol. 99, pp. 765–70

Mechanic, D. 1978. Sex, illness, illness behaviour and the use of health services. *Social Sciences and Medicine*, vol. 12, pp. 207–14

Meltzer, H., Gill, B., Petticrew, M., & Hinds, K. 1995. *The Prevalence of Psychiatric Morbidity Among Adults Living in Private Households*. HMSO, London

Melville, D. 1987. Descriptive clinical research and medically unexplained physical symptoms. *Journal of Psychosomatic Research*, vol. 31, pp. 359–65

Melzack, R. 1973. *The Puzzle of Pain*. Basic Books, New York

Meyer, E. 2000. The Neurobiology of Stress and Gastrointestinal Disease. *Gut*, vol. 47, pp. 861–9

Miilunpalo, S., Vouri, I., Oja, P., Matti, P., & Orponen, H. 1997. Self-rated health status as a health measure: the predictive value of self-reported health status on the use of physician services and on mortality in the working age population. *Journal of Clinical Epidemiology*, vol. 50[5], pp. 517–28

Milde, A. M., Enger, O., & Murison, R. 2004. The effects of postnatal maternal separation on stress responsivity and experimentally induced colitis in adult rats. *Physiology & Behavior*, vol. 81(1), pp. 71–84

Miller, P. 1953. *The New England Mind: From Colony to Province*. Harvard University Press, Cambridge

Mintel 2000a. *Ethical Medicines*. Mintel, London

Mintel 2000b. *Vitamins, Minerals and Dietary Supplements*. Mintel, London

Mintel 2003a. *Complementary Medicines UK April 2003*. Mintel, London

Mintel 2003b. *Vitamins and Mineral Supplements UK May 2003*. Mintel, London

Mintel 2004. *Leisure Shopping*. Mintel, London

Moir, A. & Jessel, D. 1989. *Brain Sex*. Michael Joseph, London

Mokdad, A. H., Bowman, B. A., Ford, E. S., Vinicor, F., Marks, J. S., & Koplan, J. P. 2001. The continuing epidemics of obesity and diabetes in the United States. *Journal of the American Medical Association*, vol. 286, pp. 1195–1200

Morris, R., Gask, L., & Ronalds, C. 1998. Cost effectiveness of a new treatment for somatised mental disorders: insight to general practioners. *Family Practice*, vol. 15, pp. 119–25

Motluk, A. 2001. Read my mind. *New Scientist*, vol. 2275, pp. 22–3

Moynihan, R., Heath, I., & Henry, D. 2002. Selling sickness: the pharmaceutical industry and disease mongering. *BMJ*, vol. 324, pp. 886–90

Mozerkey, J. 1996. *Locked In: A Young Woman's Battle with Stroke*. Golden Dog Press, Toronto

Munthe, A. 1929. *The Story of San Michele*, 1995 edn. Grafton, London

Nabiloff, B. D., Berman, S., Chang, L., Derbyshire, S. W. G., Suyenobu, B., Vogt, B. A., Mandelkern, M., & Mayer, E. A. 2003. Sex-related differences in IBS patients: central processing of visceral stimuli. *Gastroenterology*, vol. 124, no. 7, pp. 1975–7

Nader, K. 2003. Memory traces unbound. *Trends in Neuroscience*, vol. 26, pp. 65–72

Naish, J. 2004. *The Hypochondriac's Handbook*. HarperCollins, London

National Audit Office 2001. *Tackling Obesity in England*. National Audit Office, London, HC 220

Nemiah, J. C. & Sifneos, P. E. 1970a. Affect and fantasy in patients with psychosomatic disorders. In *Modern Trends in Psychosomatic Medicine*, vol. 2, O. Hill, ed. Butterworth, London

Nemiah, J. C. & Sifneos, P. E. 1970b. Psychosomatic illness: a problem of communication. *Psychother Psychosom*, vol. 18, pp. 154–60

Nesse, R. M. & Williams, G. C. 1994. *Evolution and Healing*. Phoenix, London

Nguyen-Van-Tam, J. & Logan, R. 1997. Digestive Disease. In *The Health of Adult Britain: 1841–1941*, J. Charlton & M. Murphy, eds. HMSO, London, pp. 129–39

Nowak, D., Suppli Ulrik, C., & von Mutius, E. 2004. Asthma and atopy: has peak prevalence been reached? *European Respiratory Journal*, vol. 23, pp. 359–60

O'Connor, T. G. & Rutter, M. 2000. Attachment disorder behaviour following early severe deprivation; extension and longitudinal follow-up. English and Romanian adoptees study team. *Journal of the American Academy of Child and Adolescent Psychiatry*, vol. 39, pp. 703–12

Office of Health Economics 2003. *Compendium of Health Statistics*, 12

Office of National Statistics 2001. *Living in Britain 2000*. Office for National Statistics, Social Survey Division, London

Office of National Statistics 2004a. *Focus on Gender*. Office of National Statistics, London

Office of National Statistics 2004b. *Living in Britain 2002*. HMSO, London

Olubyuide, I. O., Olawuyi, F., & Fasanmade, A. A. 1995. A study of irritable bowel syndrome, diagnosed by Manning criteria in an African population. *Digestive Diseases and Sciences*, vol. 40, pp. 983–5

Orbach, S. 2003. *Hunger Strike*. Harmondsworth: Penguin, London

Osler, W. 1892. *The Principles and Practice of Medicine: Designed for the Use of Practitioners and Students of Medicine*. Appleton, New York

Ots, T. 1990. The angry liver, the anxious heart and the melancholy spleen. *Cultural Medicine and Psychiatry*, vol. 14, pp. 21–58

Pace, F., Molteni, P., Bollani, S., Sarzi-Puttini, P., Stockbrugger, R., Porro, G. B., & Drossman, D. A. 2003. Inflammatory bowel disease versus irritable bowel syndrome: a hospital-based, case control study of disease impact on quality of life. *Scandinavian Journal of Gastroenterology*, vol. 38, pp. 1031–8

Panksepp, J. 1998. Loneliness and the social bond. In *Affective Neuroscience: The Foundations of Human and Animal Emotions*. Oxford University Press, Oxford, pp. 261–79

Parker, G. 1979. Parental characteristics in relation to depressive disorders. *British Journal of Psychiatry*, vol. 134, pp. 138–47

Parkes, E. M. 1970. *The Psychosomatic Effects of Bereavement in Modern Transient Psychosomatic Medicine.* Butterworth, London

Parkes, E. M., Benjamin, B., & Fitzgerald, R. G. 1969. Broken heart: a statistical study of mortality among widowers. *BMJ,* no. 1, pp. 740–3

Parris, M. 2002. *Chance Witness.* Penguin, London

Patterson, T. L., Smith, L. W., Smith, T. L., Yager, J., & Grant, I. 1992. Symptoms of illness in late adulthood are related to childhood social deprivation and misfortune in men but not in women. *Journal of Behavioural Medicine,* vol. 15, pp. 113–25

Payer, L. 1992. *Disease-Mongers: How Doctors, Drug Companies, and Insurers Are Making You Feel Sick.* Wiley, London

Pearce, J. M. S. 2001. Headaches in the whiplash syndrome. *Spinal Cord,* vol. 39, pp. 228–33

Pearson, D. J. 1991. Pseudo-food allergy. *Rheumatic Disease Clinics of North America,* vol. 17, no. 2, pp. 343–9

Peto, A. 1969. Terrifying eyes: a visual superego forerunner. *Psychoanalytic Study of the Child,* vol. 24, pp. 197–212

Peveler, R., Kilkenny, L., & Kinmouth, A. 1997. Medically unexplained symptoms in primary care: a comparison of self report screening questionnaires and clinical opinion. *Journal of Psychosomatic Research,* vol. 42, pp. 245–53

Phillips, M. L., Gregory, L. J., Cullen, S., Ng, V., Andrew, C., Giampietro, V., Bullmore, E., Zalaya, F., Amaro, E., Thompson, D. G., Hobson, A. R., Williams, S. C. R., Brammer, M., & Aziz, Q. 2003. The effect of negative emotional context on neural and behavioural responses to oesophageal stimulation. *Brain,* vol. 126, pp. 669–84

Pilowsky, I. 1969. Abnormal illness behaviour. *British Journal of Medical Psychology,* vol. 42, pp. 347–51

Plotsky, P. M. & Meaney, M. J. 1993. Early postnatal experience alters hypothalamic corticotrophin releasing factor (CRF) mRNA content and stress induced release in adult rats. *Molecular Brain Research,* vol. 18, pp. 195–200

Poirry, P. A. 1850. *Traite de Médicine Practique,* vol. 8, pp. 379–81

Popper, K. 1934. *The Logic of Scientific Discovery.* Hutchinson, London

Porter, R. 1999. *The Greatest Benefit to Mankind: A Medical History of Humanity from Antiquity to the Present.* HarperCollins, London

Porter, R. 2000. *Quacks; Fakers and Charlatans in English Medicine.* Tempus, Stroud

Prescription Pricing Authority 2004. *Primary Care Prescribing and Budget Setting.* Department of Health

Pujol, R. 1967. Reflexions sur la fatigue et ses aspects psychologies. *Annales médico-psychologiques,* vol. 125, pp. 23–5

Putnam, R. 2000. *Bowling Alone.* Simon and Schuster, New York

Read, N. W. 1998. Enough is enough: a response to the debate, 'Do the Rome Criteria Stand Up?' In *Functional Dyspepsia and Irritable Bowel Syndrome: New Concepts and Controversies.* Kluwer, Dordrecht

Read, N. W. 1999. The role of the psychotherapies in the irritable bowel syndrome. In *Irritable Bowel Syndrome,* 13th edn, L.A. Houghton & P. J. Whorwell, eds. Bailliere, London, pp. 437–87

Read, N. W. 2000. Bridging the gap between mind and body: do cultural and psychoanalytical concepts of visceral disease have an explanation in contemporary neuroscience? In *The Biological Basis for Mind Body Interactions*, vol. 122, E. Mayer & C. P. Saper, eds., Elsevier, Amsterdam, pp. 425–43

Repetti, R. L., Taylor, S. E., & Seeman, T. E. 2002. Risky families: family social environments and the mental and physical health of offspring. *Psychological Bulletin*, vol. 128, pp. 330–66

Ritzer, G. 2000, *The McDonaldisation of Society*. Pine Forge, California

Riva, G. 1996. The role of emotional and socio-cognitive patterns in obesity; eating attitudes in obese adolescents before and after a dietary behavioural therapy. *Psychological Reports*, vol. 78, pp. 35–46

Roberts, A. H., Kewman, D. G., Mercier, L., & Hovell, M. 1993. The power of non-specific effects in healing: implications of psychosocial and biological treatments. *Clinical Psychology Review*, vol. 13, pp. 375–91

Robinson, R. L., Birnbaum, H. G., Morley, M. A., Sisitsky, T., Greenberg, P. E., & Claxton, A. J. 2003. Economic cost and epidemiological characteristics of patients with fibromyalgia claims. *Rheumatology*, vol. 30, pp. 1318–25

Rodriguez, L. A. G. & Rugiomez, A. 1999. Increased risk of irritable bowel syndrome after bacterial gastroenteritis: cohort study. *BMJ*, vol. 318, pp. 565–6

Rosendal, M., Olesen, F., & Fink, P. 2005. Management of medically unexplained symptoms. *BMJ*, vol. 330, pp. 4–5

Rosensweig, P., Brohier, S., & Zipfield, A. 1993. The placebo effect in healthy volunteers: influence of experimental conditions on adverse events profile during phase 1 studies. *Clinical Pharmacology and Therapeutics*, vol. 54, pp. 578–83

Rotenberg, V. S. 2004. The peculiarity of the right-hemisphere function in depression: solving the paradoxes. *Progress in Neuro-psychopharmacology and Biological Psychiatry*, vol. 28, pp. 1–13

Royal College of Physicians 2003. *Allergy – the Unment Need: A Blueprint for Better Patient Care*. RCP, London

Russo, J., Katon, W., Sullivan, M., Clark, M., & Buchwald, D. 1994. Severity of somatisation and its relationship to psychiatric disorders and personality. *Psychosomatics*, vol. 35, pp. 546–56

Rutter, M. & Smith, D. J. 2004. Towards causal explanations of time trends in psychosocial disorders of young people. In *Psychosocial Disorders of Young People*, M. Rutter & D. J. Smith, eds, John Wiley and Sons Ltd, Chichester

Ryan, F. P. 2003. *Virus X: Understanding the Real Threat of the New Pandemic Plagues*. HarperCollins, London

Sacks, O. W. 1981. *Migraine*. Penguin, London

Sanchez, G. C. & Brown, T. N. 1994. Nostalgia: a Swiss disease. *American Journal of Psychiatry*, vol. 151, pp. 1715–16

Sansone, R. A., Levitt, J. L., & Sansone, L. A. The prevalence of personality disorders among those with eating disorders. *Eating Disorders: The Journal of Treatment & Prevention*, vol. 13, no. 1, pp. 7–21

Sartre, J.-P. 1957. *Being and Nothingness*. Methuen, London

Schaeffer, H. 1929. Conceptions nouvelles sur l'hystérie. *Presse Médicale*. pp. 237–9

Schmale, A. H. 1958. Relationship of separation and depression to disease. *Psychosomatic Medicine*, vol. 20, pp. 259–77

Schore, A. N. 1994. *Affect Regulation and the Origin of the Self: The Neurobiology of Emotional Development*. Lawrence Earlbaum, Hillsdale

Seckl, J. R. 2001. Prenatal stress, glucocorticoids and the programming of the brain. *Journal of Neuroendocrinology*, vol. 13, no. 2, pp. 113–28

Segal, I. & Walker, A. R. P. 1984. The irritable bowel syndrome in the black community. *South African Medical Journal*, vol. 65, pp. 73–4

Seligman, M. E. P. 1988. Boomer blues. *Psychology Today*, pp. 50–5

Selye, H. 1936. A syndrome produced by diverse noxious agents. *Nature*, vol. 138, p. 32

Selye, H. 1956. *The Stress of Life*. McGraw Hill, London

Selye, H. 1982. History and Present Status of the Stress Concept. In *Handbook of Stress: Theoretical and Clinical Aspects*, L. Goldberger & S. Breznitz, eds. Free Press, London

Shah, I. 1973. *The Exploits of the Incomparable Mullah Nasrudin*. Paladin, London

Shalev, A., Bleich, A., & Ursano, R. J. 1990. Post-traumatic stress disorder: somatic comorbidity and effort tolerance. *Psychosomatics*, vol. 31, pp. 197–203

Shanks, N., Larocque, S., & Meaney, M. J. 1995. Neonatal endotoxin exposure alters the development of the hypothalamic-pituitary-adrenal axis: early illness and later responsivity to stress. *Journal of Neuroscience*, vol. 15, no. 1, pp. 376–84

Share, M. & Carson, A. 2001. Unexplained somatic symptoms, functional syndromes and somatisation: do we need a paradigm shift? *Annals of Internal Medicine*, vol. 134, no. 9, pp. 926–9

Shevlin, M., Brusden, V., Walker, S., Davies, M., & Ramkalawan, T. 1997. Death of Diana, Princess of Wales: her death and funeral rate as traumatic stressors. *BMJ*, vol. 315, pp. 1467–8

Shore, M. 1980. Discussions, Self-Psychology and Applied Psychoanalysis. In *Advances in Self Psychology*, A. Goldberg, ed. International Universities Press, New York

Shorter, E. 1993. *From Paralysis to Fatigue: A History of Psychosomatic Illness in the Modern Era*. Free Press, New York

Showalter, E. 1997. *Hystories: Hysterical Epidemics and Modern Culture*. Picador, London

Sidford, I. 1997. General practitioners' workload in primary care led NHS: practices' consultation rates have increased by three-quarters in the past 25 years. *BMJ*, vol. 315, no. 7107, pp. 546–7

Siegel, D. 2000. *The Developing Mind: Towards a Neurobiology of Interpersonal Experience*. Guilford Press, New York

Sifneos, P. E. 1973. The prevalence of alexithymic characteristics in psychosomatic patients. *Psychother Psychosom*, vol. 22, pp. 55–73

Simini, B. 1994 (letter). *Lancet*, vol. 344, p. 1642

Simon, G. E. & VonKorff, M. 1991. Somatization and psychiatric disorder in NIMH Epidemiological Catchment Area study. *American Journal of Psychiatry*, vol. 148, pp. 1494–1500

Singer, T., Seymour, B., O'Doherty, J., Kaube, H., Dolan, R. J., & Frith, C. D. 2004. Empathy for Pain Involves the Affective but not Sensory Components of Pain. *Science*, vol. 303, no. 5661, pp. 1157–62

Skey, F. C. 1855. Clinical Lecture on Hysteric Diseases. *Lancet*, 24 February, pp. 205–7

Skultans, V. 1985. The English Malady. In *English Madness*, V. Skultans ed. Routledge & Kegan Paul, London

Smith, C. R. 1994. The course of somatisation and its effects on utilization of health care resources. *Psychosomatics*, vol. 35, no. 3, pp. 263–7

Solomon, S. 2001. Post-traumatic headache. *Medical Clinics of North America*, vol. 85

Solomon, Z. & Mukulineer, M. 1987. Combat stress reaction, post-traumatic stress disorder and somatic complaints among Israeli soldiers. *Journal of Psychosomatic Research*, vol. 31, pp. 131–7

Solomon, Z., Mukulineer, M., & Kotler, M. 1987. A two-year follow-up of somatic complaints among Israeli combat stress reaction casualties. *Journal of Psychosomatic Research*, vol. 31, pp. 463–9

Southey, R. 1951. *Letters from England.* Cresset, London

Sperry, R. W. 1987. Structure and significance of the conscious revolution. *Journal of Mind and Behaviour*, vol. 8, pp. 37–65

Spitz, R. A. 1945. Hospitalism: an enquiry in the genesis of psychiatric conditions in early childhood. In *The Psychoanalytic Study of the Child*. International Universities Press, New York, pp. 53–84

Spitz, R. A. 1965. *The First Year of Life: A Psychoanalytical Study of Normal and Deviant Development.* International Universities Press, New York

Spitz, R. A. 1972. Bridges: on anticipation, duration and meaning. *Journal of the American Psychoanalytical Association*, vol. 20, pp. 721–35

Spitz, R. A. & Wolf, K. N. 1946. Anaclitic Depression. In *The Psychoanalytic Study of the Child II*. International Universities Press, New York, pp. 313–42

Stallard, P., Velleman, R., & Baldwin, S. 1998. Prospective study of post-traumatic stress disorder in children involved in road traffic accidents. *BMJ*, vol. 317, pp. 1619–23

Stallones, R. 1980. The rise and fall of Ischaemic heart disease. *Scientific American*, vol. 243, pp. 43–9

Stanton, T. 2002. *Body Psychotherapy.* Brunner Routledge, Hove

Statistical Office of the European Communities 2002. *Health statistics: key data on health 2002; data 1970–2001*. Office for Official Publications of the European Communities, Luxembourg

Stekel, W. 1932. Eine Interessante Somatisation. *Psychoanalytische Praxis*, vol. 2, p. 148

Steptoe, A., Owen, N., Kunz-Ebrecht, S. R., & Brydon, L. 2004. Loneliness and neuroendocrine, cardiovascular, and inflammatory stress responses in middle-aged men and women. *Psychoneuroendocrinology*, vol. 29, no. 5, pp. 593–611

Stern, D. N. 1977. *The First Relationship.* Harvard University Press, Cambridge

Sternberg, E. M. 2000. Interactions between the immune and neuroendocrine systems. In *The Biological Basis for Mind Body Interactions*, vol. 122, E. Mayer & C. P. Saper, eds. Elsevier, Amsterdam, pp. 35–42

Stretch, R., Bliese, P., Marlowe, D., Wright, K., Knudson, K., & Hoover, C. 1995. Physical health symptomatology of Gulf War era service personnel from the states of Pennsylvania and Hawaii. *Military Medicine*, vol. 160, pp. 131–6

Stroud, M. 1994. *Shadows on the Wasteland.* Penguin, London

Sun, W. M., Donnelly, T. C., & Read, N. W. 1989. Anorectal Function in Normal Human Subjects: Effect of Gender. *International Journal of Colorectal Disease*, vol. 4, pp. 188–96

Tapsell, S. M. 2000. *Follow-up Study of the Health Effects of the Easter 1998 Flooding in Banbury and Kidlington.* Flood Hazard Research Centre, Enfield

Taylor, G. 1987a. *Psychosomatic Medicine and Contemporary Psychoanalysis.* International Universities Press, New York

Tennes, K. 1982. The role of hormones in mother–infant transactions. In *The Development of Attachment and Affiliative Systems*, R. N. Emde & R. J. Harmon, eds. Plenum, New York

Terr, L. C. 1983. Chowchilla Revisited: the effects of psychic trauma four years after a school bus kidnapping. *American Journal of Psychiatry*, vol. 140, pp. 1543–50

Thomas, K. B. 1994. The placebo in General Practice. *Lancet*, vol. 344, pp. 1066–7

Thomas, K. J., Nicholl, J. P., & Coleman, P. 2001. Use and expenditure of complementary medicine in England: A population based survey. *Complementary Therapies in Medicine*, vol. 9, pp. 2–11

Toffler, A. 1981. *The Third Wave.* Pan Macmillan, London

Trimble, M. R. 1981. *Post-Traumatic Neurosis from Railway Spine to Whiplash.* Wiley, New York

Trowbridge, B. 1996. *The Hidden Meaning of Illness: Disease as Symbol and Metaphor.* A.R.E.Press, Virginia Beach

Tucker, D. M., Sandstead, N. M., & Logan, G. M. 1981. Dietary fibre and personality factors in determinants of stool output. *Gastroenterology*, vol. 81, pp. 879–83

Turner, B. S. 1996a. *The Body and Society.* Sage, London

Turner, P. 1996b. UK Labour Market Trends. *Economic Review*, pp. 20–3

Uvnas-Moberg, K. 2003. *The Oxytocin Factor: Tapping the Hormone of Calm, Healing and Love.* Da Capo Press, Cambridge

Van der Kolk, B., McFarlane, A. C., & Weisaeth, L. 1996. *Traumatic Stress: The Effect of Overwhelming Stress on Mind, Body and Society.* Guilford, New York

Van Ommeren, M., Sharma, B., Poudyal, B. N., Sharma, G. K., Cardena, E., & De Jong, J. T. 2001. Trauma and loss as determinants of medically unexplained illness in a Bhutanese refugee camp. *Psychological Medicine*, vol. 31, pp. 1259–67

Veith, I. 1965. *Hysteria: The History of a Disease.* University of Chicago Press, Chicago

Venable, V. L., Carlson, C. R., & Wilson, J. 2001. The role of anger and depression in recurrent headache. *Headache*, vol. 41, pp. 21–30

Vines, G. 1998. A gut feeling. *New Scientist*, vol. 159, p. 26

Voudouris, N. J., Peck, C. L., & Coleman, G. 1990. The role of conditioning and verbal expectancy in the placebo response. *Pain*, vol. 43, pp. 121–8

Vrettos, A. 1995. *Somatic Fictions: Imagining Illness in Victorian Culture.* Stanford University Press, Stanford

Wager, T. D., Phan, K. L., Liberzon, I., & Taylor, S. F. 2003. Valence, gender and lateralisation of emotion; a meta-analysis from neuroimaging. *Neuroimaging*, vol. 19, pp. 513–31

Waldcott, G. L. 1998. The preskeletal phase of chronic fluoride intoxication. *Fluoride*, vol. 31, no. 1, pp. 13–20

Waller, G. 1991. Sexual abuse as a factor in eating disorders. *British Journal of Psychiatry*, vol. 159, pp. 664–71

Wallerstein, J. S. & Blakeslee, S. 1989. *Second Chances: Men, Women and Children a Decade after Divorce.* Ticknor and Fields, New York

Walsh, G. J. & Honan, D. J. 1954. St Augustine: the city of God. In *The Writings of St Augustine.* Fathers of the Church, New York, pp. 252–62

Wanless, D. 2003. *Building on the Best: Choice, Responsiveness and Equity in the NHS.* Stationery Office, London

Ware, N. C. & Kleinman, A. 1992a. Culture and somatic experience: the social course of illness in neurasthenia and chronic fatigue syndrome. *Psychosomatic Medicine*, vol. 54, pp. 546–60

Weber, M. 1965. *The Protestant Ethic and The Spirit of Capitalism*. Charles Scribner's Sons, New York

Weinstock, M. 1997. Does prenatal stress impair coping and regulation of the hypothalamo-pituitary adrenal axis? *Neuroscience Biobehavioural Reviews*, vol. 21, pp. 1–10

Weisberg, R., Bruce, S. E., Machan, J. T., Kessler, R. C., Culpepper, L., & Keller, M. B. 2002. Nonpsychiatric illness among primary care patients with trauma histories and posttraumatic stress disorder. *Psychiatric Services*, vol. 53, pp. 848–54

Wells, A. S., Read, N. W., Uvnas-Moberg, K., & Asler, P. 1997. Influence of fat and carbohydrate on postprandial sleepiness, mood and humour. *Physiology and Behaviour*, vol. 61, pp. 679–86

Wells, N. E. J., Hahn, B. A., & Whorwell, P. J. 1997. Clinical economics review: irritable bowel syndrome. *Alimentary Pharmacology and Therapeutics*, vol. 11, pp. 1019–30

Wessley, S., Hotopf, M., & Sharpe, M. 1998. *Chronic Fatigue and its Syndromes*. OUP, Oxford

Wessley, S. & Ismail, K. 2002. Medically unexplained symptoms and syndromes. *Clinical Medicine*, vol. 2, no. 6, pp. 501–4

Wessley, S., Nimnuan, C., & Sharpe, M. 1999. Functional Somatic Syndromes: one or many, *Lancet*, vol. 354, pp. 936–9

West, D. A. 1986. The Effects of Loneliness. *Comprehens. Psychiatry*, vol. 27, pp. 351–6

Whitehead, W. E., Palsson, O., & Jones, K. R. 2002. Systematic Review of the Comorbidity of Irritable Bowel Syndrome with other disorders: What are the causes and implications?. *Gastroenterology*, vol. 122, no. 4, pp. 1140–56

Whorwell, P. J., Prior, A., & Faraghar, E. B. 1984. Controlled trial of hypnotherapy in the treatment of severe refractory irritable bowel syndrome. *Lancet*, vol. 2, pp. 1232–4

Whytt, R. 1765. *Observations on the nature, Causes and Cure of those disorders which have been commonly called Nervous, Hypochondria or Hysteric to which are prefixed some remarks on the sympathy of nerves*, 3rd edn, J.Balfour, Edinburgh

Wickramasekere, I. 1980. A conditioned response model of the placebo effect. Predictions from the model. *Biofeedback and Self-Regulation*, vol. 5[1], pp. 5–14

Wickramasekere, I. 1998. Secrets kept from the mind but not the body or behaviour: the unsolved problems of identifying and treating somatisation and psychophysiological disease. *Biofeedback and Self-Regulation*, vol. 14, pp. 81–132

Wickramasekere, I. 1999. How does biofeedback reduce clinical symptoms and so memories and beliefs have biological consequences? Towards a model of mind-body healing. *Applied Psychophysiology and Biofeedback*, vol. 24[2], pp. 91–105

Wickramasekere, I., Davies, T. E., & Davies, S. M. 1996. Applied psychophysiology: a bridge between the biomedical model and the biopsychosocial model in family medicine. *Professional Psychology: Research and Practice*, vol. 27[3], pp. 221–33

Wickramasekere, I., Kolm, P., Pope, A. T., & Turner, M. 1998. Observations of a Paradoxical Temperature Increase During Cognitive Stress in Some Chronic Pain Patients. *Applied Psychophysiology and Biofeedback*, vol. 23[4], pp. 233–41

Winnicott, D. W. 1951. Transitional objects and transitional phenomena. In *Through Paediatrics to Psychoanalysis*. Karnac, London, pp. 229–42

Winnicott, D. W. 1964. *The Child, the Family and the Outside World*, Penguin, London

Winnicott, D. W. 1986. *Home is Where We Start From*. Penguin, London

Wittstein, I. S., Thiemann, D. R., Lima, J. A. C., Baughman, K. L., Schulman, S. P., Gerstenblith, G., Wu, K. C., Rade, J. J., Bivalacqua, T. J., & Champion, H. C. 2005. Neurohumoral Features of Myocardial Stunning Due to Sudden Emotional Stress. *The New England Journal of Medicine*, vol. 352, no. 6, pp. 539–48

Wolf, S. 1949. The effects of suggestion and conditioning on the action of chemical agents in human subjects – the pharmacology of placebos. *Journal of Clinical Investigation*, vol. 29, no. 1, pp. 100–9

Wolf, S. 1965. *The Stomach*. Oxford University Press, New York

Wolf, S. & Wolff, H. G. 1943. *Human Gastric Function. An Experimental Study of Man and his Stomach*. Oxford University Press, New York

Wolfe, F. & Cathey, M. 1983. Prevalence of primary and secondary fibrositis. *Journal of Rheumatology*, vol. 10, pp. 965–8

Wolfe, J., Proctor, S. P., & Erickson, D. J. 1999. Relationship of psychiatric status to Gulf War veterans' health problems. *Psychosomatic Medicine*, vol. 61, pp. 532–40

Wolpert, L. 1999. *Malignant Sadness: The Anatomy of Depression*. Faber and Faber, London

World Health Organisation 1999. *Making a Difference*. WHO, Geneva

Yunus, M. B. 2000. Central sensitivity syndromes: a unified concept for fibromyalgia and other similar maladies. *Journal of the Indian Rheumatology Association*, vol. 8, no. 1, pp. 27–32

Index